Adolescent Substance Abuse

A Comprehensive Guide to Theory and Practice

CRITICAL ISSUES IN PSYCHIATRY
An Educational Series for Residents and Clinicians

Series Editor: Sherwyn M. Woods, M.D., Ph.D.
University of Southern California School of Medicine
Los Angeles, California

Recent volumes in the series:

ADOLESCENT SUBSTANCE ABUSE: A Comprehensive Guide to Theory
and Practice
Yifrah Kaminer, M.D.

CASE STUDIES IN INSOMNIA
Edited by Peter J. Hauri, Ph.D.

CHILD AND ADULT DEVELOPMENT: A Psychoanalytic Introduction for Clinicians
Calvin A. Colarusso, M.D.

CLINICAL DISORDERS OF MEMORY
Aman U. Khan, M.D.

CONTEMPORARY PERSPECTIVES ON PSYCHOTHERAPY WITH LESBIANS
AND GAY MEN
Edited by Terry S. Stein, M.D., and Carol J. Cohen, M.D.

DECIPHERING MOTIVATION IN PSYCHOTHERAPY
David M. Allen, M.D.

DRUG AND ALCOHOL ABUSE: A Clinical Guide to Diagnosis and Treatment
Third Edition
Marc A. Schuckit, M.D.

ETHNIC PSYCHIATRY
Edited by Charles B. Wilkinson, M.D.

EVALUATING FAMILY MENTAL HEALTH: History, Epidemiology, and
Treatment Issues
John J. Schwab, M.D., Judith J. Stephenson, S.M., and John F. Ice, M.D.

EVALUATION OF THE PSYCHIATRIC PATIENT: A Primer
Seymour L. Hallek, M.D.

THE FREEDOM OF THE SELF: The Bio-Existential Treatment of Character Problems
Eugene M. Abroms, M.D.

HANDBOOK OF BEHAVIOR THERAPY IN THE PSYCHIATRIC SETTING
Edited by Alan S. Bellack, Ph.D., and Michel Hersen, Ph.D.

RESEARCH IN PSYCHIATRY: Issues, Strategies, and Methods
Edited by L.K. George Hsu, M.D., and Michel Hersen, Ph.D.

SEXUAL LIFE: A Clinician's Guide
Stephen B. Levine, M.D.

STATES OF MIND: Configurational Analysis of Individual Psychology, Second Edition
Mardi J. Horowitz, M.D.

A Continuation Order Plan is available for this series. A continuation order will bring delivery of each new volume immediately upon publication. Volumes are billed only upon actual shipment. For further information please contact the publisher.

Adolescent Substance Abuse

A Comprehensive Guide to Theory and Practice

Yifrah Kaminer, M.D.

Alcohol Research Center
The University of Connecticut Health Center
Farmington, Connecticut

Plenum Medical Book Company • New York and London

Library of Congress Cataloging-in-Publication Data

Kaminer, Yifrah, 1951-
    Adolescent substance abuse : a comprehensive guide to theory and
practice / Yifrah Kaminer.
        p.   cm. -- (Critical issues in psychiatry)
    Includes bibliographical references and index.
    ISBN 0-306-44692-8
    1. Teenagers--Substance use. 2. Substance abuse--Treatment.
I. Title. II. Series.
RJ506.D78K35 1994
616.86'00835--dc20   94-14604
                                                                   CIP

ISBN 0-306-44692-8

©1994 Plenum Publishing Corporation
233 Spring Street, New York, N.Y. 10013

Plenum Medical Book Company is an imprint of Plenum Publishing Corporation

Printed in the United States of America

Foreword

Alcohol and drug abuse problems take a remarkable toll worldwide. In the United States alone, the cost to the public is calculated at over $125 billion per year in health care and work hours lost. In general medical facilities an average of a quarter of all patients present with addictive disorders, many of which go undiagnosed. Furthermore, as many as two-thirds of patients with non-addictive psychiatric disorders have been found to be substance abusers, depending on the region and the clinical setting.

In terms of prevention and early treatment, there is no population more important than adolescents beginning to abuse alcohol and drugs. We know that their patterns of abuse are highly susceptible to change, and that these patterns may abate or may become aggravated and emerge as full-blown addiction. Because of this, specialists conversant with the needs of adolescents troubled by alcohol and drug use are sorely needed. Ironically, there are very few health professionals who are well-versed in this field.

This problem derives in part from the nature of psychiatric services in the principal teaching centers for child and adolescent psychiatry. In general, these tend to be either psychodynamically or psychopharmacologically oriented. Neither of these modalities, however, plays a key role in the practical treatment of adolescent substance abuse. On the other hand, abstinence-oriented social and milieu therapies, which are typically used in treating adolescent substance abusers, are not found in our teaching hospitals, and these settings are therefore less suitable for training specialists in adolescent addiction psychiatry. Conversely, treatment programs currently addressing adolescent substance abusers often need to be informed of appropriate psychiatric diagnostic and treatment modalities.

Some historical notes help to provide a context for understanding the emergence of medical interest in adolescent substance abuse. The conception of compulsive drug use as a disease process was important to the acceptance of addiction in mainstream medicine. It was propounded by E. M. Jellinek, a social scientist in the 1950s, and soon adopted by Alcoholics Anonymous. Since then, it has been supported by the emergence of a large body of psychiatric research. Our growing understanding of the genetic transmission of vulnerability to alcoholism is important in this regard, and is illustrated by adoption studies like those originally carried out by Donald Goodwin and Marc Schuckit. These demonstrate a greater prevalence of alcoholism among biological children of alcoholics than adopted ones. These initial studies were premised on a comparison of children adopted away from their families of origin, relative to their biological siblings, who were reared by their natural parents. Also important in this genetic perspective was a related body of work by Robert Cloninger on the types of alcoholism more likely to be transmitted by male and female parents, suggesting differences in the degree to which childhood environmental factors might affect the inheritance of susceptibility.

Clinical modalities have also been important in pointing to the importance of psychiatric treatment for children and adolescents. For example, family therapy has become an important modality in achieving rehabilitation for addicted patients. Peter Steinglass developed a systems orientation for looking at the families of alcoholics, emphasizing the value of restructuring the way in which substance use is embedded in patterns of family relations. Allied with the use of family members, we have developed Network Therapy to engage family and peers in providing support for patients in the context of ongoing individual therapy. Group therapy is particularly useful to address the problems of substance abuse with adolescents. Irvin Yalom was initially important in developing an empirical justification for introducing alcoholic patients into homogeneous treatment groups. His work pointed to the feasibility of developing specific focused approaches to dealing with the problems of relapse and denial raised in group settings.

Recent studies on adolescents have illustrated the characteristic nature of their substance use. For example, the predominance of overt psychopathology among middle-class youth who become heavy substance users stands in contrast to the socially determined and normative behavior of abuse in disadvantaged populations. These social factors have underlined the importance of epidemiological studies with school children, such as those carried out by Denise Kandel, and the diagnostic instruments tailored to the adolescent population developed by Yifrah Kaminer.

A recent study of medical school curriculum in addiction conducted by the American Psychiatric Association revealed that considerable curriculum time was devoted to addiction, but that important questions remained of the quality of teaching and of faculty commitment. Teachers' attitudes and institutional support are vital issues, since those inex-

perienced in caring for addicted patients are vulnerable to disillusion-
ment, particularly when they have had little exposure to the positive
consequences of long-term rehabilitation. Thus, courses oriented toward enhancing positive attitudes were rarely in evidence among the
curricula submitted. These shortcomings are highlighted by the well-
documented attitudinal problems of medical students, residents, and
graduate physicians on how to evaluate the substance abuser and refer
him or her for proper rehabilitative care.

In order to attract qualified practitioners and academics, the substance abuse field in the United States has moved toward implementing
an educational format that parallels the one accepted in medicine broadly, with an attendant format for post-residency fellows. The best established option for such training is now the Certificate of Added Qualifica-
tions. This current procedure of the American Board of Medical
Specialties entails modification of specialty certification to reflect that a
candidate has completed at least one year of full-time formal training in
a subspecialty program beyond the basic residency and has passed an
additional examination prepared by a member board. Currently there
are 122 fellows enrolled in 46 separate programs.

While these developments in fellowship training are valuable in addressing the unmet needs of many adult alcoholics and drug abusers,
they will not necessarily assure the material improvements needed for
adolescent treatment. A large infusion of substance abuse training is
needed in child psychiatry fellowships, as well as in psychology and social
work training programs related to the youth population. In particular,
multimodality substance abuse programs for adolescents must be insti-
tuted in our teaching hospitals so that future trainees will be conversant
with the best means to approach the needs of youthful substance abusers. This current volume takes an important step in synthesizing the
knowledge that is necessary for trainees placed in such settings so that
they will have available to them the full complement of pre-clinical and
clinical information needed to approach their patients. It is invaluable
for graduate clinicians and for researchers as well.

Because of this, the current volume provides a unique and advantageous perspective to the trainees and practitioners in the adolescent
substance abuse field. It offers a sophisticated perspective on addiction
treatment techniques developed in recent years, with a sensitivity to the
social and developmental needs of the adolescent. In addition, it provides an important and well-integrated perspective on the psychiatric
issues that play an important role in the treatment of such patients.

MARC GALANTER, M.D.
New York University School of Medicine

Special thanks to Eileen McMurrer, M.Ed., for her invaluable contribution in researching and reviewing the extensive literature cited herein, and for special editorial assistance on the various evolutions of this book

Acknowledgments

Many thanks to Tim Rivinus for his support and for contributing to the
Emergency Manual section of the treatment chapter;
To Ralph Tarter and Tom McLellan, my mentors, from whom I learned
what I know and also what I still have to learn about substance abuse
and its treatment;
To Roger Weiss for exposing me to the field with patience and humor;
To Marc Galanter, Richard Frances, and Ed Khantzian for their camara-
derie and professional grasp of the importance of adolescent sub-
stance abuse specialization;
To Oscar Bukstein for walking with me in the trenches;
To the devoted and caring professionals at the Western Psychiatric Insti-
tute and Clinic in Pittsburgh, PA, and the E. P. Bradley Hospital in
Providence, RI, who experienced with me the best and worst of
treating our kids;
To Doug Zeidonis for hooking me into writing this book;
To James McGuire for being himself;
To Missy Tatum for her faith in me, her attention to detail, and her
enormous patience;
And to my wife, to whom I am addicted.

Contents

PART II. INTERVENTIONS: PREVENTION OF ADOLESCENT
SUBSTANCE USE AND ASSESSMENT AND TREATMENT OF
PSYCHOACTIVE SUBSTANCE USE DISORDERS

PART I

Understanding Adolescent Substance Use

CHAPTER 1

Introduction

For a period of several months, my colleagues and I discussed this question: Is there a need for a new book on adolescent substance use (ASU)* and adolescent psychoactive substance use disorders (APSUDs)† in the 1990s? In order to justify such an endeavor, we asked ourselves these questions:

1. Is APSUD sufficiently distinct from adult PSUD to warrant a separate volume, given the early stage in which the study of adolescent substance abuse finds itself?
2. What are the essential topics that should be included in such a book so that the volume is complete and updated without indulging in an encyclopedic retrospective data collection?
3. In fact, how do we shy away from philosophical and ideological controversies that divide the various camps of addictionologists and yet include those pieces of experience and attitude that will benefit the reader interested in ASU and APSUDs?

With regard to the first question, before the 1970s, addictionologists at large followed the same split path that divided child and adolescent psychiatry from general psychiatry and adolescent medicine from internal medicine: They related to an adolescent as a "miniature adult,"

---

*The term "adolescent substance use" (ASU) refers to the nonpathological use of, experimentation with, or occasional irregular use of psychoactive substances, i.e., use that does not meet the criteria in the *Diagnostic and Statistical Manual of Mental Disorders,* 4th edition (DSM-IV), for Substance-Related Disorders according to a consequence-oriented, problem-based classification system of the American Psychiatric Association (1994).
†The term "adolescent psychoactive substance use disorder" (APSUD) refers to a pathological use of drugs that has become a regular feature of the adolescent life-style. Such use includes abuse and dependence according to DSM-IV.

ignoring adolescence as a developmental phase. They failed to recognize that although there are areas of symptoms in common between APSUDs and adult PSUDs, there are significant differences between adolescents and adults and blanket imitation of traditional adult substance abuse treatment for adolescents is developmentally inappropriate and therefore may be ineffective.

What are these differences? Many adolescents, especially those in early and middle adolescence, have yet to achieve the stage of Formal Operational Thinking as defined by Piaget (1962). Incomplete attainment of this cognitive capacity leads to major difficulties in understanding and internalizing abstract values and concepts that are so important in the addiction field (e.g., denial, higher power, responsibility, "triggers"). There are many frustrated addiction specialists who struggle with adolescent substance abusers without acknowledging that the adolescent is not resisting treatment but simply cannot understand it and has not been engaged on his or her own terms. Added to this incomprehension is the existence among many adolescent substance abusers of concomitant high-risk behaviors (Jessor & Jessor, 1977), psychiatric problems, learning disabilities, impulse control and attention problems, and serious family and school problems, which makes the treatment challenge even greater.

Adolescents with APSUDs also differ from adult patients in having a shorter history of substance use disorder. Tolerance, craving, withdrawal, and withdrawal avoidance are less common and, in most cases, less severe. The need for detoxification is relatively rare, and long-term physical side effects are usually not yet manifested. Therefore, typical descriptions from the adult PSUD jargon such as hitting "rock bottom," "once a junky, always a junky," and a simplistic cause–effect disease model without additional developmental stage-oriented interventions do not apply well to adolescents.

More than any other age group, adolescents make use of role modeling and imitation and yield to peer pressure as part of the process of achieving independence and identity. These concepts apply to the initiation of ASU and transition and maintenance from ASU to APSUD, as well as to regression, cessation, and relapse cycles of APSUD. Adolescent culture is often based on actions, immediate gratification, an "all-or-nothing" approach to life, intense peer involvement and testing of relationships, self-esteem, interpretation of social status, academic success, and vocational readiness (Erikson, 1968). It is important to consider the adolescent's false sense of invulnerability, narcissistic approach to life, and lack of fully developed empathy, which often lead to an assumption that adults cannot understand adolescents and therefore cannot help them. These factors require treatment oriented to the "here and now" for dually diagnosed adolescents, their families, and their caretakers, who are less interested in the end result of their substance abuse in a couple of decades than in the relationship between substance abuse and their present social, academic, family, and legal lives. Furthermore, adolescent substance-abuse treatment settings also require a complex network that often involves schools, family courts, the juvenile justice system, and state departments of social, youth, and child and family services.

Research on ASU and APSUD started to gain momentum in the 1970s, when epidemiological and etiological issues became the foci of investigation. Treatment-related issues were not systematically explored until the 1980s; consequently, and unfortunately, the literature examining APSUDs still lags behind the adult data. However, significant progress has been made in improving the understanding of the etiology and pathogenesis of psychopathology in children and adolescents. PSUDs and other high-risk behaviors appear to constitute part of a larger picture that originates in biological vulnerabilities characterized by primary temperament phenotypes exposed to continuous interactions with the environment. The constant dynamic bilateral transaction between the infant in distress and the caretaker's responses, which mediate each other, defines the liability of the phenotype to move back and forth beyond and under the threshold range for deviant behavior (Tarter & Mezzich, 1992). The continuing psychosocial interactions of the developing infant, child, and adolescent enable us to identify the history of ongoing psychopathological processes at any age.

The assessment of the individual's relative psychological vulnerability and resilience, and the exploration of amenability for intervention, enable the design of intervention-matching (prevention or treatment) that may alter the natural course of the behavior or disorder (ASU or APSUD).

With regard to the second and third questions we posed ourselves, the biopsychosocial model is followed, accompanied by the developmental transactional perspective (Sameroff & Chandler, 1975), and the approach is as scientific as possible. Factual data take the "front seat," clinical experience comes as the second-best alternative, and anything else (theories, models, philosophies) is treated respectfully but cautiously, in a critical, objective manner. The foremost goal remains to suggest the latest and best in the quality of care of ASU and APSUDs by adherence to the updated knowledge.

I hope that the sequence of the chapters and their integral organization will make the reading of the book enjoyable. It is also my wish that the large body of information gathered in the book will stimulate improved clinical and research efforts concerning APSUDs.

REFERENCES

American Psychiatric Association (1994). *Diagnostic and Statistical Manual of Mental Disorders,* 4th ed. Washington, DC: American Psychiatric Association.

Erikson, E. H. (1968). *Identity: Youth and Crisis.* New York: Plenum Press.

Jessor, R. J., & Jessor, S. L. (1977). *Problem Behavior and Psychosocial Development: A Longitudinal Study of Youth.* New York: Academic Press.

Piaget, J. (1962). *The Moral Judgment of the Child.* New York: Collier.

Sameroff, A. J., & Chandler, M. J. (1975). Reproductive risk and the continuum of caretaking casualty. In F. D. Horowitz (Ed.), *Review of Child Development Research,* Vol. 4 (pp. 187–244). Chicago: University of Chicago Press.

Tarter, R. E., & Mezzich, A. C. (1992). Ontogeny of substance abuse. In M. Glantz & R. Pickens (Eds.), *Vulnerability to Drug Abuse* (pp. 149–178). Washington, DC: American Psychological Association.

CHAPTER 2

Terminology and Classification

Major efforts expended in recent decades toward developing a consequence-oriented, problem-based, clinically valid classification system have resulted in the inclusion of a large number of syndromes in the *Diagnostic and Statistical Manual of Mental Disorders,* 4th edition (DSM-IV), of the American Psychiatric Association (1994), or the generally comparable *International Classification of Diseases,* 10th edition (ICD-10), which has been developed to succeed the 9th edition (ICD-9) published by the World Health Organization (1980). However, for many of these disorders, including substance-related disorders, there are relatively limited data on key dimensions that are necessary for validating their designation as distinct disorders.

The importance of diagnostic classifications rests in the communicative reliability of this system between professionals. Also, an ideal diagnostic label is expected to indicate the course of the disorder, the most likely prognosis, and the best available treatment (Schuckit, Zisook, & Mortola, 1985). The purpose of this chapter is twofold: (1) to review the evolution of the diagnostic conception of PSUD up to the crystallization period of the new DSM-IV (American Psychiatric Association, 1994) and ICD-10 criteria and to investigate its application for adolescent psychoactive substance use disorder (APSUD); (2) to explore whether APSUD is sufficiently distinct from adult PSUD to merit a separate diagnostic entity. In other words, is APSUD a disorder with specific features that can be measured to provide clinical utility and predictive validity that are different from the present hypothesized model of adolescent–adult PSUD continuum?

The following sections present a review of data both for and against such designation.

7

2.1. EVOLUTION OF THE NOSOLOGY OF PSYCHOACTIVE SUBSTANCE USE DISORDER

The same diagnostic criteria for PSUD are at present indiscriminately utilized for adolescents as well as adults. The research on the development of an operational definition of PSUD has lacked age-population specificity. Lack of clarity, uniformity, and standardization in the terminology used for substance use disorders in general was demonstrated in the 1980s (Rinaldi, Steindler, Wilford, & Goodwin, 1988). This inconsistency is probably related to an array of concepts and terms in active use as well as disagreements among the variety of professional disciplines involved in the field (Rinaldi et al., 1988).

The state of the art regarding the validity of APSUD is also unclear, because it has not been thoroughly investigated, nor has its clinical utility and specificity been negated.

2.1.1. Early Phase of the Conception of Terminology for Substance Use Disorders

The quest for lucid terminology for the pathological use of drugs before the 1970s resulted in the first broadly conceived American nomenclature, DSM-I (American Psychiatric Association, 1952). Alcoholism and drug dependence appeared as subsets of sociopathic personality disturbance (a diagnostic category that also included antisocial behavior and sexual deviations). DSM-II (American Psychiatric Association, 1968) did not represent significant progress from DSM-I. During the same period, Jellinek (1952, 1960) emphasized the reintroduction and expansion of the disease model. Meyer (1986) pointed out that the antecedents of the disease model can be traced to the writings of Benjamin Rush and Thomas Trotter in the 18th and 19th centuries and to the publications of members of the American Association for the Study of Alcohol and Other Narcotics about a century ago. The aforenamed physicians and association identified "withdrawal," "craving," and "loss of control" as necessary components of physical addiction, which is sine qua non to the disease model. Also, in 1902, Charles Towns described an "addictive triad": increased craving, growing tolerance, and withdrawal syndrome when the drug is withheld (Musto, 1973). Jellinek presented five species of alcoholism, but only gamma and delta were regarded as addictive diseases characterized by "physiological vulnerabilities" (Meyer, 1986).

For the gamma alcoholic, the addictive process was characterized by "loss of control" while drinking. The delta alcoholic was defined by an "inability to abstain entirely," but without loss of control. The validity of

Jellinek's descriptive, unitary formulation failed the test of scientific empiricism (Mendelson & Mello, 1966; Merry, 1966); however, the disease model has been adopted by self-help as well as professional groups (Alcoholics Anonymous, 1955; American Medical Association, 1977; National Council on Alcoholism, 1972).

An international contribution was established in 1964 when the World Health Organization (WHO) recommended the use of the concepts "physical" and "psychic" dependence, although the boundaries of these concepts remained vague (Kleber, 1990).

2.1.2. DSM-III Substance Use Disorders

The categorical approach to pathological use of drugs resulted in DSM-III (American Psychiatric Association, 1980), in which the terms "abuse" and "dependence" were the pivotal concepts in the section entitled "Substance Use Disorders."

Necessary for the diagnosis of dependence in DSM-III were tolerance or withdrawal or both, in keeping with the Jellinek model. Substance abuse in DSM-III, on the other hand, focused on impairment in other life domains as a result of use.

The division of substance abuse disorders into these two categories has been supported by several research groups (Filmore, 1988; Hasin, Grant, & Endicott, 1990; Roizen, Cahalan, & Shanks, 1978). Recently, Hasin et al. (1990) reported a 4-year longitudinal epidemiological study of male drinkers. At follow-up, 70% of the subjects who were initially classified as alcohol abusers were either still abusers or classified as remitted and only 30% progressed to alcohol dependence. This finding contrasted significantly with the commonly held assumption that abuse is usually a prodromal phase to dependence and thus supported the distinction between abuse and dependence. Furthermore, this distinction was reported to be moderately predictive of disorder severity and treatment outcome (Hermos, Locastro, Glynn, Bouchard, & DeLarby, 1988; Rounsaville, Dolinsky, Babor, & Meyer, 1987). Other predictors, however, including age of onset and intensity of alcohol or drug use (Schuckit et al., 1985), family history of substance abuse–dependence (Buydens-Branchey, Branchey, & Noumair, 1989), and number and severity of comorbid conditions, especially antisocial personality, have predicted both severity and outcome at least as robustly (Nathan, 1991).

The progress in terminology attributed to DSM-III was captured by Nathan (1991, p. 356), who stated that

DSM-III moved away from the implicit moralizing that burdened those positions of DSM-I and DSM-II devoted to substance abuse and dependence, the sexual deviations, and antisocial behavior. It did so, in part, by allocating a separate category to the substance use disorders, thereby eliminating the guilt by association implicit in their DSM-I and DSM-II placement. In addition, the text of the DSM-III highlighted research findings that implicated sociocultural and genetic factors in the etiology of these disorders, thereby emphasizing the role scientists and clinicians had begun to play in their study and treatment.

Criticism of DSM-III criteria for abuse–dependence has mainly addressed its inflexibility in accounting for the heterogeneity among identified patients and problems with specificity and sensitivity (Rounsaville, 1987; Rounsaville, Spitzer, & Williams, 1986; Schuckit et al., 1985). Rounsaville (1987) identified the following seven key problems: (1) There is a lack of reference to coexistent features commonly manifested in these disorders. (2) The conceptualization of substance use disorders is not theory-driven. (3) The use of tolerance as a criterion for dependence is not specified. (4) The relation between abuse and dependence is inconsistent and illogical in several substance categories in DSM-III. (5) Blackouts are incorrectly defined in the alcohol abuse and dependence criteria. (6) The limiting, time-linked phrases (e.g., one month duration, intoxicated throughout the day) were not derived empirically and, in many instances, do not accord with clinical experience. (7) Quantity and frequency of drug use are inconsistent features of the criteria.

Nathan (1991) pointed out that the dependence criteria include and sometimes mix two different concepts: psychological dependence, characterized by a pathological pattern of use, and physiological dependence, demonstrated by a substance-specific withdrawal syndrome.

Kleber (1990) noted that there was no provision in DSM-III for severity of dependence. Also, there is no distinction between dependence and long-term medical use of an opiate or sedative that results in tolerance and that, with abrupt cessation, is likely to result in withdrawal. According to DSM-III, opiate and sedative dependence with no abuse are considered psychiatric disorders, whereas similar states related to chronic use of antihypertensive drugs or tricyclic antidepressants are not (Kleber, 1990).

2.1.3. Substance Dependence Syndrome and DSM-III-R Psychoactive Substance Use Disorders

An alternative to the traditional categorical approach to the diagnosis of substance use disorders emerged in England in the mid-1970s. The alcohol dependence syndrome (ADS) (Edwards & Gross, 1976) first proposed as a clinical description of alcoholism has since been elaborated and generalized as a substance dependence syndrome (SDS) to a variety of drugs (Edwards, 1986; Edwards, Arif, & Hodgson, 1981).

The syndrome has been included in the WHO *International Classification of Diseases,* 9th edition (ICD-9, 1980) and has also been incorporated in DSM-III-R (American Psychiatric Association, 1987). The ADS is a dimensional conceptualization of alcoholism that is based on primary symptoms combined with behaviors that characterize pathological drinkers. Along each of the seven dimensions of the syndrome, persons vary widely. The SDS concept was attractive to the drafters of DSM-III-R because it appears to address most of the seven key problems of DSM-III identified by Rounsaville (1987). Recent empirical data support the coherence of SDS in cocaine users (Bryant, Rounsaville, & Babor, 1991) and the relationships of SDS to related disabilities across various classes of drugs (Hasin, Grant, Harford, & Endicott, 1988).

DSM-III-R differs from DSM-III not only conceptually but also by the following changes: (1) The cluster of disorders was entitled Psychoactive Substance Use Disorders (PSUD). (2) The format of the criteria has been changed to a diagnostic index so that no single symptom is required for a diagnosis of dependence. Also, the criteria for dependence have been broadened to include cognitive and behavioral symptoms. (3) The category of abuse was reduced to a residual one. (4) A system has been provided for denoting severity of dependence as "in remission," "mild," "moderate," or "severe" (American Psychiatric Association, 1987). Nine criteria for substance dependence have been defined; any three or more of these criteria are required to make the diagnosis, allowing for a number of possible combinations of criteria that qualify as a disorder.

Some concerns raised regarding DSM-III-R criteria were these: (1) They were designed without subjecting them to empirical testing in comparison with DSM-III criteria. (2) Reducing abuse to a residual category negates some empirical evidence to the contrary (Hasin et al., 1990). (3) DSM-III-R criteria establish an additional shift from the traditional approach to addictions and thereby complicate the ability of various disciplines in the field to communicate.

2.1.4. DSM-IV Substance-Related Disorders

It is difficult to make frequent shifts of gear from one classification system to the next. The work group on substance use disorders that prepared the DSM-IV criteria recognized this problem and followed two general guidelines. First, an objective of promoting clinical and research continuity was established, so that any further alterations in the diagnostic nomenclature will be made most carefully. Second, an effort was made to have DSM-IV be as compatible as possible with the forthcoming WHO ICD-10, by comparing DSM-III, DSM-III-R, ICD-10, and the criteria proposed for DSM-IV substance use disorders in field trials (Schuckit, Helzer, Crowley, Nathan, Woody, & Davis, 1991). It was also recommended that before changes in diagnostic scheme are acceptable, any future work group will have to consider data indicating a high likelihood that an altered approach has real benefits over what now exists in DSM-IV.

In the DSM-IV criteria, abuse does not represent a residual category as it does in DSM-III-R. Instead, abuse is diagnosed according to a distinct and specific set of behaviors. The requirement that the disturbance must have persisted for at least 1 month was deleted; instead, a period of 1 year must be evaluated. Dependence incorporates the DSM-III-R emphasis on compulsive use as well as the DSM-III reliance on impairment in social and occupational functioning and pathological use. Tolerance or withdrawal symptoms or both may be manifested, but are not required for the diagnosis of dependence by DSM-IV criteria. DSM-IV criteria for substance dependence present only a minor departure from DSM-III-R criteria. The criteria for severity have been substituted with course modifiers, the remission category has been expanded, and there is a requirement to specify whether physiological dependence is present and whether a patient is on agonist therapy or in a controlled environment.

Since the introduction in 1980 of DSM-III criteria for substance use disorders, a tremendous effort has been devoted to elucidating the following issues: (1) the thresholds of specific symptoms for dependency and abuse, (2) subtyping according to the presence or absence of tolerance and withdrawal, (3) clustering of symptoms, (4) severity ratings and the nature of remissions, and (5) the importance of social consequences. Also, it is generally recognized that a drug-free period of 4–6 weeks is needed before a person can be reliably diagnosed with a psychiatric disorder.

In summary, it remains to be seen whether the DSM-IV criteria will be able to satisfy the vigorous standards required for a stable and valid nomenclature that will also enjoy longevity.

2.1.5. Application of the Evolution of the Terminology of Substance Use Disorders for Adolescents

The terminology of substance use disorders has been developed for adults with little or no empirical evidence for its appropriateness for adolescents. The era of DSM-I, DSM-II, and Jellinek's criteria for alcoholism was the "Stone Age" in the evolution of reliable and valid terminology in child and adolescent psychiatry and in adolescent medicine. In retrospect, it appears that even if an adolescent-centered approach had been adopted, a disease model or a deficient-morality model or both would have been imposed on adolescents with substance use disorders. Actually, every model that has emphasized the physical manifestations of pathological use of alcohol or other drugs has done very poor service in reflecting what characterizes adolescents with substance use disorders.

The advancement in terminology represented by the introduction of DSM-III criteria for substance use disorders in 1980 was acknowledged by experts in the field. Some of the key problems identified by Rounsaville (1987) appeared to be even more relevant to the nature of APSUDs than to adults. First, relying on physical evidence of dependence, the DSM-III diagnosis of substance dependence could rarely be applied to adolescents due to the scarcity of related physiological and clinical sequelae (Vingilis & Smart, 1981; Filstead, 1982). Second, there was a lack of clear reference either to comorbid disorders or to the nature of the relationships between substance use disorders and presumed related problems. Third, the issue of severity of dependence was either not recognized or simply not tackled.

The progression to DSM-III-R and the application of a dimensional approach to PSUD have been in general more "adolescent friendly" (i.e., from the descriptive perspective) than DSM-III. These criteria recognize the high variability in psychoactive substance use patterns while preserving the dependence syndrome regardless of age groups and without special emphasis on physiological consequences.

The abuse category appears to represent either a mild-severity form or an early (prepathological) phase of dependence (Peyser & Gitlow, 1988). However, formatting a severity system for the dependence category and reducing the saliency of abuse to a residual category have serious implications for allocating resources to the treatment of adolescents with PSUDs. Politicians and service providers may erroneously draw conclusions that the "War on Drugs" is being won simply by increasing the threshold for dependence (i.e., dealing only with adolescents diagnosed with moderate and severe forms and ignoring the "in remission" and "mild" forms) and by the connotation of residual category in reference to substance abuse.

Professionals working with adolescents may find the conceptual framework of DSM-IV more favorable for the terminology regarding APSUDs, although no special attention has been given to this age group during the conception of DSM-IV. The improved nosological appropriateness is being reflected especially around the categorized distinction between dependence and abuse (the latter better characterizes the majority of adolescents with PSUDs). Also, although DSM-IV is more physiologically oriented than DSM-III-R, tolerance, withdrawal, and withdrawal avoidance are accepted but not essential for the diagnosis of dependence. Therefore, individuals could be diagnosed as dependent whether or not they have a number of physiological symptoms or impairments in other life domains as defined in DSM-IV. In conclusion, the special status accorded tolerance and withdrawal in DSM-IV is good news for prevention and treatment planning for APSUDs, although the applicability of the entire nosological paradigm is still unproven.

2.1.6. The Quest for Adolescent Psychoactive Substance Use Disorder as a Distinct Diagnostic Entity

Individuals, institutes, and disciplines unrelated to mental health have tried to develop terminology for children and adolescents with substance use and related problems. The terms "experimental" and "recreational" use of drugs have typically referred to nonpathological use. However, the boundaries of these terms have never been clear regarding such parameters as chronology, quantity, frequency, or consequences. The differences between other popular terms such as "heavy," "extensive," "problem" drinking, and numerous other ill-defined terms also have yet to be elucidated (Kaminer, 1991).

Before the 1980s, research on the typology of "drinking behavior" among undergraduate students focused on classification according to two dimensions of alcohol use: quantity and frequency. A large-scale survey among 7,000 students in New England conducted by Wechsler and McFadden (1979) represented a relatively cumbersome approach to nosology. Students were classified as "light" drinkers if they reported that they usually drank no more than 3 cans of beer or 2 glasses of wine or 2 "drinks" (each containing 1.5 oz) of distilled spirits per occasion. Those classified as "medium-light" drinkers usually drank no more than 4 cans of beer, 3 glasses of wine, or 3 drinks; "medium-heavy" drinkers usually drank 5–6 cans of beer, 4 glasses of wine, or 4 drinks; and "heavy" drinkers usually consumed more than 6 cans of beer, 5 or more glasses of wine, or 5 or more drinks.

Students were also divided into the following four groups based on how often they usually drank any type of alcohol: (1) less than monthly, (2) 1–3 times a month, (3) 1 or 2 times a week, and (4) more than twice a week. Students who said they never drank alcohol, or who did not drink during the year prior to the study, were classified as abstainers. These quantity and frequency measures combined to provide a typology of the following six categories of drinking behavior: (1) abstainers, (2) infrequent–light (those who drank a light amount less than once a week or a medium-light amount less than once a month), (3) frequent–light (those who drank a light amount at least once a week or a medium-light amount more than twice a week, (4) intermediate (students who drank a medium-light or medium-heavy amount at least once a month but not more than twice a week), (5) infrequent–heavy (students who drank a medium-heavy amount less than once a month or a heavy amount less than once a week), and (6) frequent–heavy (those who drank a medium-heavy amount more than twice a week or a heavy amount at least once a week) (Wechsler & McFadden, 1979).

The National Institute for Alcohol Abuse and Alcoholism tried to define problem drinking by adolescents as drinking to the point of being drunk 6 or more times a year, or having negative consequences from alcohol use 2 or more times a year, or both. Negative consequences include such problems as impaired relationships with family or peers, legal problems, academic or behavior difficulties or both at school, and driving while intoxicated. The American Academy of Pediatrics (1987) endorsed these definitions.

A review of the literature on problem drinking reveals that the concept has been operationalized in four distinct ways: heavy intake (quantity and frequency) of alcohol or use intensity, frequent intoxications, use of alcohol for escape reasons, and the experiencing of specific negative consequences while drinking or as a result of drinking (White, 1987).

Last, many current treatment programs for adolescents with PSUDs are run by professionals who usually follow the steps and traditions of Alcoholics Anonymous (AA); consequently, the terminology used is AA-oriented. No effort to distinguish between different age groups of substance users is expected from self-help-oriented treatment facilities or groups.

2.1.7. Findings in Studies of Course and Outcome

The study of the natural history and clinical course of disorders is one avenue for investigating the extent of continuity between child–adolescent and adult psychopathology. Mood disorders and anxiety disorders are frequently diagnosed as comorbid among individuals with PSUDs (Bukstein, Brent, & Kaminer, 1989). The nature of the continuity between childhood and adulthood manifestations of each of these disorders and the relationships between anxiety, depression, and PSUD have been extensively researched (and are reviewed in Chapter 5). The methodologically sound research of PSUDs in adults (retrospective studies) and in adolescents with PSUDs (retrospective and longitudinal prospective studies) has followed strategies similar to those utilized in studies of disorders of mood or anxiety or both (Angst & Vollrath, 1991; Kandel & Davies, 1986; Nurcombe, Seifer, Scioli, Tramontana, Grapentine, & Beauchesne, 1989; Vollrath & Angst, 1989; Werry, 1991).

Several studies show evidence of discontinuity of alcohol consumption by those labeled as problem drinkers in adolescence and again in early adulthood, as well as lack of a predictive relationship between young adult drinking status and later problem drinking (Cahalan & Cisin, 1976; Filmore, 1974). Also, Blane (1979) reported that frequent heavy drinking and related problems in adolescents appear to be self-limiting and are not highly predictive of alcoholism in adults. It appears that these studies share a maturational-process-oriented paradigm.

In contrast to the aforementioned reports, other studies provide important information regarding the stability of heavy self-reported problem drinking or of problems related to alcohol use, or of both, from adolescence to early adulthood (Anderson & Magnusson, 1988; Wechsler & Rohman, 1981; White, 1987). White (1987) indicated that traditional measures of problem drinking represent at least two distinct dimensions: intensity of use and use-related problems. A follow-up of more than 1,000 adolescents for up to 10 years revealed that use of a particular drug class in that period most strongly predicted the continued use of this same class of drugs in young adulthood (Kandel, Davies, Karus, & Yamaguchi, 1986).

The different results of these two groups of studies regarding the stability and predictive validity of PSUDs are due to various methodological limitations. These limitations include high rates of sample attrition, lack of blindness to an earlier diagnosis, underscored psychiatric comorbidity and polysubstance abuse, lack of normal and/or psychiatric control, uncertainty regarding the reliability of reports about the illegal aspects of psychoactive substance use (e.g., the underage status of adolescents regarding cigarettes and alcohol use), and significant differences between adolescent substance use patterns and their related problems compared to adults (i.e., lack of a consensus on how best to measure problem drinking among adolescents).

The last limitation has attracted special interest. Blane (1979) argued that teenage drinking problems are often related to acute intoxication episodes rather than to a chronic condition as in adult alcoholics. Also, adolescents often encounter problems with their parents because of alcohol consumption even if drinking does not result in either intoxication or other problems. Such conflicts may reflect cultural, religious, or familial values as well as other psychosocioeconomic factors, not to neglect mentioning that any psychoactive substance use by an adolescent is illegal.

Two important questions need to be answered in order to conclude whether findings in studies of the course and outcome of adolescent substance use and APSUDs can clarify the age-group-distinction dilemma. First, are the substance-abuse-related problems of adolescent substance abusers really related? Second, do substance-use-related problems form a valid basis for diagnosis? In some studies of problem drinking among adolescents, a direct relationship has been reported between the number of problems experienced and the volume of alcohol consumed (Polich & Orvis, 1979). On the other hand, several studies indicate limited correlations between measures of consumption and measures of problems in adolescents (Rachal et al., 1980; White, 1987) and in adults (Sadava, 1985).

It seems that the answer to the first question is qualitatively positive based on a categorical approach (DSM-III-oriented). It is also quantitatively positive based on a dimensional approach (DSM-III-R-oriented). A response to the categorical approach would indicate that intensity of drinking and alcohol-related problems are strongly related. The dimensional approach will modify the answer by adding that intensity of drinking and number of problems represent at least two distinct dimensions of problem drinking (White, 1987). A comparison to references in the adult literature shows variable levels of agreement about the relationship between the abuse of different drugs (i.e., cocaine, opiates, and alcohol) and related problems, this agreement in general validating to a high degree the multidimensional approach of the SDS (Hasin et al., 1988; Kosten, Rounsaville, Babor, Spitzer, & Williams, 1987; McLellan, Luborsky, Woody, O'Brien, & Kron, 1981).

The presence of various dysfunctions (e.g., academic, familial, legal) as a basis for the diagnosis of PSUD is especially problematic in view of the high prevalence of comorbidity with other psychiatric disorders (Bukstein et al., 1989). The clustering of signs and symptoms that are part of the diagnostic criteria does not, in itself, constitute a disorder (especially not in polysymptomatic adolescents). Also, according to the problem-behavior theory, the persistent-deviant problem behavior is part of a larger schema that also includes substance use (Jessor & Jessor, 1977) and is not the result of substance abuse as depicted in the disease model.

The age of onset of heavy alcohol use has recently been established to correlate better with alcohol-related problems than does the duration of heavy drinking (Lee & DiClimente, 1985). Furthermore, the age of onset has been found to be crucial not only to the clinical course of alcoholism but also to onset-based alcoholism typologies (Parrella & Filstead, 1988).

Many classifications appear to have a common theme: There is among alcoholics a subgroup of patients who have a high genetic loading for alcoholism, who start abusing alcohol in their teens, whose alcoholism has a severe course, and who have a high frequency of coexisting psychiatric problems among which aggressive tendencies, impulsivity, and antisocial behavior have been prominent (Buydens-Branchey, Branchey, & Noumair, 1989). A second type of alcoholic is characterized by later onset, fewer childhood risk factors, less severe dependence, fewer alcohol-related problems, and less psychopathological dysfunction. It appears that Type A and Type B alcoholism (Babor et al., 1992), late- and early-onset subtypes (Buydens-Branchey, Branchey, & Noumair, 1989), alcoholism Type 1 (milieu-limited) and Type 2 (male-limited) (Cloninger, 1987), and gamma and delta alcoholism (Jellinek, 1952, 1960) support a dichotomous typology and have more similarities than differences.

There are two important differences between the typologies proposed by Cloninger (1987) and those proposed by Babor et al. (1992), and these differences deserve mention here: First, Cloninger's Type 1 alcoholic is characterized by binge drinking, as well as by significant anxiety and depressive symptoms. The Type A alcoholic, in contrast, is characterized by less binge drinking and fewer anxiety and depressive symptoms. Second, Cloninger's Type 2 characteristics were found not to be prevalent in female alcoholics, while in the study by Babor et al. (1992), both Type A and Type B were identified in both male and female alcoholics. The most likely explanation for these differences is the different methodological approaches employed: The typology of Cloninger (1987) was based on genetic epidemiological data, while the typology developed by Babor et al. (1992) was based on clinical assessment.

According to the interpretation of a biopsychosocial approach, a genetic predisposition combined with childhood antecedents predisposes vulnerable subjects to a more virulent form of alcoholism (Babor et al., 1992). Individuals diagnosed with Type B alcoholism have not been concluded to be a homogeneous group. It is likely that individuals with and without antisocial personality disorder (ASPD) compose the group and those with ASPD may or may not have a history of anxiety or mood disorder (Babor et al., 1992). Application of this empirically derived typology to treatment matching has been reported recently (Litt, Babor, DelBoca, Kadden, & Cooney, 1992). Type B alcoholics had better outcomes with coping-skills treatment and poor results with interactional therapy, while Type A fared better conversely. These differences were maintained for a 24-month follow-up period, with Type B patients experiencing more psychosocial dysfunction and drinking problems than Type A. This study may suggest that in matching patients to treatment, ASPD should be considered as an important factor (Litt et al., 1992).

The age of onset of alcoholism has been reported to be related not only to a specific type of alcoholism but also to a biological marker (Buydens-Branchey, Branchey, Noumair, & Leiber, 1989). Early-onset alcoholics had a significant association between a low ratio of plasma tryptophan (a serotonin precursor) to other amino acids competing for brain entry and measures of depression and aggressivity. This finding suggests a preexisting deficit in serotonin that could lead to alcoholism later in life. The typological distinction drawn by these investigators from clinical descriptions closely resembles the typology of Babor et al. (1992) in the areas of familial alcoholism, antisocial behavior, and co-morbid mood disorder.

In summary, although it appears that an early (adolescent) onset of one subtype of alcoholism has been reported, it is not distinct from the same subtype in adulthood. However, implications for prevention and treatment are crucial (as is elaborated in the following relevant chapters). Finally, it is noteworthy to refer to family history of alcoholism and other psychopathologies as a factor in the etiology, course, and development of comorbid psychosocial problems and sequelae (Nathan, 1990). However, for nosological purposes, family history per se has not yet been sufficient.

2.2. CONCLUSION

The state of the art of APSUD does not support a distinct adolescent-oriented category separate from the present DSM-III-R/IV-oriented terminology. Also, severity and chronicity do not appear to account for differences in age-related symptomatology, and their impact on meeting the criteria of PSUD phenomenology (besides medical complications) is limited. However, these conclusions do not preclude such a development in the future, especially following more empirical research regarding some key questions for which there are no data: (1) What is the natural history of PSUDs in children and adolescents? (2) What are the nature and magnitude of spontaneous recovery among adolescents? (3) What are the magnitude and nature of the effects of experimentally controlled use of alcohol and other psychoactive substances in adolescents? It is clear that such research may be constrained by legal restrictions and may therefore have to be postponed until these individuals reach adulthood. Lack of such research limits our understanding about subgrouping of adolescents with APSUDs. Any further development in adolescent substance abuse prevention and treatment will have to rely on age-appropriate generated nosology and data. Finally, the potential for the existence of "good prognosis APSUD" needs to be explored, particularly following Hasin et al.'s (1990) findings that most alcohol abusers did not progress to alcohol dependence. Most adolescents with alcohol abuse do not fit Babor's (1992) or Cloninger's (1987) description of a "malignant" course alcoholism. Therefore, it is reasonable to suggest that there are at least two different types of alcoholism in adolescence. It appears that PSUD with conduct disorder, with or without depressive symptomatology, shares considerable similarities with Type B or Type 1, and alcohol abuse or dependence without comorbid conduct disorder may be comparable to Type A or Type 1.

REFERENCES

Alcoholics Anonymous (1955). *Twelve Steps and Twelve Traditions*. New York: AA World Services.

American Academy of Pediatrics: Committee on Adolescence (1987). Alcohol use and abuse: A pediatric concern. *Pediatrics, 74*, 450–452.

American Medical Association: Committee on Alcoholism (1977). *Manual on Alcoholism*. Chicago: American Medical Association.

American Psychiatric Association (1952). *Diagnostic and Statistical Manual of Mental Disorders*, 1st ed. Washington, DC: American Psychiatric Association.

American Psychiatric Association (1968). *Diagnostic and Statistical Manual of Mental Disorders*, 2nd ed. Washington, DC: American Psychiatric Association.

American Psychiatric Association (1980). *Diagnostic and Statistical Manual of Mental Disorders*, 3rd ed. Washington, DC: American Psychiatric Association.

American Psychiatric Association (1987). *Diagnostic and Statistical Manual of Mental Disorders*, 3rd ed., rev. Washington, DC: American Psychiatric Association.

American Psychiatric Association (1994). *Diagnostic and Statistical Manual of Mental Disorders*, 4th ed. Washington, DC: American Psychiatric Association.

Anderson, T., Magnusson, D. (1988). Drinking habits and alcohol abuse among young men: A prospective longitudinal study. *Journal of Studies on Alcohol, 49*, 245–252.

Angst, J., & Vollrath, M. (1991). The natural history of anxiety disorders. *Acta Psychiatrica Scandinavica, 84*, 446–452.

Babor, T. F., Hofmann, M., DelBoca, F. K., Hesselbrock, V., Meyer, R. E., Dolinsky, Z. S., & Rounsaville, B. (1992). Types of alcoholics. I. Evidence for an empirically derived typology based on indicators of vulnerability and severity. *Archives of General Psychiatry, 49*, 599–608.

Blane, H. (1979). Middle-aged alcoholics and young drinkers. In H. Blane & M. Chafetz (Eds.), *Youth, Alcohol and Social Policy* (pp. 5–38). New York: Plenum Press.

Bryant, K. J., Rounsaville, B. J., & Babor, T. F. (1991). Coherence of the dependence syndrome in cocaine users. *British Journal of Addiction, 86,* 1299–1310.

Bukstein, O. G., Brent, D. A., & Kaminer, Y. (1989). Comorbidity of substance abuse and other psychiatric disorders in adolescents. *American Journal of Psychiatry, 146,* 1131–1141.

Buydens-Branchey, L., Branchey, M. H., & Noumair, D. (1989). Age of alcoholism onset. I. Relationship to psychopathology. *Archives of General Psychiatry, 46,* 225–230.

Buydens-Branchey, L., Branchey, M. H., Noumair, D., & Lieber, C. S. (1989). Age of alcoholism onset. II. Relationship to susceptibility to serotonin precursor availability. *Archives of General Psychiatry, 46,* 231–236.

Cahalan, D., & Cisin, I. H. (1976). Drinking behavior and drinking problems in the U.S. In B. Kissin & H. Begleiter (Eds.), *The Biology of Alcoholism,* Vol. 4 (pp. 77–115). New York: Plenum Press.

Cloninger, C. R. (1987). Neurogenetic adaptive mechanisms in alcoholism. *Science, 236,* 410–416.

Edwards, G. (1986). The alcohol dependence syndrome: A concept as a stimulus for enquiry. *British Journal of Addiction, 81,* 171–183.

Edwards, G., Arif, A., & Hodgson, R. (1981). Nomenclature and classification of drug and alcohol related problems. *Bulletin of the World Health Organization, 59,* 225–242.

Edwards, G., & Gross, M. M. (1976). Alcohol dependence: Provisional description of a clinical syndrome. *British Medical Journal, 1,* 1058–1061.

Filmore, K. M. (1974). Drinking and problem drinking in early adulthood and middle age. *Quarterly Journal of Studies on Alcohol, 35,* 819–840.

Filmore, K. M. (1988). *Alcohol Use across the Life course: A Critical Review of 70 Years of International Longitudinal Research.* Toronto: Addiction Research Foundation.

Filstead, W. J. (1982). Adolescence and alcohol. In E. M. Pattison & E. Kaufman (Eds.), *Encyclopedic Handbook of Alcoholism* (pp. 156–178). New York: Gardner Press.

Hasin, D. S., Grant, B. F., & Endicott, J. (1990). The natural history of alcohol abuse: Implications for definitions of alcohol use disorders. *American Journal of Psychiatry, 147,* 1537–1541.

Hasin, D. S., Grant, B. F., Harford, T. C., & Endicott, J. (1988). The drug dependence syndrome and related disabilities. *British Journal of Addiction, 83,* 45–55.

Hermos, J. A., Locastro, J. S., Glynn, R. J., Bouchard, G. R., & DeLarby, L. O. (1988). Predictors of reduction and cessation of drinking in community-dwelling men: Results from the normative aging study. *Journal of Studies of Alcohol, 49,* 363–368.

Jellinek, E. M. (1952). Phases of alcohol addiction. *Journal of Studies on Alcohol, 13,* 673–684.

Jellinek, E. M. (1960). *The Disease Concept of Alcoholism.* New Brunswick: Hillhouse Press.

Jessor, R., & Jessor, S. L. (1977). *Problem Behavior and Psychosocial Development: A Longitudinal Study of Youth.* New York: Academic Press.

Kaminer, Y. (1991). Adolescent substance abuse. In R. J. Frances & R. I. Miller (Eds.), *Clinical Textbook of Addictive Disorders* (pp. 320–346). New York: Guilford Press.

Kandel, D. B., & Davies, M. (1986). Adult sequelae of adolescent depressive symptoms. *Archives of General Psychiatry, 43,* 255–262.

Kandel, D. B., Davies, M., Karus, D., & Yamaguchi, K. (1986). The consequences in young adulthood of adolescent drug involvement. *Archives of General Psychiatry, 43,* 746–754.

Kleber, H. D. (1990). The nosology of abuse and dependence. *Journal of Psychiatric Research, 24,* 57–64.

Kosten, T., Rounsaville, B., Babor, T., Spitzer, R., & Williams, J. (1987). Substance use disorders in DSM-III-R: Evidence for the dependence syndrome across different psychoactive substances. *British Journal of Psychiatry, 151,* 834–843.

Lee, G. P., & DiClimente, C. C. (1985). Age of onset versus duration of problem drinking on the alcohol use inventory. *Journal of Studies on Alcohol, 46,* 398–402.

Litt, M. D., Babor, T. F., DelBoca, F. K., Kadden, R. M., & Cooney, N. L. (1992). Types of alcoholics. II. Application of an empirically derived typology to treatment matching. *Archives of General Psychiatry, 49,* 609–614.

McLellan, A. T., Luborsky, L., Woody, G. E., O'Brien, C. P., & Kron, R. (1981). Are the "addiction-related" problems of substance abusers really related? *Journal of Nervous and Mental Disease, 169,* 232–239.

Mendelson, J. H., & Mello, N. K. (1966). Experimental analysis of drinking behavior of chronic alcoholics. *Annals of the New York Academy of Sciences, 133,* 820–845.

Merry, J. (1966). The "loss of control" myth. *Lancet, 1,* 1257–1258.

Meyer, R. E. (1986). Old wine, new bottle: The alcohol dependence syndrome. *Psychiatric Clinics of North America, 9,* 435–453.

Musto, D. F. (1973). *The American Disease: Origins of Narcotic Controls.* New Haven: Yale University Press.

Nathan, P. E. (1990). Integration of biological and psychosocial research on alcoholism. *Alcoholism: Clinical and Experimental Research, 14,* 368–374.

Nathan, P. E. (1991). Substance use disorders in DSM-IV. *Journal of Abnormal Psychology, 100,* 356–361.

National Council on Alcoholism (1972). Criteria for the diagnosis of alcoholism. *American Journal of Psychiatry, 129,* 127–135.

Nurcombe, B., Seifer, R., Scioli, A., Tramontana, M. G., Grapentine, L., & Beauchesne, H. R. (1989). Is major depressive disorder in adolescence a distinct diagnostic entity? *Journal of the American Academy of Child and Adolescent Psychiatry, 28,* 333–342.

Parrella, D. P., & Filstead, W. J. (1988). Definition of onset in the development of onset-based alcoholism typologies. *Journal of Studies on Alcohol, 44,* 85–92.

Peyser, H. S., & Gitlow, S. E. (1988). Substance abuse category in DSM-III-R (letter). *American Journal of Psychiatry, 145,* 279–280.

Polich, J. M., & Orvis, B. R. (1979). *Alcohol Problems: Patterns and Prevalence in the U.S. Air Force.* Santa Monica, CA: Rand Corp.

Rachal, J. V., Guess, L. S., Hubbard, R. L., Maisto, S. A., Cavanaugh, E. R., Waddell, R., & Benrud, C. H. (1980). *Adolescent Drinking Behavior,* Vol. 1. Research Triangle Park, NC: Research Triangle Institute.

Rinaldi, R. C., Steindler, E. M., Wilford, B. B., & Goodwin, D. (1988). Clarification and standardization of substance abuse terminology. *Journal of the American Medical Association, 259,* 555–557.

Roizen, R., Cahalan, D., & Shanks, P. (1978). Spontaneous remission among untreated problem drinkers. In D. B. Kandel (Ed.), *Longitudinal Research on Drug Use: Empirical Findings and Methodological Issues* (pp. 197–221). Washington, DC: Hemisphere Press.

Rounsaville, B. J. (1987). An evaluation of the DSM-III substance-use disorders. In G. Tischler (Ed.), *Treatment and Classification in Psychiatry* (pp. 175–194). New York: Cambridge University Press.

Rounsaville, B. J., Dolinsky, Z. S., Babor, T. F., & Meyer, R. G. (1987). Psychopathology as a predictor of treatment outcome in alcoholics. *Archives of General Psychiatry, 44,* 505–513.

Rounsaville, B. J., Spitzer, R. L., & Williams, J. (1986). Proposed changes in DSM-III substance use disorders: Description and rationale. *American Journal of Psychiatry, 143,* 463–468.

Sadava, S. W. (1985). Problem behavior theory and consumption, and consequences of alcohol use. *Journal of Studies on Alcohol, 46,* 392–397.

Schuckit, M. A., Helzer, J., Crowley, T., Nathan, P., Woody, G., & Davis, W. (1991). Substance use disorders: DSM-IV in progress. *Hospital and Community Psychiatry, 42,* 471–473.

Schuckit, M. A., Zisook, S., & Mortola, J. (1985). Clinical implications of DSM-III diagnosis of alcohol abuse and alcohol dependence. *American Journal of Psychiatry, 142,* 1403–1408.

Vingilis, E., & Smart, R. G. (1981). Physical dependence on alcohol in youth. In Y. Israel, F. B. Gleser, & H. Kalant (Eds.), *Research Advances in Alcohol and Drug Problems,* Vol. 6 (pp. 197–215). New York: Plenum Press.

Vollrath, M., & Angst, J. (1989). Outcome of panic and depression in a seven-year follow-up: Results of the Zurich study. *Acta Psychiatrica Scandinavica, 80,* 591–596.

Wechsler, H., & McFadden, M. (1979). Drinking among college students in New England. *Journal of Studies on Alcohol, 40,* 969–996.

Wechsler, H., & Rohman, M. (1981). Extensive users of alcohol among college students. *Journal of Studies on Alcohol, 42,* 145–155.

Werry, J. S. (1991). Overanxious disorder: A review of its taxonomic properties. *Journal of the American Academy of Child and Adolescent Psychiatry, 30,* 533–544.

White, H. R. (1987). Longitudinal stability and dimensional structure of problem drinking in adolescence. *Journal of Studies on Alcohol, 48,* 541–550.

World Health Organization (1980). *International Classification of Diseases,* 9th ed. Geneva: World Health Organization.

CHAPTER 3

Epidemiology of Adolescent Substance Use and Adolescent Psychoactive Substance Use Disorders

It has been reported that in the early 1990s, the general downward trend in the prevalence of drug use that started in 1980 has continued (Johnston, O'Malley, & Bachman, 1992). Despite this encouraging report, which implies that adolescents continue to move away from the use of drugs (especially alcohol, marijuana, and cocaine), a considerable number of youngsters continue to use illicit drugs.

The measurement of adolescent substance use (ASU) and adolescent psychoactive substance use disorders (APSUDs) is complicated by the facts that the desired information pertains to illegal behavior related to age or drugs of use, or both, and that subpopulations of interest may not volunteer to cooperate. A cardinal source of information is the Annual National High School Seniors Survey, which has been conducted since 1975 (Johnston et al., 1992). In 1991, 15,500 seniors from 136 high schools in the United States were surveyed. Also in 1991, national samples of 8th and 10th graders were added to the study for the first time.

The survey explores drug use among different racial/ethnic subgroups of high school seniors and documents the extent to which drug use varies between the sexes. Other key issues reported are trends in attitudes and beliefs about drugs, especially regarding perceived harmfulness, perceived availability, and personal disapproval of drug use.

The study, subtitled also "Monitoring the Future," includes neither the estimated 20% of high school dropouts nor absentees on the day of survey at each school. However, the stability of the reports generated over 17 consecutive years provides a good measurement of trends in that seniors who are frequently truant are similar in many respects to dropouts (Bachman, Wallace, O'Malley, Johnston, Kurth, & Neighbors, 1991). Given that drug use is higher among dropouts, it is likely that the inclusion of dropouts would tend to raise the observed prevalence rates for all drugs and all subgroups. Eighth-grade students represented the junior high school population and 10th-grade students as well as seniors represented the high school population. These subpopulations may reduce the impact of school dropouts on prevalence estimates.

On the basis of the 1991 survey, the trends of drug use of most psychoactive substances studied may be divided into two groups. Group 1 included drugs such as the three most commonly used ones, alcohol, marijuana, and cocaine, with the addition of the category defined as "Other Stimulants." This group shows a consistent trend of reduction in use, including annual prevalence, 30-day prevalence, and, most important, 30-day prevalence daily use (Table 3.1).

Group 2 includes most of the other illicit drugs, the use rates of which either are down, by less than statistical significance, or have remained fairly stable at a low level of use. These drugs include mainly inhalants, crystal methamphetamine ("ice"), heroin, phencyclidine (PCP), sedatives, and anabolic steroids. Cigarette smoking and the use of lysergic acid diethylamide (LSD) by adolescents deserve specific attention due to an arrest in the mild decline trend of the former and the increase in use of the latter (Table 3.2).

3.1. TRENDS IN THE USE OF SPECIFIC DRUGS PER SUBPOPULATIONS

3.1.1. Cigarette Smoking

The decline in use in 30-day prevalence and daily use prevalence among seniors in the last 10 years amounts only to 10% and 1.8%, respectively. The rate of smoking among males dropped slightly more than among females, resulting in a modest reversal of the sex differences (in contrast to the situation with most other drugs used). In the last 10 years, rates for females' daily use, as well as in the category of a half-pack or more per day, have been slightly higher than among males.

Among 8th graders, 44% have already tried cigarettes. Initiation of use when they were 6th graders was reported by 20%. Smoking in the

Table 3.1
Downward Trends in Usage Prevalence of Marijuana, Alcohol, Cocaine, and Other Stimulants[a]

Drug	Annual prevalence[b]				30-Day prevalence				30-Day prevalence daily use			
	Highest[c]	Lowest[c]	1991	Δ88–91[d]	Highest[c]	Lowest[c]	1991	Δ88–91[d]	Highest[c]	Lowest[c]	1991	Δ88–91[d]
Marijuana	1979 / 50.8	1990 / 27.0	23.9	−9.2	1978 / 37.1	1990 / 14.0	13.8	−4.2	1978 / 10.7	1990 / 2.2	2.0	−0.7
Alcohol	1979 / 88.1	1990 / 80.6	77.7	−7.6	1978 / 72.1	1990 / 57.1	54.0	−9.9	1979 / 6.9	1990 / 3.7	3.6	−0.6
									1981[e] / 41.4	1990[e] / 32.2	29.8	−4.9
Cocaine	1985 / 13.1	1990 / 5.3	3.5	−4.4	1985 / 6.7	1990 / 1.9	1.4	−2.0	1985–6 / 0.4	1990 / 0.1	0.1	−0.1
Other stimulants adjusted	1982 / 20.3	1990 / 9.1	8.2	−2.7	1982 / 10.7	1990 / 3.7	3.2	−1.4	1983 / 0.8	1990 / 0.2	0.2	−0.1

[a]Based on data within the public domain (Johnston et al., 1992). The figures cited are the percentages of seniors who used the drugs in the periods noted.
[b]The year denotes the years of graduation.
[c]The highest and lowest percentages are stated for the most recent year before 1991.
[d]Δ = Change.
[e]Five or more drinks at one sitting within the past 2 weeks.

Table 3.2

Trends in Usage Prevalence of Cigarettes, Inhalants, Heroin, Other Opiates, Sedatives, LSD, and Steroids[a]

	Annual prevalence[b]				30-Day prevalence				30-Day prevalence daily use			
	Highest[c]	Lowest[c]	1991	Δ88–91[d]	Highest[c]	Lowest[c]	1991	Δ88–91[d]	Highest[c]	Lowest[c]	1991	Δ88–91[d]
Cigarettes	1977[e]	1989[e]			1976	1989			1976–7	1988		
	75.7	64.4	63.1	−3.3	38.8	28.6	28.3	−0.4	28.8	18.1	18.5	+0.4
									1976[f]	1988[f]		
									19.4	10.6	10.7	+0.1
Inhalants adjusted	1979	1981			1987	1981–3			1985–7	1978		
	8.9	6.1	6.9	+0.1	3.5	2.5	2.6	−0.4	0.4	0.1	0.5	+0.2
Heroin	1975	1990			1975	1990			1989	1990		
	1.0	0.5	0.4	−0.1	0.4	0.2	0.2	0.0	0.1	0.0	0.0	0.0

Other opiates	1977	1990			1977	1990			1989	1979		
	6.4	4.5	3.5	−1.1	2.8	1.1	1.1	−0.5	0.2	0.0	0.1	0.0

Sedatives	1975	1989–90			1975	1990			1975	1989–90		
	11.7	3.6	3.6	−0.1	5.4	1.4	1.5	+0.1	0.3	0.1	0.1	0.0

LSD	1975	1990			1981	1984			1990	1989		
	7.2	5.4	5.2	+0.4	2.5	1.5	1.9	+0.1	0.1	0.1	0.1	0.0

Steroids[g]	1989	1990			1990	1989			1990	1989		
	1.9	1.7	1.4	−0.5	1.0	0.8	0.8	0.0	0.2	0.1	0.1	−0.1

[a] Based on data within the public domain (Johnston et al., 1992). The figures cited are the percentages of seniors who used the drugs in the periods noted.
[b] The year denotes the year of graduation.
[c] The highest and lowest percentages are stated for the most recent year before 1991.
[d] Δ = Change.
[e] Lifetime prevalence (no report on annual prevalence).
[f] Half a pack or more per day.
[g] Data collection started in 1989.

past 30 days is reported by 14% of these students and daily use by 7% (Table 3.3).

Native American seniors have had the highest rates for use of cigarettes, as compared to other ethnic/racial subpopulations. White seniors were rated second, followed by Hispanic, black, and Asian-American subgroups (Bachman et al., 1991). Daily smoking by white seniors dropped by about 25% in the last decade, as compared to a decline by almost two thirds among African-American seniors.

3.1.2. Alcohol

The proportions of seniors who had drunk in the last 30 days dropped 3% from the 1990 level and 18% from a decade ago. The rate of decline of binge drinking was about 2% in 1991 and about 10% as compared to 1981. The 30-day prevalence declined more than 3% and daily use was reduced by only 0.1% in the last year. The sex differences in alcohol use have narrowed. Gender differences in annual prevalence have been virtually eliminated. The proportions of males admitting to binge drinking continued to decline in the 1980s, whereas the decline in binge drinking by females was more modest, resulting in a continued narrowing of the gap between the sexes. Reports on various types of alcoholic beverages indicate that the largest sex difference is attributed to heavy use of beer by males. Hard liquor is consumed only slightly more by males than by females. Females tend to drink more wine coolers than male seniors, and wine is equally used by both sexes.

Drinking in the past year is reported by 54% of 8th graders, 27% report having gotten drunk at least once (Table 3.3), and 13% admitted to binge drinking during the 2-week period prior to the survey. More than 8% started drinking before or in the 6th grade.

Alcohol use among the white and Native American subgroups is higher than among other ethnic/racial subpopulations. Rates of daily drinking were the highest among 12th-grade Native Americans and were nearly as high among Mexican Americans and white seniors. Within each of these groups, daily drinking is about 2–4 times as likely among males as among females. African-American, Hispanic, and Asian-American females are more likely to abstain from alcohol than are white females.

3.1.3. Marijuana

This is the most widely used illicit drug among high school seniors. Between the years 1990 and 1991, the reported annual use of marijuana dropped 3%; the 30-day prevalence declined only slightly, 0.2%, as com-

Table 3.3
A Comparison of Drug Usage Percentage for 8th, 10th, and 12th Graders in 1991[a]

	Lifetime			Annual			30-Day			Daily		
	Eighth	Tenth	Twelfth	Eighth	Tenth	Twelfth	Eighth	Tenth	Twelfth	Eighth	Tenth	Twelfth
Drug ≈ N:	17,500	14,800	15,000	17,500	14,800	15,000	17,500	14,800	15,000	17,500	14,800	15,000
Marijuana/hashish	10.2	23.4	36.7	6.2	16.5	28.9	3.2	8.7	13.8	0.2	0.8	2.0
Inhalants	17.6	15.7	17.6	9.0	7.1	6.6	4.4	2.7	2.4	0.2	0.1	0.2
Inhalants adj.	—	—	18.0	—	—	6.9	—	—	2.6	—	—	0.5
Amyl/butyl nitrites	—	—	1.6	—	—	0.9	—	—	0.4	—	—	0.2
Hallucinogens	3.2	6.1	9.6	1.9	4.0	5.8	0.8	1.6	2.2	0.1	0.0	0.1
Hallucinogens adj.	—	—	10.0	—	—	6.1	—	—	2.4	—	—	0.1
LSD	2.7	5.6	8.8	1.7	3.7	5.2	0.6	1.5	1.9	0.0	0.0	0.1
PCP	—	—	2.9	—	—	1.4	—	—	0.5	—	—	0.1
Other psychs	1.4	2.2	3.7	0.7	1.3	2.0	0.3	0.4	0.7	0.0	0.0	0.1
Cocaine	2.3	4.1	7.8	1.1	2.2	3.5	0.5	0.7	1.4	0.1	0.1	0.1
"Crack"	1.3	1.7	3.1	0.7	0.9	1.5	0.3	0.3	0.7	0.0	0.0	0.1
Other cocaine	2.0	3.8	7.0	1.0	2.1	3.2	0.5	0.6	1.2	0.0	0.0	0.1
Heroin	1.2	1.2	0.9	0.7	0.5	0.4	0.3	0.2	0.2	0.0	0.0	0.0
Stimulants adj.	10.5	13.2	15.4	6.2	8.2	8.2	2.6	3.3	3.2	0.1	0.1	0.2
"Ice"	—	—	3.3	—	—	1.4	—	—	0.6	—	—	0.1
Tranquilizers	3.8	5.8	7.2	1.8	3.2	3.6	0.8	1.2	1.4	0.0	0.0	0.1
Alcohol												
Any use	70.1	83.8	88.0	54.0	72.3	77.7	25.1	42.8	54.0	0.5	1.3	3.6
≥5 Drinks in last 2 weeks	—	—	—	—	—	—	—	—	—	12.9	22.9	29.8
Cigarettes												
Any use	44.0	55.1	63.1	—	—	—	14.3	20.8	28.3	7.2	12.6	18.5
≥1/2 Pack/day	—	—	—	—	—	—	—	—	—	3.1	6.5	10.7
Steroids	1.9	1.8	2.1	1.0	1.1	1.4	0.4	0.6	0.8	0.0	0.1	0.1
Smokeless tobacco	22.2	28.2	—	—	—	—	6.9	10.0	—	0.2	0.2	—
Been drunk	26.7	50.0	65.4	17.5	40.1	52.7	7.6	20.5	31.6	0.2	0.2	0.9

[a] Based on data within the public domain (Johnston et al., 1992).

pared to 2.6% between 1989 and 1990. The daily use of marijuana also dropped 0.2% as compared to 0.7% between the years 1989 and 1990. The absolute and ratio differences between the sexes have narrowed slightly during the 1980s.

Of 8th graders, 10% reported ever using marijuana, and 6% admitted to use within the preceding year. More than 2% used the drug in the 6th grade. Further, 3% admitted to marijuana use during the 1-month period before the survey, and 0.2% reported daily use during the last 30 days.

Marijuana has been referred to as a "gateway" drug (Kandel, 1982). Indeed, the single best predictor of cocaine use is frequent use of marijuana during adolescence. Only 1% of those not regularly using any drug and 4% of legal drug users had experimented with opiates, cocaine, and hallucinogens, as compared to 26% of marijuana users (Kandel, 1982).

Annual prevalence rates for marijuana are highest among Native American females and males, and nearly as high among white males and females and Mexican American males. The lowest annual rates are reported by Latin-American females, African-American females, and Asian-American males and females (Bachman et al., 1991). Monthly and daily rates maintain the same racial and ethnic distinctions. Male–female differences are more pronounced among African Americans and Hispanics.

3.1.4. Cocaine

The annual use among seniors fell more than 30% and 30-day use declined about 25% between the years 1990 and 1991. Daily use remained very low at 0.1%. Crack cocaine use among seniors dropped from 1.9% to 1.5% annual prevalence between 1990 and 1991, respectively, from a peak of 4.1% in 1986. The ratio of male–female prevalence rates in cocaine use narrowed further during the recent downturn in use. Both sexes also showed a decline in crack use.

Relatively few students initiate cocaine or crack use by the 8th grade (2.3% lifetime prevalence).

Prevalence rates for cocaine are highest among male and female Native Americans and white and Hispanic male seniors. Black females report less cocaine use than other females. African-American and Hispanic male cocaine use prevalence is double that for females from the same ethnic/racial groups.

3.1.5. LSD

This drug reached an all-time low for lifetime, annual, and 30-day prevalence in the mid-1980s. Since then, there appears to be some upward drift in use (see Table 3.2).

LSD use may be found at all grade levels, with 2.7% lifetime prevalence and 30-day prevalence of 0.6% among 8th graders.

3.1.6. Phencyclidine (PCP)

This drug is a hallucinogen, the use of which is infrequently reported by seniors. However, a mild increase in annual and 30-day use since 1990 warrants continuous monitoring of its use.

3.1.7. Stimulants Adjusted

This category excludes the inappropriate reporting of nonprescription stimulants, crystal methamphetamine ("ice"), and doctor-prescribed stimulants. A steady decline in all trends in prevalence was reported.

Since 1982, females have shown slightly higher or equivalent rates of stimulant use, due to their more frequent use of amphetamines for the purpose of weight loss. Both sexes have shown a decline in the use of stimulants since 1984. More than 10% of 8th graders reported lifetime use of drugs from this category; also, 2.6% and 0.1% of 30-day use and daily use, respectively, were recorded.

Another stimulant with some hallucinogenic effects is 3,4-methylenedioxymethamphetamine (MDMA), known also as "ecstasy." It was reported to be used by only 0.6% and 0.1% of seniors (annual use and 30-day prevalence, respectively).

"Ice" use has also been infrequent, and its 30-day prevalence in 1990 and 1991 was 0.6%.

3.1.8. Heroin

The use of this drug among seniors is very low (Table 3.2), but actually it is slightly higher in the lower grades than in the 12th grade. Johnston et al. (1992) explain this phenomenon with the observation that few of the eventual school dropouts have left school by the 8th or 10th grade, whereas most have left by the 12th grade. Lifetime prevalence is 1.2% for both 8th and 10th grades, compared with 0.9% for seniors (Table 3.3).

3.1.9. Anabolic Steroids

These agents were added to the survey in 1989. Since then, there has been a very gradual decline in lifetime and annual prevalence. Among males, who account for most of the steroid use, the proportions using in the prior year were 2.8% in 1989, 2.6% in 1990, and 2.4% in 1991.

While the use of anabolic steroids is relatively low at all grade levels, there is very little difference among the grades (Table 3.3). For just the boys in the 8th, 10th, and 12th grades, the corresponding rates are 3%, 3.1%, and 3.5%.

Risk groups for exposure are athletes and bodybuilders, who use steroids to enhance their ability and to be aggressive (Kashkin & Kleber, 1989), and wrestlers concerned with making their weight class.

In another recent study of adolescent users of anabolic steroids, it was reported that about 250,000 seniors have used these substances at least once and that those adolescents who became chronic users were more likely to use other drugs as well. Many of these adolescents reported having shared needles (Durant, Rickert, Ashworth, Newman, & Slavens, 1993).

3.1.10. Inhalants

The use of inhalants in the form of such compounds as glues, aerosols, and gasoline is relatively more common at young ages. More than 17% of 8th graders have tried an inhalant, and 30-day prevalence exceeds 4%. Annual and 30-day prevalence tend to decrease in the higher grades.

3.2. SUMMARY OF DRUG USE TRENDS ACCORDING TO GRADE, SEX, AND ETHNIC/RACIAL VARIABLES

3.2.1. Grade

With the exception of cigarettes and alcohol use, little drug use is initiated by the 6th grade. Also, only heroin and inhalant use were found to be slightly higher in the lower vs. the higher grade surveyed. The use of other drugs increased with grade (Table 3.3). Early initiation of use of a given drug predicts subsequent abuse of that substance, as well as a more extensive and persistent involvement in use of other drugs (Kandel, 1982).

There are reports specific to the use of alcohol indicating that the earlier a child begins to use alcohol, the more likely he or she is to become intensely involved in heavy drinking and combination drug use and to manifest problem behaviors (Barnes & Welte, 1986; Jessor & Jessor, 1977; Windle, 1991).

3.2.2. Sex

Males are more likely to use most illicit drugs, and the differences tend to be largest at the higher frequency levels. Consistent with past and present research, gender differences in drug use among students have dwindled (Barnes & Welte, 1986; Johnston et al., 1992). Two categories of drugs, stimulants and cigarettes, show parity of use between males and females. The sexes also attain near parity on tranquilizer use. In all ethnic/racial groups, fewer females than males report drug use.

3.2.3. Ethnic/Racial

Native American seniors have had the highest rates for use of marijuana, cocaine, alcohol, cigarettes, inhalants, hallucinogens, heroin, other opiates, stimulants, and sedatives and tranquilizers not taken under a doctor's order. African- and Asian-American students have the lowest rate of use for these drugs. White and Hispanic seniors had the second and third highest respective rates of drug use. Differences between groups in dropout rates and willingness to report drug use were recorded, and their possible impact on the results need to be discussed. Dropout rates are far above average among Native American youth and well above average among Hispanic students. Dropout rates among African Americans are not much higher than those for whites, and Asian Americans have the lowest dropout rates. These dropout rates could have increased the gaps between the rates of drug use among the various groups.

The willingness of African-American and Hispanic youths to report drug use is lower than that of white youths (Bachman et al., 1991); however, this underreporting is known to occur most often at the lowest levels of use (Mensch & Kandel, 1988). Bachman et al. (1991) conclude that there are "two worlds" of drug use within the African-American community, the extremes of abstinence at one end and heavy use/abuse at the other. Also, it was reported that there is an inverse correlation of drug use rates between whites and African Americans along the age axis. That is, the higher rate of drug use among white youths compared to African-American adolescents dwindles in early adulthood, and by middle adulthood, the rates among African Americans supersede those among whites.

Blanton, Anthony, and Schuster (1993) note that racial and ethnic group comparisons sometimes carry the risk of reinforcing prejudices and drawing public attention away from more important factors such as community characteristics and social similarities. These authors reported that group comparisons in crack cocaine smoking provide evidence that given similar social and environmental conditions, crack use does not strongly depend on race-specific personal factors.

3.3. TRENDS IN ATTITUDES AND BELIEFS ABOUT DRUGS AMONG SENIORS

The study of youth attitudes and beliefs about drugs was hypothesized to be related to changing patterns in the demand for drugs. Significant changes in the perception of the potential hazards associated with drug use are believed to be correlated with the trends of drug use delineated earlier in this chapter and are presumed to continue to have impact on the epidemiology of drug use, especially among adolescents.

Three sets of attitude and belief questions have been investigated in the "Monitoring the Future" Survey (Johnston et al., 1992). One set concerns seniors' views about the harmfulness of drugs; the second inquires about the level of disapproval of each senior surveyed regarding various drug use. The third set surveys attitudes regarding the perceived availability of drugs.

3.3.1. Perceived Harmfulness and Disapproval Rates

The general trend of increase in the rates of these variables continued in the last decade. Several drugs showed a continuation of increase in perceived risk among seniors in 1991; these include marijuana, amphetamines, and barbiturates. Others showed little change, such as cocaine and heroin. The disapproval rate of drugs is at very high levels.

Cocaine and heroin emerged as being perceived by seniors as the most harmful drugs. Although the rates of harmfulness are linearly correlated with frequency of use (e.g., once or twice, occasionally, or regularly), the disapproval rate for even the experimental use of these drugs was in the 90% range.

LSD, amphetamines, and barbiturates were perceived as being less harmful than cocaine and heroin; however, their rates of disapproval were very slightly less than those for the latter drugs.

Experimental or occasional use of marijuana or alcohol was perceived as harmful by about 40% and 30% respectively. The rate of disapproval has been much higher (by 40–50% for each drug).

Thus, it appears that disapproval rates are very high for regular use of all drugs and experimental or occasional use of most drugs. Regarding ethnic/racial differences, it was reported that black seniors are more likely than white seniors to perceive high risks and to disapprove of various forms of drug use.

3.3.2. Perceived Availability

A decrease in perceived availability of all drugs was reported in 1991. Since 1989, a trend of increased difficulty in getting drugs such as cocaine, amphetamines, barbiturates, and PCP was reported by seniors. The investigators of "Monitoring the Future" believe that one reason for this decline in perceived availability is that fewer seniors have friends who use drugs. Marijuana is reported as the most readily available illegal drug. It was indicated that, after marijuana, amphetamines, tranquilizers, and barbiturates are most available to seniors. Cocaine, LSD, and PCP follow in that order.

3.4. CONCLUSION

The figures cited herein serve at best as a periodic "snapshot" of adolescent drug use. It is not known how many of the seniors are polydrug users. Also, no clear clinical significance can be drawn from the survey conducted by Johnston et al. (1992). A very cautious generalization may conclude that adolescents identified as daily users are at a very high risk for developing APSUDs.

The lack of data regarding the involvement of school dropouts in ASU and PSUDs is a reason for concern. The growing involvement of these children and adolescents in organized drug dealing and selling should be addressed. Assessment followed by planned intervention is imperative before more youth become involved in gang activities that carry increased risk for morbidity and mortality due to violence and PSUD-related medical complications.

REFERENCES

Bachman, J. G., Wallace, J. M., O'Malley, P. M., Johnston, L. D., Kurth, C. L., & Neighbors, H. W. (1991). Racial/ethnic differences in smoking, drinking and illicit drug use among American high school seniors 1976–1989. *American Journal of Public Health, 81,* 372–377.

Barnes, G. M., & Welte, J. W. (1986). Patterns and predictors of alcohol use among 7th–12th grade students in New York State. *Journal of Studies on Alcohol, 47,* 53–62.

Blanton, M. L., Anthony, J. C., & Schuster, C. R. (1993). Probing the meaning of racial/ethnic group comparisons in crack cocaine smoking. *Journal of the American Medical Association, 269,* 993–997.

Durant, R. H., Rickert, V. I., Ashworth, C. S., Newman, C. N., & Slavens, G. (1993). Use of multiple drugs among adolescents who use anabolic steroids. *New England Journal of Medicine, 328,* 922–926.

Jessor, R., & Jessor, S. L. (1977). *Problem Behavior and Psychosocial Development: A Longitudinal Study of Youth.* New York: Academic Press.

Johnston, L. D., O'Malley, P. M., & Bachman, J. G. (1992). *Details of Annual Drug Survey.* Ann Arbor: A release by the University of Michigan News and Information Services. January 27.

Kandel, D. B. (1982). Epidemiological and psychosocial perspective on adolescent drug use. *Journal of the American Academy of Child Psychiatry. 20,* 328–347.

Kashkin, K. B., & Kleber, H. D. (1989). Hooked on hormones? An anabolic steroid addiction hypothesis. *Journal of the American Medical Association, 262,* 3166–3170.

Mensch, B. S., & Kandel, D. B. (1988). Underreporting of substance use in a national longitudinal youth cohort. *Public Opinion Quarterly, 52,* 100–124.

Windle, M. (1991). Alcohol use and abuse: Some findings from the national adolescent student health survey. *Alcohol Health & Research World, 15,* 5–10.

CHAPTER 4

Etiology and Pathogenesis of Adolescent Substance Use and Adolescent Psychoactive Substance Use Disorders

There is a growing consensus in the literature that children of alcoholics (COAs) or of parents with other psychoactive substance use disorders (PSUDs) are more prone to PSUDs and PSUD-related problems than are children of nonabusers (Cotton, 1979; Hill, Steinhauer, Smith, & Locke, 1991). Also, PSUDs and other psychiatric disorders such as antisocial personality disorder (ASPD) and mood disorders tend to cluster in families (Merikangas, Leckman, Prusoff, Pauls, & Weissman, 1985). COAs are at least 4–5 times more likely to become alcoholics than are children of nonalcoholic parents (Goodwin, 1985). Variables that are most reliably associated with heightened risk of alcoholism are family history of alcoholism and history of antisocial behavior in adolescence (Nathan, 1988). Indeed, based on more than 100 studies reviewed by Cotton (1979), the strong familial aggregation of alcoholism is one of the most robust findings in medical research.

There is no universal consensus regarding an etiological model of PSUD that may apply to the different subpopulations. Present evidence points to the importance of multiple factors such as genetic–biological, developmental, and environmental processes.

The most demonstrative and influential empirical study recognizing the heterogeneity of the population of alcoholics was derived from an investigation of the importance of biological vs. environmental etiology of alcoholism by Cloninger, Bohman, and Sigvardsson (1981). They concluded that some alcoholics may have developed alcoholism because of environmental causes (Type 1: milieu-limited), whereas others may have been influenced by a strong genetic vulnerability for an early-onset (Type 2: male-limited) alcoholism.

The growing understanding of the importance of the heterogeneity of patterns of psychoactive substance use, abuse, and dependence—each potentially having multiple etiologies—and reports that perhaps only 30% of the variance of familial transmission of alcoholism is attributable to genetic factors (Merikangas, 1990; Pickens, Svikis, McGue, Lykken, Heston, & Clayton, 1991) support the increasing interest in studies that investigate the interaction of biological and environmental factors according to a biopsychosocial paradigm.

Investigators from various fields, such as molecular and clinical genetics, pathophysiology, and neuropsychopharmacology, as well as psychopathology and sociobehavioral science, have participated in efforts to improve understanding of the etiology and pathogenesis of PSUDs.

There are distinct advantages in taking a broad-spectrum approach to this endeavor, since doing so favors the widely accepted multifactorial paradigm of addiction (Nathan, 1990). However, it is important to acknowledge the likelihood that each factor carries a different etiological and/or pathogenetic relative weight.

Donovan (1986, p. 1) stated:

> Most researchers acknowledge multifactorial etiology in their introductions but then use the investigatory techniques with which they are most expert, techniques generally unidimensional in scope. The research results are then biased toward a unidimensional etiological explanation.

Although there has been rapid growth in the literature on adolescent substance use (ASU) and adolescent PSUDs (APSUDs), research on this population is still in its infancy. Also, due to the longer history of research on adult alcoholism (as compared with that of research on abuse of other psychoactive substances), the relative magnitude and depth of studies on the etiology and pathogenesis of alcoholism are greater. These facts are especially noteworthy because, when appropriate in this discussion, relevant adult-oriented literature on alcoholism is presented and relied on as a basis for generalization. However, it is crucial to remember that although alcohol abuse/dependence is a subset of PSUD, results should be generalized cautiously and their limitations noted.

This chapter examines the vast literature pertaining to multiple determinants of risk and invulnerability to APSUDs (i.e., genetic–

biological, developmental, environmental) as well as to the transition from ASU to APSUD. The importance of distinguishing between normative and pathological use of psychoactive substances is illuminated in terms of developmental task perspective. The biopsychosocial approach utilized in this chapter helps to emphasize that because the initiation of ASU, the transition to PSUD, and the maintenance of PSUD and related behaviors may be predicted by somewhat different etiological pathways, different therapeutic interventions (e.g., prevention, treatment) may be implemented along the life span. Attempts to separate genetic–biological contributions to the development of ASU and PSUDs from developmental and environmental factors may appear to be forced and artificial, if not impossible. However, for the sake of clarity, such an attempt is made in this chapter, as reflected by the subheadings. Diagnostic terminology in this chapter is derived from DSM-III-R (American Psychiatric Association, 1987) or DSM-IV (American Psychiatric Association, 1994) whenever possible. Other definitions used are according to pre-DSM-III-R classifications reported by the publication cited.

4.1. IS THERE—AND, IF THERE IS, WHAT IS— NORMATIVE ADOLESCENT SUBSTANCE USE?

While any illicit drug use may be viewed as illegal and therefore as a form of abuse (including age-group-restricted agents such as tobacco and alcohol for adolescents), this viewpoint appears to be detached from reality. The majority of adolescents who engage in ASU do not escalate to APSUD. Even the majority of COAs (about two thirds of them) do not develop alcoholism even if there is one sibling who has already been diagnosed as alcoholic (Wilson & Crowe, 1991).

It is imperative to examine ASU as a normative phenomenon in order to develop a frame of reference that will distinguish this behavior from mild forms of PSUD (i.e., abuse), although such a distinction may seem somewhat contrived.

Adolescence has long been recognized as a phase of transition (Erikson, 1968) during which biological, psychological, and sexual maturation is accelerated, cognitive capacities approach their peak, and adult social roles are experimented with. In order to establish independent and autonomous identity, the adolescent is expected to test and modify behaviors and attitudes in reciprocity especially with his or her immediate environment (e.g., family, peer group, role models). This maturation process may involve initiation of experimentation and occasional use of psychoactive substances, usually in very specific culturally accepted circumstances (e.g., alcohol use on weekends and cigarette smoking with the peer group). Such experimentation may be considered normative behavior in terms of prevalence and developmental task perspective (Newcomb & Bentler, 1988).

The socialization model of substance use posits that behavioral norms, values, and beliefs commonly held by peer groups encourage substance use by adolescents (Huba, Wingard, & Bentler, 1980). Indeed, experimentation with psychoactive substances was reported as an indication of psychological health in a longitudinal study of a large adolescent cohort followed from the early 1980s. Shedler and Block (1990) reported that youngsters who had experimented with psychoactive substances were psychologically healthier than either frequent users or abstainers. This study demonstrated that given the cultural norms within the time frame in which it was conducted, ASU was the rule rather than the exception.

4.2. DETERMINANTS OF RISK AND INVULNERABILITY FOR ADOLESCENT PSYCHOACTIVE SUBSTANCE USE DISORDERS FROM A DEVELOPMENTAL PERSPECTIVE

Examination of risk and protective factors for any psychopathology at a very early age is advantageous because the researcher has an opportunity to understand the genesis of many psychological characteristics before the effects of caretaking and large environmental determinants have had an impact on the developing neonate or infant (Seifer & Sameroff, 1987).

Two issues of importance must be noted before the literature on this topic is reviewed: (1) definitions of risk or vulnerability factors and of protective or invulnerability factors and (2) understanding the methodology of research models used to study these factors, especially the selection of subjects and their demographic characteristics.

4.2.1. Definitions

Clayton (1992) defined a risk factor for drug abuse as

an individual attribute, individual characteristic, situational condition, or environmental context that increases the probability of drug use or abuse or a transition in level of involvement with drugs (p. 15).

According to the same author, a protective factor

. . . inhibits, reduces, or buffers this probability (p. 16).

In the context of this emphasis on risk for unfavorable outcomes, there has been a growing interest in the converse issue of what determines favorable outcome in children who are defined as vulnerable to a particular disorder by virtue of their personal characteristics (e.g., genetic vulnerabilities, temperament) or environmental influences (e.g., family, peers) or both. The at-risk children who show good outcome are called "invulnerable" (Seifer & Sameroff, 1987).

4.2.2. Research Models

Most studies on the etiology and development of PSUDs are retrospective, and many were conducted among chronic alcoholics and other adults who manifested long-standing PSUDs with memory, cognitive, and social deficits as well as medical complications attributed to alcoholism (Tarter & Edwards, 1986). Even when examining competent adults at the end of a developmental path, one loses the ability to study the developmental process and to distinguish between etiological factors and those that are caused by or are merely associated with the outcome (Seifer & Sameroff, 1987). Most risk models in ASU and APSUD are based on a single factor that defines child vulnerability, such as parental mental illness, parental alcoholism, parental antisocial personality, or childhood trauma. It seems that it is necessary to define the meaning of risk between two extremes. At one pole is a rigid set of single factors (e.g., the severity and chronicity of risk factors may be better predictors of poor outcome than a diagnosis), and at the other end there is an operational definition that includes any factor related to unfavorable outcome (Seifer & Sameroff, 1987).

Clayton (1992) presented four possible assumptions about risk and protective factors:

1. A single risk or protective factor can have multiple outcomes.
2. Several risk or protective factors can have an impact on a single outcome.
3. Psychoactive substance abuse itself may have important effects on risk and protective factors.
4. The relationship of risk and protective factors to each other and to transitions in psychoactive substance abuse may be influenced by age-graded norms.

4.2.3. Context of Development and Levels of Organization

An approach to understanding human development has been suggested by Sameroff and Chandler (1975):

It is proposed that a systems model of hierarchies of organization may best define the components of developmental processes. The three levels of most interest for the present question of defining risk would be the individual organism, the immediate family, and the cultural context that the family inhabits. The interplay of all three levels must be considered if one is to understand developmental processes and outcomes. In the case of research on risk factors, there is conflict as to which level produces the primary vulnerability (Seifer & Sameroff, 1987, p. 66).

Subsequent sections in this chapter are organized according to this paradigm in order to better understand the factors that determine vulnerability to APSUD and the factors that contribute to the progression from ASU to APSUD.

4.3. GENETIC–BIOLOGICAL RISK FACTORS

How early do risk factors appear? Following a genetic–biological approach, one would assume that risk factors are constitutional and may be detected even before the child is born using the techniques of molecular genetics. If that is the case, taking the spectrum of alcohol consumption through alcohol dependence, for example, then what is inherited? Drinking habits? Alcoholism per se? A suspectibility to alcoholism? Related comorbidity? Or are there any other possibilities? Also, do the behaviors related to the phenomenon of alcohol drinking or the full-blown disorder result from the impact of one or more genes? What genes may be responsible for the coexpression of additional comorbidities?

To answer these intriguing questions, three main designs for behavioral genetic studies have been utilized: (1) Twins who have identical genomes have been studied in comparison to twins who share only half their genes. (2) Adopted-away COAs constituted the population for a second research method. (3) Genetic markers associated with alcoholism or other PSUDs or both have been sought, especially in high-risk populations (particularly in COAs).

4.3.1. Studies of Twins

Research has suggested that individuals differ in their susceptibility to alcoholism. There is strong supporting evidence for a genetic influence in alcoholism from animal research (Li, Lumeg, McBride, & Murphy, 1987) and from human studies (Cadoret, O'Gorman, Troughton, & Heywood, 1986).

The concordance for alcoholism has been reported by Kaij (1960) to be higher among monozygotic (MZ) than dizygotic (DZ) twins. This Swedish investigator found that the more severe the alcoholism, the greater the difference. A Finnish study (Partanen, Bruun, & Markkanen, 1966) found that the differences between identical and fraternal twins with regard to alcohol problems were confined primarily to young alcoholics, but there was no difference in the total sample. Hrubre and Omenn (1981) confirmed the findings by Kaij (1960) of a higher concordance for alcoholism among MZ than DZ twins and also obtained evidence pointing to a genetic vulnerability to alcoholic liver, to cirrhosis, and to medical complications involving the heart, brain, and pancreas. In contrast, a British study (Clifford, Fulker, Gurling, & Murray, 1981) found no differences between MZ and DZ twins. A recent Finnish study (Kaprio, Koskenvuo, Langinvainio, Romanov, Sarna, & Rose, 1987) evaluated genetic influences on alcohol use and abuse of a large cohort of 2,819 pairs of adult twin brothers. None of the drinking measures (frequency, quantity, and density) was associated with zygosity; however, significant genetic variance was found for each of the drinking measures, with heritability estimates ranging from 0.36 to 0.4. No genetic influence was found for alcohol-induced passouts.

The studies reviewed above point to a genetic influence on alcohol use patterns, but their findings are not clear-cut with respect to a genetic basis for alcoholism. The higher concordance may apply only to the severe forms of alcoholism.

Considerably fewer studies focusing on genetic precursors for drug abuse have been conducted as compared with the research on alcoholism. However, a genetic component of vulnerability to drug abuse has also been suggested in studies on both twins (Pickens et al., 1991) and adoptees (Cadoret et al., 1986). Pickens et al. (1991) conducted the only twin study of drug abuse and reported that the drug-abuse concordance rate for male MZ twins was 2 times higher than that for DZ twins.

Heritability data suggest large environmental influences on any gene's behavioral expression. Consequently, multigenerational family linkage studies may lose power when affected family members abuse substances principally because of environmental influences (Uhl, Persico, & Smith, 1992). Indeed, there is concern as to how representative twins are of the general population due to the infrequent occurrence of twin births. Also, the potential effects of shared environment on the behavioral development of twin brothers may contribute to the higher resemblance on which the genetic interpretation depends. Clifford et al. (1981) suggested that at least 20% of the variance in alcohol consumption is attributable to the influence of shared family experiences and noted that frequency of social contact is demonstrably greater among MZ twins. It was reported that MZ twins tend to affect each other's drinking habits more than DZ twins, although, not surprisingly, the effect of social interaction is age-dependent. The highest correlation for alcohol use among MZ twin brothers is 0.58 during late adolescence and early adulthood, a period by the end of which their drinking habits have been fully developed (Kaprio et al., 1987).

4.3.2. Adoption and Cross-Fostering Studies

Another approach used to differentiate genetic from environmental factors in studying the etiology of ASU and APSUDs is the adoption, or separation, paradigm, which has already been utilized in research on disorders such as schizophrenia and mood disorders (Cadoret et al., 1986). The adoption paradigm may contribute information to the question of which factors differentially place an individual at risk for ASU vs. PSUD, thus limiting the need to extrapolate from the literature of one condition to the other.

The process of adoption usually separates children from their biological parents soon after birth when placements are arranged in adoptive homes. Thus, the biological parents provide the genetic load that the child receives, but little or no environmental impact. The adoptive parents furnish essentially all the environmental input.

The first adoption study on alcoholism was conducted by Roe (1944), who studied a small sample of 27 children of alcoholic parents. Only 1 subject of this sample and 2 of the control group abused alcohol, suggesting no genetic impact on drinking behavior. It is noteworthy that no criteria were given for a diagnosis of alcoholism.

Later studies reached different conclusions. About 25% of the sons of alcoholics, even if reared away from their biological parents, will develop alcoholism (Cloninger et al., 1981; Goodwin, Schulsinger, Hermansen, Guze, & Winokur, 1973). Cloninger et al. (1981) showed that children who are reared by alcoholic adoptive parents are no more likely to become alcoholic themselves than are other children. In contrast, Goodwin et al. (1973) reported a 33% incidence of alcoholism among adopted-away sons of Danish alcoholic fathers, an incidence approximately 5 times higher than among adopted-away sons of nonalcoholic parents. Alcoholism in adopted-away daughters of Danish alcoholics was not significantly increased above the incidence in adopted controls. These findings and other findings reviewed in this section are difficult to compare because of the different clinical characteristics by which alcoholism was defined, and the differences in adoptive placements and in age at final placement.

Wilson and Crowe (1991) point out that while the 26% increase in incidence of alcoholism found by Goodwin et al. (1973) is a useful figure for estimating the probability of future alcoholism among sons of alcoholics, it is also noteworthy that about two thirds of the sons of alcoholics investigated in this study did not become alcoholics.

The findings of Cadoret (1992) from adoption studies reiterated the importance of two risk factors indigenous to the biological parent: (1) alcohol problems, defined as the presence of one or more recorded social or medical problem(s) due to drinking; (2) delinquency/criminality, defined as adjudication of delinquency as an adolescent or conviction of a felony as an adult. These parental conditions appear to be instrumental in determining the transition from use to abuse. Cadoret et al. (1986) suggested in an earlier study that some underlying biochemical route may be involved both in substance abuse and in problem or deviant behavior. They have summarized the findings of this adoption study by suggesting two independent genetic pathways to substance abuse, one through ASPD inherited from biological parents with an antisocial behavior/disorder and the other from biological parents with alcohol problems to offspring who do not manifest ASPD but do develop ASU or APSUD. However, Cadoret (1992) indicates that the contribution of environmental factors to the expression of any type of genetically transmitted alcoholism is significant with or without aggressive, delinquent, or antisocial behavior.

Perhaps the most intriguing research employing an adoption paradigm is represented in articles published by Cloninger and colleagues in the 1980s (Bohman, Sigvardsson, & Cloninger, 1981; Cloninger et al., 1981; Cloninger, 1987; Cloninger, Sigvardsson, & Bohman, 1988). Cloninger and colleagues studied the neurobiology of motivation and learning by trying to identify subtypes of alcoholism and suggested quantifiable personality traits that may be related to neurobehavioral aspects of various brain systems activated by monoamine modulators. Cloninger et al. (1981) studied 862 Swedish men aged 23–43 years who were adopted prior to age 3 by nonrelatives (the average age at final placement in the adoptive home was 3 months). The subjects were born out of wedlock; information about biological parents was available from public sources. On the basis of data obtained from the community Temperance Board, the adopters were classified according to the severity of their alcohol abuse (none, mild, moderate, or severe). The results of the study identified two types of alcohol abuse that have different genetic and environmental causes: Type 1 (milieu-limited) and Type 2 (male-limited) alcoholism. Type 1 depends on the gene–environment for its clinical expression. Type 2, as its name implies, is highly heritable from father to son and is characteristic of most men in hospital treatment samples. Cloninger (1987) related Type 1 to the gamma alcoholic group (loss-of-control drinkers) of Jellinek (1960) and Type 2 to Jellinek's delta group (those with the inability to abstain from alcohol). Type 2 is also characterized by early onset before age 25, usually in adolescence, and is accompanied by antisocial aggressive behavior. Type 1 is manifested by males and females usually after 25 years of age. There is most probably a spectrum of alcohol disorder phenotypes wherein Type 1 and Type 2 represent the extreme poles of the disorder. Cloninger (1987) reported that three personality traits differentiate the two subtypes of alcoholism: novelty-seeking, harm avoidance, and reward dependence. Type 1 is low on novelty-seeking and high on the other traits, while Type 2 is the opposite, as reflected by alcohol-seeking behavior associated with impulsivity, risk-taking, and a tendency toward antisocial behavior.

Critiques by Schuckit and Irwin (1989) and Irwin, Schuckit, and Smith (1990) pointed out that an early age of onset and ASPD may be responsible for the characteristics of Type 2, meaning that this is not a heritable subtype of alcoholism. However, these criticisms are not supported by research results that confirm the hypothesis of Cloninger (1987) that personality traits may be associated with alcoholism subtypes. These results include studies regarding the typology of alcoholism (see Chapter 2). Finally, early onset of alcohol abuse is a poor prognostic sign (Kandel, 1982) that also may indicate increased incidence of ASPD, depression, and attempted suicide in adolescence and early adulthood (Buydens-Branchey, Branchey, & Noumair, 1989).

4.3.3. Biological Markers

One approach used to characterize the inheritance of alcoholism has been to look for markers of vulnerability (e.g., genetic, behavioral) to later development of alcoholism across the life span. Identifying such markers is of importance in detecting individuals at risk and thus in guiding efforts at primary prevention. Use of such markers is also of benefit in subdividing the alcoholism phenotype into more biologically homogeneous forms (Dinwiddie, 1992). Understanding the etiology and pathogenesis of alcoholism and other PSUDs across different phases of life is necessary, because as individuals age, their cumulative use of psychoactive substances may increase. In some instances, the marker of interest may even be changed by alcohol consumption (Hill et al., 1991).

The current state of knowledge does not permit a conclusion as to whether every potential marker reported in the literature indeed qualifies to be one or is merely a correlate of risk associated with or caused by alcoholism outcome or related problems or both (Nathan, 1990). The markers reviewed below have received growing attention especially since the early 1980s and include biological as well as neurobiohavioral and psychosocial ones.

4.3.3.1. Genetic Studies of Dopamine Receptors

The brain's dopaminergic reward system in the mesolimbic–mesocortical area attracted the interest of investigators who reported on the ability of psychoactive substances to activate these systems. Molecular geneticists detected the gene for the dopamine D_2 receptor (DRD_2) on chromosome 11, and Blum et al. (1990) provided initial evidence that DRD_2 might have an influence on susceptibility to alcoholism. The findings of Blum et al. (1990) need to be viewed with caution because of the small size of the sample of deceased alcoholics whose brain tissue was the source of the DNA investigated. Also, in view of the presumed heterogeneity of alcoholism and its likely polygenic causes, it is unlikely that one gene has the power to identify almost 70% of alcoholics (Gordis, Tabakoff, Goldman, & Berg, 1990).

Two alleles of the D_2 receptors named A_1 and A_2 were detected on chromosome 11 by Blum et al. (1990). The A_1 allele was reported to be related to alcoholism. Ethnic/racial variations were reported regarding this allele (i.e., the frequency of the A_1 allele in African Americans is significantly higher than in whites). This finding suggests that cohort selection from various minority groups may influence the result of such a study.

Uhl et al. (1992) reviewed six studies concerning this matter that were published after the report of Blum et al. (1990). Alcoholics displayed approximately twice the amount of A_1 displayed by control populations. The severity of alcoholism appeared to be directly correlated with such an association. The overall odds ratio for all studies combined was 2.2. The A_1 allele has also been found to be associated with Tourette's syndrome, attention-deficit hyperactivity disorder, and autism. Subjects with histories of polysubstance abuse also yielded elevated A_1 and more significant B_1 frequencies (Smith et al., 1992).

Another recent publication reported that genetics plays a role in determining smoking behavior according to a study of male twins (Carmelli, Swan, Robinette, & Fabsitz, 1992). The study indicated significant familial influences on smoking behavior, but not on smoking intensity. Three components of smoking behavior (never smoked, current smoking, and quitting) were moderately influenced by genetic factors. The authors concluded that smoking could be viewed as a collection of forms of behavior rather than a single habit.

In conclusion, the pattern of alcoholism inheritance does not fit a single-gene (Mendelian) pattern of inheritance such as in color blindness or Huntington's chorea. No single gene is postulated to control such a complex behavior as is manifested in alcoholism. Observed rates of alcoholism are not consistent with a simple polygenic model either (assuming a number of genes of approximately equal impact) (Dinwiddie, 1992). It is suggested on the basis of present knowledge that alcoholism is heterogeneous and polygenic with incomplete penetrance. In addition, Gordis et al. (1990) suggest that there may be phenocopies mixed into the same families as the genetically influenced alcoholism (i.e., alcoholism of a nongenetic type that is clinically identical to genetically influenced variants).

The genetic contribution to alcoholism and other PSUDs is an increased vulnerability, namely, the predisposition to these disorders as supported by twin and adoption studies (Cloninger, 1987; Pickens et al., 1991). Also, it is suggested that caution be exercised in concluding that genetic markers that have been found may be the ultimate answer to an accurate subtyping of alcoholics or high-risk populations. Finally, evidence to date suggests that if the allele modifies risk for alcoholism, it does so in a nonspecific way, possibly by modulating the phenotypic expression of alcoholism. However, it is still inconclusive whether the A_1 allele is a modifier or only a potential marker. Further rigorous and replicable research is needed in this domain.

4.3.3.2. Neurophysiological Components

4.3.3.2.1. Event-Related Potential (ERP). This potential is a unique neurophysiological characteristic associated with information processing. Studies of ERP amplitude of nonalcoholic sons of alcoholic fathers revealed a smaller ERP amplitude as compared with sons of nonalcoholic parents (Begleiter, Porjesz, Bihari, & Kissin, 1984). These workers concluded that ERP deficits identified in high-risk populations may be useful as phenotypic markers.

P300 is an ERP component that occurs with a latency of 300 msec when a simple auditory stimulus is used to elicit a response. It is thought to reflect memory-updating operations during information processing. The amplitude of the P300 component was reduced in a nonclinical sample of offspring of alcoholics (Begleiter et al., 1984). Hill et al. (1991) reported results that are in agreement with those of Begleiter and colleagues in a three-generation pedigree study of children in families with a high density of alcoholism. Analysis of these children's neurophysiological characteristics in comparison to those of normal controls revealed that because children in the high-risk group and the control group were of comparable age, a potential developmental lag or deficiency among the first group is possible, thus limiting the investigators' ability to allocate significance to targeted stimuli. Begleiter and Porjesz (1990) reported that their subjects came from families in which the alcoholism was found to occur only in males and was highly heritable, of early onset, and characterized by a severe course with associated criminality and was thus consistent with alcoholism Type 2 according to the Cloninger (1987) formulation.

Studies on sons of alcoholics revealed increased high-frequency brain waves measured by electroencephalogram (EEG) activity and an increased slow alpha response to alcohol (Pollock et al., 1983). The effort to distinguish between subgroups of alcoholics was bolstered by reported findings that Type 1 and Type 2 alcoholics differ in neurophysiological measures such as EEG activity, as summarized by Cloninger (1987). Abstinent Type 1 alcoholics at rest were found to be hypervigilant and apprehensive with much anticipatory worrying; their resting EEG showed minimal brain activity in the slow alpha frequency range, excessive beta activity, and poor synchrony. A gender difference was revealed in that the alcoholic probands with minimal alpha EEG activity were women with characteristic Type 1 alcoholic features. In response to alcohol, individuals with such EEG patterns showed a marked increase in alpha activity and subjectively reported a sense of calm alertness that they regard as a pleasant relief of tension.

In contrast, abstinent Type 2 alcoholics at rest are hypovigilant, distractible, impulsive, and easily bored. They also show increasing amplitudes of EEG potentials evoked by visual stimuli of increasing intensity.

Hill et al. (1991) implemented the visual ERP paradigm of Begleiter et al. (1984) among high-risk children as compared to a normal control group. Preliminary results from the visual tasks administered suggest that these two groups show opposite effects. Control children show large P300 for the more difficult as compared with the easy condition. The difficult condition requiring more attention to the task appears to normalize the responses of the high-risk children. Hill et al. (1991) concluded that in three-generation pedigrees who received ERP assessment, the processing of both auditory and visual stimuli met with performance difficulties, especially in the least challenging situations.

4.3.3.2.2. Soft Neurological Signs. It was reported that compromised neurological development may be indicated by the presence of greater static ataxia (upper body sway) in sons of alcoholics (Hegedus, Tarter, Hill,

Jacob, & Winsten, 1984). These high-risk children were found to sway more than children of controls (Hill et al., 1991). This finding of a soft neurological sign is of significant importance because the children studied in the Hill report averaged 11 years of age and had not begun to experiment with alcohol or other psychoactive substances.

Other soft neurological signs reported in sons of alcoholics include decreased memory associated with decreased P300 and decreased capacity to assess significance and sufficient encoding (Hegedus, Alterman, & Tarter, 1984). Cognitive impairment and lower ratings in children's performance in language, psychomotor skills, and other adaptive functioning have also been reported (Tarter, Hegedus, Goldstein, Shelly, & Alterman, 1984). Adult alcoholics manifest a higher than expected proportion of either left-handedness or ambidexterity (Tarter & Edwards, 1986). The specificity of these disturbances has not been determined, and overall they probably reflect incapacity in self-regulation and goal-directed behavior.

Cardiac reactivity or responsivity to stimuli is another intriguing potential marker. Hill et al. (1991) reported that the mean heart rate of all the adult members in their study (affected or unaffected) was elevated with respect to controls. This particular finding was not related to recent consumption of alcohol, cigarettes, or caffeine. Adult individuals from affected families show a significantly smaller difference in their response to certainty and uncertainty under conditions of minimal task demand. It is suggested that this result represents decreased attentional processing. Analysis of the data regarding cardiac reactivity in the children of the families studied by Hill et al. (1991) has not yet generated unequivocal results.

Finally, the issue of attention deficit and hyperactivity that is often reported as a risk factor/marker is addressed in Section 4.4. Attention deficit and hyperactivity as a disorder and its relationship to PSUD are reviewed in Chapter 5.

4.3.3.2.3. Neurotransmitters. Investigations of neuropsychological and physiological precursors or markers of alcoholism conducted with sons of alcoholics and nonalcoholics suggest some possible biological differences that may increase vulnerability to alcoholism. Decreased activity of the neurotransmitter monoamine oxidase, which can be measured in platelets, was found among alcoholics and their first-degree relatives. This decrease was suggested as a marker for heightened risk status (Alexopoulos, Lieberman, & Frances, 1983). Alcoholics and other individuals with impulsive–aggressive behavior have been reported to have low cerebrospinal fluid (CSF) levels of serotonin and dopamine and their metabolites. Goodwin (1985) has suggested that children of alcoholics may be deficient in serotonin or may have an increased level of serotonin in the presence of alcohol. The "addictive cycle"—a pattern in which a person initially drinks to feel good and then later has to resume drinking after an abstinence period in order to stop feeling bad—may result from such an imbalance of serotonin. This model requires that alcohol would have a biphasic effect, causing subsequent underactivity of the reward system. However, alcohol has been reported to interfere with the metabolism of serotonin by inhibiting the amino acid tryptophan (a serotonin precursor) (Buydens-Branchey, Branchey, Noumair, & Lieber, 1989).

The age of onset of alcoholism has been reported to be related not only to a specific type of alcoholism, such as Type 2, but also to serotonin as a biological marker. Buydens-Branchey, Branchey, & Noumair (1989) reported that early-onset alcoholics had a significant association between a low tryptophan ratio to neutral amino acids in blood and depressive and aggressive tendencies. This finding also supports the report by Goodwin (1985) that a deficit in serotonin is a marker for future development of alcoholism. The role of serotonin in behavioral inhibition is reviewed in Section 4.3.3.3. It has also been hypothesized that alcohol has a biphasic effect on the synthesis of prostaglandins (Horrobin, 1980), suggesting that prostaglandins may serve as markers.

Goodwin (1985) also offers an overproduction model, i.e., the hypothesis that a genetic propensity to alcoholism involves the production of endogenous substances that facilitate addiction. It has been reported that endogenous morphinelike compounds were found in the brains of alcoholics (Davis & Walsh, 1970) and in the CSF of alcoholics in greater quantities than in nonalcoholics after alcohol ingestion (Borg, Kvande, Magnusson, & Sjoquist, 1980). Recent findings on the treatment of alcoholism support this theory. O'Malley, Jaffc, Chang, Schottenfeld, Meyer, and Rounsaville (1992) reported that the opiate antagonist naltrexone blocks the reinforcing properties of alcohol.

Cloninger (1987) reviewed the subject of neurogenetic adaptive mechanisms in alcoholism and emphasized the importance of personality variables in understanding susceptibility to alcohol-seeking behavior (which characterized Type 2) and loss of control over drinking (which characterized Type 1). The heritability of adaptive personality traits involves a complex interaction between brain-system-related personality dimensions and neurotransmitters. The environmental factors involved include relevant stimuli and behavioral responses. The assessment of Cloninger (1987) has been that genetic and environmental factors have roughly equal importance in determining behavioral responses.

Cloninger's hypothesis and its relevance to the quest for biological markers indicating an inheritance of suspectibility for alcoholism typologies is reviewed here in detail due to its importance for prevention and treatment. The possibility of identifying such markers is especially significant for adolescents with vulnerability for early-onset Type 2 alcoholism.

4.3.3.3. Personality Dimensions

The three major brain systems that influence stimulus–response characteristics are behavioral activation (novelty-seeking), behavioral inhibition (harm avoidance), and behavioral maintenance (reward dependence). Their respective principal monoamine neuromodulators are dopamine, serotonin, and norepinephrine.

Novelty-seeking refers to "a heritable tendency toward frequent exploratory activity and intense exhilaration in response to novel or appetitive stimuli" (Cloninger, 1987, p. 413). Dopaminergic cells possibly act as a final common pathway for activation of exploratory behavior by mammals. That low doses of ethanol have an excitatory effect on neurons of the mesolimbic area, particularly from the ventral tegmental area to the nucleus accumbens, suggests that this action of ethanol may provide a pharmacological reward that would facilitate alcohol-seeking behavior. Dopamine agonists, such as amphetamines and cocaine (as well as alcohol, opiates, and opioid neuropeptides), facilitate dopaminergic transmission and behavioral activation. Dopamine blockers, such as haloperidol, reduce exploratory behavior and lead to "anhedonia (reduced responsiveness to positive reinforcement)" (Cloninger, 1987, p. 413). Long-term alcohol intake produces behavioral tolerance to the depressant effects of high doses of ethanol, but not to these activating effects of low doses.

Harm avoidance refers to "a heritable tendency to respond intensely to aversive stimuli and their conditioned signals, thereby facilitating learning to inhibit behavior in order to avoid punishment, novelty, and frustrative omission of expected rewards. Harm avoidance may involve variation in the behavioral inhibition system, which includes the septo-hippocampal system" (Cloninger, 1987, p. 414). Serotonergic and cholinergic projections are involved in the function of this system. "The septo-hippocampal system is thought to function as a comparator, checking predicted against actual events, and then interrupting behavior when the unexpected is encountered. Ascending serotonergic projections from the dorsal raphe nuclei to the substantia nigra inhibit nigro-striatal dopaminergic neurons and are essential for conditioned inhibition of activity by signals of punishment and frustrative nonreward" (Cloninger, 1987, p. 414).

Ethanol, benzodiazepines, and other antianxiety drugs block the expression of behavioral inhibition acquired by operant conditioning. These antianxiety effects are thought to be a consequence of inhibition of serotonergic neurons by γ-aminobutyric acid.

"In human subjects, serotonergic activity, as measured by cerebrospinal fluid concentrations of its metabolites, is strongly correlated with harm avoidance. Increased serotonergic activity also inhibits dopaminergic activity, so that dopamine and serotonin turnover are strongly correlated in human subjects and other mammals. Consequently, high harm avoidance is expected to inhibit alcohol seeking behavior and to accelerate the development of behavior tolerance and psychological dependence on alcohol" (Cloninger, 1987, p. 414). The expectation is consistent with the findings in clinical and family studies that low harm avoidance is associated with alcohol-seeking behavior (such as in Type 2) and high harm avoidance is associated with susceptibility to loss of control (such as in Type 1).

Reward dependence is hypothesized to "involve variation in behavioral maintenance or resistance to extinction of previously rewarded behavior. This resistance to extinction is hypothesized to result from facilitation of paired-associate learning by a brain system that is activated primarily at the onset of reward or the offset of punishment, thereby facilitating formation of conditioned signals of reward or relief from punishment" (Cloninger, 1987, p. 414). Norepinephrine seems to modulate the general level of neuronal activity or response to other inputs and may play a critical role in neuromodulation of this system, especially in the learning of new paired associations.

In human subjects, short-term reduction of norepinephrine release by a presynaptic agonist (e.g., clonidine) or destructive lesion of the locus coeruleus in the pons (the origin of major ascending noradrenergic pathways), as in alcohol-induced Korsakoff's amnestic syndrome, impairs paired-associate learning. Arginine, vasopressin, and norepinephrine metabolites are reduced in the CSF of patients with Korsakoff's syndrome.

It is noteworthy that the locus coeruleus is inhibited by increased serotonergic activity at the onset of punishment or the offset of rewards. Also, social approval or disapproval (e.g., of alcohol use) plays a significant role in behavior-related paired-associate learning.

Individuals with low basal noradrenergic activity show more severe depressivelike responses to separation and have greater increases in norepinephrine release after receiving low doses of ethanol.

Cloninger (1987) concluded that the tridimensional structure of personality suggests three systems that are neuromodulated by specific monoamines and are genetically regulated independently, even though they interact with each other.

4.3.3.4. Endocrinological Studies

Studies of the endocrinological profile of alcoholics along the hypothalamic–pituitary–thyroid axis revealed that 31% of male alcoholics who were abstinent for 2–29 years had a persistent blunted response of the pituitary to thyrotropin-releasing hormone (Loosen, Wilson, Dew, & Tipermas, 1983).

To respond to the dilemma of whether blunting is a preexisting hereditary condition that can serve as a marker or is a consequence of long-term exposure to ethanol, Moss, Guthrie, and Linnoila (1986) studied a small sample of children of alcoholics and controls from nonalcoholic families aged 8–17 years. The sons of alcoholic families had significantly higher basal and peak thyrotropin levels than did the control boys. The daughters showed no difference from the control girls.

It is noteworthy that analyses of triiodothyronine, prolactin, and growth hormone concentrations revealed no differences between the index children and the controls.

This is the first report of male-limited neuroendocrine difference between sons of alcoholics and controls from nonalcoholic families. This result is in contrast to the findings in adult abstainers. Further studies are needed in order to elucidate the significance of these findings.

4.3.3.5. Aggression as a Potential Biological Marker

The search for biological markers for alcoholism and other PSUDs includes investigation of traits and behaviors that may predispose to these addictions. As an example, cortisol appears to be a biological marker for impulsivity as well as a possible marker for secondary drug abuse among adults (King, Curtis, & Knoblich, 1992).

ASPD and PSUDs are common in alcoholics and their relatives. Also, aggression is considered to be an antecedent of PSUDs.

King et al. (1992) investigated the relationship of biological factors in sociopathy to drug abuse behavior. Their paradigm has some significant similarities and few differences in comparison to the neurogenetic adaptive paradigm of alcoholism proposed by Cloninger (1987). They have examined three conceptual models—aversive arousal, incentive motivation, and aggression—and have identified biological markers and personality traits that characterize these models. The importance of their paradigm in addition to the similarities to Cloninger's model is especially poignant in the conceptualization of the aggression model.

The aversive arousal system "mediates the behavioral and autonomic responses of an organism to either the expectation or delivery of aversive stimuli" (King et al., 1992, p. 116). Cortisol is the biological marker identified with this system, and low levels characterize the associated temperamental factor (impulsivity). The personality traits and behavioral manifestations that characterize this system are similar to those of the novelty-seeking system of Cloninger (1987), in which the principal neuromodulator is dopamine.

Developmental work has found that behaviorally inhibited shy children have high levels of salivary cortisol taken at baseline (Kagan, Resnick, & Snidman, 1988). In contrast to these findings, violent individuals have lower levels of urinary cortisol than nonviolent individuals, thus supporting findings in animal studies (Virkkunen, 1985).

These low levels of glucocorticoids in animals and humans reflect a temperamental variable that may predispose a person to ASU and APSUDs. Shyness is an inhibitory behavior that represents a state of high arousal and appears to be relatively stable during infancy and childhood (as identified by high levels of cortisol) and therefore may be a protective factor.

The incentive motivation system is similar in many respects to the behavioral activation (novelty-seeking) of Cloninger (1987), with dopamine as the identified marker.

The aggression model is the most intriguing one. Aggression is not a unitary behavior but a constellation of adaptive behaviors that are situationally determined and are amenable to topological classification and neurobiological manipulation (Moss & Tarter, 1993). Serotonin and its metabolite 5-hydroxyindole acetic acid (5-HIAA) have been linked to impulsive aggression in psychiatric patients (Coccaro, 1989). King et al. (1992) focused on a metabolite of phenylethylamine, phenylacetic acid (PAA), as another marker for aggressive behavior. Low levels of 5-HIAA in the CSF and low levels of plasma PAA correlated strongly with aggressive behavior.

4.3.4. Ethnic Differences in Heritability

The Oriental flushing reaction is an aversive reaction to alcohol consumption that is relatively common among individuals of Mongoloid ancestry (Chan, 1986). The prevalence of this manifestation of intolerance to alcohol among Asians is estimated to be between 47% and 85% as compared to only 3–29% of Caucasians. A typical flushing reaction is similar to the one provoked by taking disulfiram with alcohol (an aversive pharmacological therapy for alcohol abuse) and includes objective symptoms such as cutaneous flushing, increase in skin temperature and pulse rate, and decrease in blood pressure (Miller et al., 1987). Subjective symptoms include nausea, dizziness, anxiety, headaches, and sleepiness (Miller et al., 1987).

The importance of understanding the etiology and nature of this intolerance to ethanol may be critical, for the following reasons: (1) Increased tolerance to alcohol has been associated with the development of alcoholism (Goodwin, 1985; Schuckit, 1984). (2) The low prevalence of alcoholism among the Oriental population has been attributed to an intolerance to ethanol that may provide protection against the onset of alcoholism (Chan, 1986).

The exact mechanism of the Oriental flushing reaction is not known, although many studies have indicated a deficiency in aldehyde dehydrogenase, which may account for elevated levels of acetaldehyde in the blood (Chan, 1986). The histamine receptors have also attracted attention, although the role of histamine in the expression of intolerance to alcohol is not clear (Miller et al., 1987). The importance of identifying a potential protective marker against alcohol use or alcoholism within specific populations is significant and warrants continued investigation.

It is important to note also that the vulnerability to alcoholism may be expressed not only in the sober state, but also during alcoholic intoxication (Tarter & Edwards, 1986). Such state-related markers that could differentiate persons on the basis of family history of alcoholism include a decrease in stress attributable to the dampening effect of alcohol (Sher & Levenson, 1982). This effect is manifested as decreased subjective feelings of intoxication (similar to an innate tolerance) at equivalent blood alcohol levels and a lower stress response as measured by prolactin levels after drinking (Schuckit, Parker, & Rossman, 1983).

4.3.5. Gender Differences in Heritability

Alcohol use, abuse, and dependence appear to be less prevalent among females. According to the Epidemiological Catchment Area (ECA) study of three cities in the United States, there is a 4:1–7:1 male excess for the lifetime prevalence of alcohol abuse or dependence (Robins et al., 1984). Sons of alcoholics are at 2–3 times greater risk than daughters of alcoholics. Biological and environmental protective factors are responsible for the reduced risk for females. The evidence for a genetic influence on the development of alcoholism in women is less conclusive than for men. A common belief is that disapproval of female intoxication by both men and women serves as an environmental protective factor (Gomberg, 1993).

In the Swedish study of adopted sons and daughters of alcoholics and nonalcoholics (Bohman et al., 1981), only 2.8% of the adopted daughters of alcoholic parents became alcoholics. If the mother was alcoholic, the risk factor increased to 10.3%. It is noteworthy that alcoholic mothers in comparison with alcoholic fathers have more alcoholic sons (28% vs. 23%) and daughters (10% vs. 4%). A stereotypical belief is that alcoholism in the mother is more destructive than alcoholism in the father; however, there is little evidence to support this supposition.

The association between the inability to terminate drinking binges once started (loss of control) that characterizes alcoholism Type 1 (milieu-limited) and the female sex is especially intriguing, since women are not represented in Type 2 (male-limited) alcoholism, which is based on greater genetic predisposition (Cloninger, 1987). It appears that this association is based on variables, such as personality traits, that have a sex-influenced expression but are heritable regardless of the parental or offspring gender (Cloninger, 1987). Males with a positive family history for alcoholism are more likely than women with a similar family background to become problem drinkers and to develop alcohol- and substance-related problems at an earlier age (Pandina & Johnson, 1990).

The gender-related phenotypical differences are also of importance because male relatives of hospitalized alcoholic women have been distinguished with 80% accuracy from those of alcoholic men by the discriminant function that characterizes Type 1 vs. Type 2 alcoholism (Cloninger, 1987). It is noteworthy that even though alcoholism is less common in women than in men, male and female alcoholics have equal numbers of alcoholic relatives.

The development of metabolic tolerance in sons of alcoholics and the identification of gender differences led to the investigation of other pathophysiological avenues in the search for markers (Schenker & Speeg, 1990).

Gender-related research suggests that the pathophysiological consequences of short-term (intoxication) and long-term alcohol abuse are greater for women than for men at equivalent consumption levels. Women are at higher risk of suffering from the harmful effects of alcohol (e.g., alcoholic liver disease develops more readily in women than in men) (Lex, 1985). This phenomenon can be attributed to increased bioavailability of ethanol resulting from decreased gastric oxidation of ethanol, which is the result of decreased gastric alcohol dehydrogenase activity and first-pass gastric metabolism (Frezza, Di-Padova, Pozzatto, Terpin, Baraona, & Lieber, 1990). In contrast, sons of alcoholics may have a high level of alcohol dehydrogenase, resulting in decreased sensitivity to alcohol compared to controls.

Alcoholic women are more likely to have an additional psychiatric diagnosis than men (65% vs. 44%), as reported in the ECA study (Helzer & Pryzbeck, 1988). A study of the causes of comorbidity of alcoholism and major depression in women was conducted with 2163 female twins from a population-based registry (Kendler, Heath, Neale, Kessler, & Eaves, 1993). It was concluded that the comorbidity is substantial and appears to result largely from genetic factors that influence the risk of both disorders. However, there are genetic factors that influence the risk of major depression but do not influence the risk of alcoholism, and vice versa. Gomberg (1993) reported that there is a relationship between depression, antisocial personality, and age at onset among women alcoholics. She concluded that there is a relationship between antisocial personality behaviors and early onset of alcoholism for both sexes.

4.4. TEMPERAMENT AND A DEVELOPMENTAL MODEL OF PSYCHOPATHOLOGY AND PSYCHOACTIVE SUBSTANCE USE DISORDER

For individuals diagnosed in adolescence and adulthood with PSUD, it is very difficult to untangle the effects of psychoactive substances on their current personality from their personality prior to the transition from ASU to PSUD. Longitudinal studies looking at the development of ASU and PSUDs need to take into consideration the temperament of the individual as determined by neurobiological processes that can be identified and measured very early in life. Also, the understanding of the interaction between the temperament (nature) and the immediate environment in early life (nurture) is critical for elucidating the development of any psychopathology.

Temperament can be defined according to Allport (1961, p. 34) as

the characteristic phenomena of an individual's nature, including his susceptibility to emotional stimulation, his customary strength and speed to response, the quality of his prevailing mood, and all the peculiarities of fluctuation and intensity of mood, these being phenomena regarded as dependent on constitutional makeup, and therefore largely hereditary in origin.

Temperament comprises the primary psychological characteristics of the newborn from which personality and other complex behavior develop. Basic differences in temperament between individuals are attributed to the activity and neuromodulation of neurogenetic adaptive mechanisms (Cloninger, 1987). Situational variables (e.g., developmental, experiential, cognitive) will elicit differences in any given paradigm along the life span; however, the relative contribution of temperament to the variation in behavior diminishes with age because of consequences of experience and the biological maturation process (Tarter & Mezzich, 1992). Viewed from a developmental perspective, temperament may be more influential if the onset of psychopathology is to occur at an early age (e.g., Type 2 alcoholism as compared to Type 1).

There are nine features of temperament and three temperamental constellations (Thomas & Chess, 1984). The components are: (1) activity level, (2) rhythmicity, (3) approach or withdrawal, (4) adaptability, (5) threshold or responsiveness, (6) intensity of reaction, (7) quality of mood, (8) distractibility, and (9) attention span and persistence.

The constellations include: (1) the "easy child," (2) the "difficult child" at the opposite end of the temperamental spectrum, and (3) the "slow-to-warm-up child," a category between the first two. Most but not all children fit into one of these groups with variations within each category. It is important to clarify that an extreme rating does not represent psychopathology, but rather indicates the wide range of behavioral styles of normal children (Thomas & Chess, 1984).

Thomas and Chess (1984, p. 8) also coined the concept "goodness of fit," which implies that

> the properties of the environment and its expectations and demands are in accord with the neonate or infant's own capacities, motivations, and style of behaving. When this consonance is present optimal development is possible. Conversely "poorness of fit" involves dissonance so that distorted development and maladaptive functioning occur.

Sameroff and Chandler (1975) introduced an ecological approach to explain the genesis of functional and dysfunctional behavior that they called the "developmental transactional perspective." The developmental axis of the paradigm reflects the fact that every behavior is developed on the basis of processes that have identifiable histories and a potentially predictable course and outcome. Sameroff and Chandler (1975) discussed the interaction between what they termed a "reproductive risk" and a "continuum of caretaking casualty." The child's level of distress is in part mediated by the caretaker's response, which in turn is mediated by the child's response to caretaking. This is an ongoing dynamic sequence that exemplifies the developmental transaction process.

In essence, the interplay among the individual, the immediate family, and the cultural context that the family inhabits defines the potential risk for APSUDs.

Difficult temperament in early childhood as characterized by slow adaptability, social withdrawal, negative mood, high intensity of emo-

tional reactions, and dysrhythmia is related to heightened risk for conduct disorders in childhood, delinquency, and an increased risk for alcoholism and PSUDs in adolescence (Lerner & Vicary, 1984; Maziade,
Caron, Cote, Boutin, & Thiverge, 1990). Tarter and Mezzich (1992)
noted that poor marital adjustment, even prior to the child's birth, may
influence the subsequent emergence of a difficult temperament in offspring. Marriages are often dysfunctional and conflictual when one or
both partners are alcoholic, and children perceived as difficult are subjected to more coercive and aversive child-rearing strategies (Lee &
Bates, 1985). Conversely, "easy" children elicit positive reactions even
from alcoholic parents, thus reducing their risk for maladjustment in
adolescence (Werner, 1986).

4.4.1. First Year of Life

During the first year, high-risk children may experience self-
regulatory problems and early infant–parent relationship difficulties
through a disrupted attachment process. Attachment refers to the social
bond between child and caregiver, which is an important process for the
establishment of a child's sense of security (Bowlby, 1969, 1980). Three
patterns of attachment have been identified: secure, insecure–avoidant,
and insecure–ambivalent/resistant (Ainsworth, Blehar, Waters, & Wall,
1978; Main & Solomon, 1986). The presence of problematic maternal
drinking patterns prior to and during pregnancy was related to observed negative attachment patterns in 1-year-olds, infant patterns of
insecurity being associated with higher maternal alcohol use (O'Connor,
Sigman, & Brill, 1987). Johnson, Sher, and Rolf (1991) commented that
it is difficult to determine the specific factors that underlie the observed
association between heavy maternal alcohol consumption and insecure
attachment. The association could be attributable to fetal alcohol effects,
inherited temperamental characteristics, or dysfunctional parent/care-
giver–infant interaction. Glantz (1992) concluded that the poor attachment and impaired self-regulation characteristic of the high-risk child's
infancy period lays the foundation for developing serious dysfunctions
later in life.

4.4.2. Early Childhood

Early childhood is a developmental phase characterized by a continuous effort to control the environment, and to explore the immediate
environment while the caretaker serves as a guide and base for emotion-

al refueling. Children at risk who feel insecure and who are temperamentally difficult may start to exhibit tantrums, as well as refusals and oppositional behaviors. These children may be perceived negatively by parents. In a conflictual or dysfunctional home environment, many of the children who also manifest a high level of activity may start to develop disruptive aggressive behaviors identified as early as 4 years of age (Tarter & Mezzich, 1992). Children who are subjected to aggression of various forms (e.g., verbal, physical, disciplinary) are more likely than other children to perpetrate aggression. A conduct disorder (CD) may typically ensue from an aggressive disposition in childhood. Indeed, viewed from the perspective of child and adolescent psychiatry, a CD is the most frequently diagnosed comorbid condition in children having hyperactivity, ranging from 40% to 70% of cases (Szatmari, Boyle, & Offord, 1989).

CD in children and adolescents accompanied by early onset of alcohol use is one end point of deviant psychological development. Tarter and Mezzich (1992) stated in their discussion of the development of several intermediary behavioral phenotypes for emerging behavior traits (aggressivity, CD, antisocial personality) that they link the temperament phenotype of high behavioral activity level to alcoholism. These phenotypes, termed "liability promoters," are composed of the combined effects of genetic and environmental factors that determine the probability of developing alcoholism at any time in life. Once the liability threshold is exceeded, the presence of psychopathology may be determined. Tarter and Mezzich argue that simplistic end-point typologies of alcoholism (e.g., primary, Type 2) do not capture the dynamic person–environment interactions that occur during development, which are necessary for understanding the etiology of PSUDs.

4.4.3. Late Childhood and Preadolescence

The period of prelatency and latency years, approximately between the ages of 5 and 12, is characterized by the increasing relative weight of extrafamily environmental factors. Adaptation of the high-risk child to a school environment and peers is the first developmental challenge for adjustment outside the home. Martin, Nagle, and Paget (1983) reported that the temperament traits of persistence, distractibility, and behavioral activity level explained 20–30% of the variance on a measure of "constructive self-directed activity" among children in the first grade. The magnitude of expression of these temperament traits correlated significantly with achievement test scores. The performance level in kindergarten and elementary school has been reported by several researchers to correlate with temperament traits of persistence, approach or withdrawal, and distractibility (Tarter & Mezzich, 1992).

These studies also imply an association between temperament traits and the quality of adjustment in school. Individual differences in temperament traits influence academic performance and social adjustment in the school environment. Maladjusted kids are at risk for experiencing teacher and peer group discrimination and rejection and may ultimately become school dropouts. These factors contribute to the potential for behaviors and psychopathology associated with alcohol abuse.

Several longitudinal research studies have related observations of subjects at early latency to subsequent involvement with psychoactive substances (Glantz, 1992). Lerner and Vicary (1984) reported that "difficult" temperament and aggressiveness, when accompanied by shyness, is predictive of future ASU.

Shedler and Block (1990) also pointed out early-latency age period children who manifested behaviors that represented temperamental deviations and that were associated with frequent drug use in late adolescence. Children who were characterized as insecure and lacking adequate social and coping skills when evaluated at age 11 were described as being "visibly deviant from their peers, emotionally labile, inattentive and unable to concentrate, not involved in what they do, and stubborn" (p. 618).

As the child matures, peer influences on behavior increase and to a certain extent replace part of the parental control (a trend that continues until its peak in adolescence, when the individual's disengagement from parental influence has become a key developmental milestone). The peer network may operate in the same direction as the family's or in the opposite direction. That is, it may interact so as to increase or decrease the risk for onset of alcohol and other psychoactive substance use. It does not come as a surprise, therefore, that ASU is most commonly initiated during this transition phase from parental to peer influence.

The high-risk child is likely to be associating at the mid- to late-latency age period with other kids whose self-image, social role models, and other perceptions of life domains (e.g., family, school, peers) are similar to his or hers. This behavior has been termed assortative pairing. These are early aspects of the problem-behavior process (Jessor, 1987). Also, parents and older siblings may have additional influence on the child's initiation of the use of gateway drugs (Kandel, 1982). As Glantz noted (1992, pp. 409–410), "The high risk child is unlikely to be strongly influenced by any protective factors. He or she is unlikely to be involved in any group that reinforces conformity and traditional values, such as a religious organization."

4.4.4. Temperament and Specificity of Psychopathology

An important question emanating from this discussion concerns the process that determines the specificity of a youngster's developing a certain psychopathology. Tarter (1991) reviewed this subject and presented the following model: Highly active children, as noted previously, may receive less supervision and communication from parents than normally active children. Consequently, environmental exploration, consisting of novelty- or sensation-seeking, is more likely to occur in such children. This seeking, in turn, may expose them to more situations in which alcohol and other psychoactive drugs are available.

It is noteworthy that children who have difficult temperaments are at about 2.5 times increased risk for developing psychopathology by adolescence as compared to children with normative temperaments. About half the cases of difficult temperament develop into clinical disorders by adolescence (Maziade et al., 1990). However, although the expression of temperament tends to be relatively stable during development, its phenotypes are modifiable, especially at a young age. Protective factors such as having high intelligence and a supportive family may delay or protect children with difficult temperaments from adverse outcomes, particularly externalizing and disruptive behavior disorders.

Thus, although deviations of temperament expression predispose to psychopathology, the specific psychopathology is determined by the interactions with the environment. Corrective experiences—provided through improved consonance between the individual and the environment regardless of the ever-changing demands, stresses, and inevitable conflicts—have an impact on the liability threshold of the expression of psychopathologies.

4.4.4.1. Temperament Traits and Externalizing Disorders

In consolidating the updated knowledge concerning temperament traits, Tarter and Mezzich (1992) derived five basic dimensions: behavior activity level, attention span–persistence, emotionality, sociability, and soothability. Deviations within each of these dimensions have important associations with risk for alcoholism.

Behavior activity level and attention span–persistence are two temperament dimensions that have been most strongly implicated as being associated with vulnerability to alcoholism (Tarter & Mezzich, 1992). These dimensions are presumably traits that all individuals have but at varying levels. A trait becomes a liability only when its heightened severity is beyond a critical value. When the threshold is exceeded, the individual may qualify for a diagnosis such as attention deficit disorder with or without hyperactivity (American Psychiatric Association, 1987). As Tarter and Mezzich noted, it is important not to view a trait as a dichotomous variable (e.g., normal vs. hyperactive); even subthreshold levels of elevated behavior activity level are relevant for elucidating a vulnerability to PSUDs.

Externalizing disorders such as conduct disorder and attention deficit hyperactivity disorder (ADHD) have been linked with later alcoholism. Studies of alcoholism suggest a neuropsychological dysfunction as the underlying mechanism (Tarter, 1982). It was reported that sons of alcoholic biological fathers are also more likely than other children to be hyperactive, even when they are reared by adoptive nonbiological parents (Cantwell, 1972; Morrison & Stewart, 1973). Behavioral activity regulation of adolescent substance abusers in treatment [consisting of the general activity, sleep activity, and flexibility rigidity scales of the Dimensions of Temperament Scale—Revised (DOTS-R)] correlated with drug-use severity and associated psychosocial problems (Tarter, Laird, Kabene, Bukstein, & Kaminer, 1990).

Among alcoholics, the number of childhood hyperactivity characteristics, combined with a score measuring severity of psychosocial immaturity, accounts for almost half the variance on a scale measuring alcoholism severity (Tarter, 1982).

An extended discussion of clinical implications of the relationship between ADHD and PSUDs is provided in Chapter 5. Whereas high behavioral activity has received attention, particularly in the research on alcoholic men, evidence supports an important role for other temperament traits that are relevant to the development of externalizing disorders and PSUDs/alcoholism (Tarter & Mezzich, 1992). These traits are low attention span and persistence, low sociability, and low soothability (return to homeostasis). These deviations in temperament traits are implicated in Type 2 alcoholics and as a liability for predisposition to psychopathology.

4.4.4.2. Antisocial Behavior/Personality

Boys are more likely to be antisocial in childhood than girls and are more likely to develop antisocial personality as adults than are girls. This finding is unlike the relationship between heavy drinking and alcoholism, which has been found to be the same regardless of sex (Cloninger, Christiansen, Reich, & Gottesman, 1978). Male and female criminality occurs in the same families, as would be expected if the familial causes of antisocial personality are the same in both men and women. This finding indicates that the familial factors (genetic and environmental) responsible for the development of antisocial personality are largely the same in women as in men (Cloninger et al., 1978). "Although a marked preponderance of men occur in alcoholism, antisocial personality and criminality, they exemplify fundamentally distinct mechanisms underlying the phenotypic differentiation of men and women" (Cloninger et al., 1978, p. 947).

Cadoret, O'Gorman, Troughton, and Heywood (1985) concluded that there may be specificity of inheritance for antisocial behavior and alcoholism. It was also found that having antisocial parents did not increase alcohol abuse in offspring, nor was there an increase in antisocial personality in adoptees with biological relatives with problem drinking. Conversely, as reviewed by Hawkins, Lishner, Catalano, and Howard, (1986), there appears to be a strong correlation between antisocial behavior and APSUDs. Robins (1978) found that the greater the variety, frequency, and seriousness of childhood antisocial behavior, the more likely antisocial behavior is to persist into adulthood. Delinquency has generally been found to occur prior to drug use. Loeber (1985) suggested that different etiological paths may be associated with age of initiation of substance use and that there is an inverse correlation between age of initiation of substance use and antisocial behavior.

There is disagreement as to the relative strength of early childhood predictors of PSUD and the importance of the severity of antisocial behavior vs. family dysfunction.

Dropping out of school is a phenomenon that increases the risk of becoming a substance abuser and engaging in deviant behaviors, including illegal behavior and drug trafficking and selling. About 50% of juveniles in the justice system who committed violent crimes were under the influence of psychoactive substances (Clayton, 1992).

4.5. PSYCHOSOCIAL AND ENVIRONMENTAL CHARACTERISTICS OF THE INITIATION AND MAINTENANCE OF ADOLESCENT SUBSTANCE USE AND THE TRANSITION TO ADOLESCENT PSYCHOACTIVE SUBSTANCE USE DISORDERS

Already in the late 1970s, as many as 42 authors had reported studies covering a wide range of contemporary theories (mainly psychosocial hypotheses) about initiation and continuation of drug use and eventual transition from use to abuse. Lettieri, Sayers, and Pearson (1980) compiled these reports into NIDA Research Monograph and grouped them according to the following classes of theories: (1) theories on one's relationship to self [e.g., an ego/self theory of substance dependence—a contemporary psychoanalytic perspective (E. J. Khantzian)]; self-esteem and self-derogation theory of drug abuse (H. B. Kaplan) (2) theories on one's relationship to others [e.g., a social–psychological framework for studying drug use (R. Jessor and S. Jessor)]; (3) theories on one's relationship to society [e.g., the natural history of drug abuse (L. N. Robins)]; and (4) theories on one's relationship to nature [e.g., a genetic approach (M. A. Schuckit)].

In the 1980s, significant research was conducted on the risk and protective factors for transitions from psychoactive substance use to abuse and dependence (Clayton, 1992).

Clayton (1992) provided a thorough review of the state of the art regarding transitions in drug abuse with emphasis on risk and protective factors. He expanded beyond the simplistic etiological model of ASU and APSUDs derived from the transmission-of-infectious-disease postulate (i.e., the host–agent–environment concept). Clayton (1992) cited a list of specific risk factors accepted partially or fully by most researchers of ASU and APSUD etiology and pathogenesis (Bry, McKeon, & Pandina, 1982; Hawkins & Catalano, 1989; Labouvie, Pandina, White, & Johnson, 1986; Newcomb, Maddahian, & Bentler, 1986). These factors are grade point average, lack of religiosity, psychopathology, poor relationship with parents, early alcohol use, low self-esteem, lack of conformity, sensation-seeking, perception of availability, and perception of norms concerning drug use. Hawkins and Catalano (1989) accepted the four general domains of risk factors (psychological, parental, school, and peer-related) and added three more domains: (1) contextual and environmental factors (laws and norms, availability of drugs, extreme economic deprivation, neighborhood disorganization, school organizational factors); (2) neurophysiological factors (ADHD, cognitive impairment from neural damage, intelligence, hormonal imbalances); and (3) intergenerational transmission (living with parents and siblings who abuse alcohol or other drugs or both).

It is recognized that some risk factors are multidimensional (e.g., religiosity) and that there may be a different relative weight to each risk factor or to any combination of them. However, the research on this topic is still sparse and far from providing any conclusive empirical evidence concerning these assumptions.

4.5.1. Transitions in Adolescent Substance Use

Kandel (1975) introduced the "gateway" theory, which suggests that there are at least four distinct developmental stages in the initiation of legal and illegal drug use by children and adolescents, such use progressing through (1) beer or wine, (2) cigarettes or hard liquor, (3) marijuana, and (4) other illicit drugs. A fifth stage, problem drinking, may take place between marijuana and other illicit drug use (Kandel, 1982). Clayton (1992) suggested that the etiological models of transition must move further from the first event of use and focus on the following types of transitions, which reflect different dimensions of use and abuse: (1) initiation, (2) continuation, (3) maintenance and progression within drug classes, (4) progression across drug classes, and (5) regression, cessation, and relapse cycles.

1. *Initiation* is the transition from being a nonuser to being a user, ignoring, for the most part, the frequency, quantity, pattern of use, and other dimensions.
2. *Continuation* is the following transition in ASU that may lead to PSUD. Very little work has been conducted on this phase between experimentation and maintenance of use. Clayton (1992, p. 23) noted that "there is a need to understand whether an aversive first experience with a drug reduces, increases, or has little or no effect on continuation of use of a particular drug."
3. *Maintenance and progression* within a class of psychoactive substances is the third transition in drug abuse. Maintenance needs to be understood within the norms of a peer group or subculture; for example, college students are particularly at risk for excessive consumption of alcohol and problematic drinking. The frequency and quantity of drinking and the behavior related to drinking are usually determined by the group. Transition within a class of drugs may be presented by progression from snorting cocaine or opioids to injection.
4. *Progression across drug classes* is characterized by polysubstance abuse and dependence as the end point of this continuum. According to Kandel (1975, 1982), most adolescents who use illicit drugs progress through marijuana. It is relatively unusual for an adolescent to use cocaine or heroin without first experimenting with marijuana. In fact, 26% of marijuana users will progress to the next stage, compared to only 4% who have never experimented with marijuana. Kandel (1982) reported that 25% of the total youth population proceeded through all four developmental stages of drug use by the mid-20s, while two thirds of young people pass through the first three stages. According to the paradigm of Kandel (1975), "It is crucial to keep in mind that position on a particular point in the sequence does not indicate that the young person will necessarily progress to other drugs higher up in the sequence. Participation in each stage is a necessary but not

sufficient condition for participation in a later stage" (Kandel, 1982, p. 335).

5. *Regression, cessation, and relapse cycles* constitute the fifth transition.

The bipolar operation of risk and protective factors creates different configurations that are important for each of the processes noted in these transitions. Clayton (1992) suggested that these transitions are appropriate for each substance and that research on the etiology of polysubstance abuse must take into account the different stages of transitions being experienced for each drug used by a person.

4.5.2. Risk Factor Domains

It is not possible to thoroughly review here the extensive literature, including "dozens" of theories about the etiology and pathogenesis of ASU and APSUDs (Lettieri et al., 1980). However, an effort will be made in the following sections to cover three pivotal psychosocial risk factor domains: psychological, family, and peers.

4.5.2.1. Psychological Risk Factors

Considerable research has been directed at understanding the impact of intrapersonal and interpersonal aspects on the development of ASU and APSUDs. The motivational model of alcohol use presents drinking as a final common pathway to a decision-making process based on the individual motivation (Miles-Cox & Klinger, 1988). Alcohol expectancies in the form of positive or negative affective consequences usually interact with various factors such as current life situations and past experiences with drinking (Goldman, 1989). This model recognizes that there are multiple factors that influence drinking and suggests ways in which they are channeled through an emotional and motivational system and their decision-theory applications.

Sensation-seeking deserves another look in this chapter, only this time from a psychological perspective. Zuckerman (1979, p. 17) defined sensation-seeking as "the need for varied, novel, and complex sensations and experiences and the willingness to take physical and social risks for the sake of such experiences." The general construct is described as having four dimensions: experience-seeking, thrill- or adventure-seeking, disinhibition, and boredom susceptibility. Sensation-seeking as a construct and as a compilation of separate dimensions (the relationship of which is not yet fully clear) has been related to alcohol and drug use and criminality in adolescents and young adults (Cloninger, 1987). Sensation-seeking dimensions have been partially incorporated into a construct termed "arousability" and have been examined with other constructs from the emotions–feelings regulation field such as affectivity.

Overall, Clayton (1992) commented that the research on sensation-seeking is complex and has yielded different results for men and women and that the construct needs to be further explored.

The use of psychoactive substances as coping mechanisms to deal with distress is well documented in epidemiological studies and has face validity when users and abusers are asked about their motivation for this behavior (Khantzian, 1985).

Links from emotional distress to adolescent psychoactive substance use were also investigated (Swaim, Oetting, Edwards, & Beauvais, 1989). Emotional-distress and self-medication models (Khantzian, 1985) predict that the individual who is emotionally distressed through anxiety, depression, or some other psychological problem may try to alleviate the discomfort with the use of drugs. Swaim et al. (1989) reported that with the exception of a small residual path directly from anger to drug use (accounting for less than 5% of the variance), the emotional-distress hypothesis for adolescents has not been confirmed.

The research on psychological risk factors reviewed herein has potential implications for the improvement of the identification of youth at risk and the implementation of interventions.

4.5.2.2. Psychoactive Substance Use and Developmental Lag

Baumrind and Moselle have hypothesized that pathological psychoactive substance use during the developmental stage of childhood and adolescence impairs psychosocial development in such a way as to cause developmental arrest or regression (Baumrind & Moselle, 1985; Rivinus, 1992). Six factors relative to developmental arrest have been identified:

1. Psychoactive substance use obscures and impedes role definitions and transitions between work and play by adolescents as defined by Piaget (1962).
2. Psychoactive substance use promotes a false perception of reality and blurs reality-testing during a critical period. Choices made independent of family and mentors require a fully rounded sense of reality-testing. The development of this process throughout adolescence is impeded by psychoactive substance use to such an extent that reality-testing remains dwarfed.

3. Psychoactive substance use reinforces an egocentric view of the world, promotes grandiose views, and leaves the young person alternating between a hypertrophied internal locus of control and a feeling of complete external locus of control and helplessness.
4. Psychoactive substance use allows young people to avoid confrontation with environmental, vocational, and academic demands and responsibilities.
5. Psychoactive substance use isolates the individual from wider cultural goals, creating a subgroup that is highly culturally relative, negative, and rebellious.
6. Psychoactive substance abuse gives an illusory sense of liberation, freedom, and emancipation while in fact causing dependent and regressive parent–child interactions and dependency on social systems at large to rescue the "lost" or delinquent adolescent. Rivinus (1992) has pointed out that psychoactive substance use can be a false detour and become a transitional object from which little separation is permitted during a number of adolescent developmental crises and stages.

4.5.2.3. Familial Risk Factors

Clayton (1992) noted that one of the questions in the "Monitoring the Future" studies of drug abuse among high school seniors (Johnston, O'Malley, & Bachman, 1989) asks about family structure. There were 64 different family structures or types of household composition that emerged from the study, thus raising the need to change our perception of what is meant by the term family in this era.

It is noteworthy that there is a higher percentage than ever before of single-parent families characterizing a large segment of American families, especially among African Americans. Kellam, Simon, and Ensminger (1983) discovered in a study of African-American families that counter to common belief, it was not the absence of the father that was predictive of later drug use, but rather the aloneness of the mother. The presence of an additional adult almost entirely nullified the likelihood of delinquency and subsequent drug use.

Needle, Su, and Doherty (1990) studied the impact of changes in family structure on the prediction of youth substance abuse in a prospective longitudinal study. Different outcomes among boys vs. girls were reported. Boys were affected more than girls, especially when parental divorce took place during adolescence. Remarriage of the custodial parent benefited boys more than girls with regard to ASU. This study underscores that family disruption is not a discrete event, but an ongoing process (Clayton, 1992).

According to Kandel (1982), three major different aspects of parental characteristics predict initiation of ASU: parental drug behaviors, parental attitudes about drugs, and various aspects of parent–child interactions. These factors vary in importance at different stages of drug involvement. The risk of children from an alcohol- or drug-abusing family increases when: initiation of parental drinking and other potentially harmful behaviors (e.g., antisocial behavior) becomes part of the children's behavioral repertoire; a controlling parental style is utilized, including rules against the use of drugs by their offspring while they continue to abuse (usually ineffective); and when marijuana use is tolerated (Jessor & Jessor, 1977).

The availability of alcohol and other psychoactive substances at home and poor role modeling regarding drug and alcohol use behavior by parents, other adults in the family, and older siblings has a powerful effect on the developing child. The process is explained, according to the social-learning theory (Bandura, 1977), by social reinforcement of values and behaviors. The earlier a child is exposed to the dysfunctional drug- and alcohol-oriented parenting, the greater is the predicted risk. Parent–child interactions are of great importance. Lack of perceived closeness to parents is an especially strong predictor of initiation of use of drugs other than marijuana (Kandel, 1982). Ahmed, Bush, Davidson, and Iannotti (1984) have reported on a measure termed "salience"—the number of household users of a substance and the degree of children's involvement in parental substance-taking behavior. This measure was found to be a good predictor of both expectations of use and actual abuse of alcohol, cigarettes, and marijuana. Ahmed et al. (1984) reported on the characteristics of these families, which include: high stress; poor and inconsistent family management skills; increased separation, divorce, death, and prison terms; and decreased family activities.

Disruptive effects of parental drinking on family life are multiple. Consequences such as marital distress, health problems, legal or vocational problems or both, and financial instability present adaptive challenges (Johnson et al., 1991). Disrupted parenting includes an inability to promote social competence by monitoring and assigning consequences to the child's behavior. A deficit in parenting skills can increase the likelihood that the child will develop disruptive behaviors and social and academic deficits (Johnson et al., 1991). A recent study compared the disciplinary practices with respect to 10- to 12-year-old boys of substance-abusing fathers (SA+) and a control group of sons of non-substance-abusing fathers (SA−) (Tarter, Blackson, Martin, Loeber, &

Moss, 1993). Sons of SA+ fathers scored higher on traits characterizing a difficult temperament, and discipline was less effective in their households. These results demonstrate behavioral characteristics and a temperament style that predisposes these boys to future maladjustment.

Disrupted family rituals, emotional neglect within the family, isolation from the community, and a rejecting, stigmatizing label of the child of an alcoholic decrease opportunities for religious and cultural activities and may perpetuate deviant behavior (Rivinus, 1991).

Adolescents who are diagnosed with APSUDs report more negative life events than adolescents who are nonusers; however, when adolescents with APSUDs are compared with nonabusing adolescents, they report a comparable number of stressful life experiences if they both have substance-abusing parents (Brown, 1989). Also, it is noteworthy that adolescents with substance abuse in only one family generation experienced more emotional distress than those with substance-use patterns consistent across generations.

4.5.2.3.1. Family Violence and Childhood Trauma. The majority of present studies suggest increased prevalence of alcoholism among parents who abuse children (Johnson et al., 1991). However, the empirical literature on parental alcoholism, family violence, and childhood psychopathology is less conclusive (West & Prinz, 1987). An important research study on this subject investigated a large cohort of 18- to 21-year-old Danish males with respect to the relationship between parental alcoholism and childhood antecedents of antisocial behavior (Pollock, Briere, Schneider, Knop, Mednick, & Goodwin, 1990). Young males with alcoholic fathers did not report or exhibit more antisocial behavior than a control group; however, when parental alcoholism was controlled, self-reported history of being physically abused by a parent as a child was predictive of five of the six antisocial-behavior variables utilized for the assessment of this behavior. Pollock et al. (1990, p. 1292) concluded that their data support the notion that "parental alcoholism and physical abusiveness toward children may represent relatively independent phenomena."

Alcoholism is more strongly related to child maltreatment than any other parental psychiatric disorder, and the relationship between alcoholism and spouse abuse appears to be even stronger than that between alcoholism and child abuse (Famularo, Stone, Barnum, & Wharton, 1986). It seems that although the exact nature of causality is not yet clear, any form of experiencing family violence (e.g., passive or active, physical or sexual) may lead to childhood and adolescent predisposition to psychopathology and may result in the development of mood disorders, posttraumatic stress disorders, anxiety disorders, conduct disorders, and cluster B personality disorders. High rates of child physical and sexual abuse were reported in the general population, and even higher rates were found in juvenile detention centers and among psychiatric patients (Dembo, Dertke, LaVoie, Border, Washburn, & Schmeidler, 1987).

Children and adolescents with a history of abuse may become victims or aggressors or both in the presence of other peers (thus enlarging the cycle of violence and trauma) and dysfunctional in their performance and behavior in other life domains such as school attendance and precocious and irresponsible sexual behavior.

4.5.2.3.2. Parental Alcoholism—PSUD and Offspring Psychopathology. The relationship between parental or multigenerational alcoholism and childhood psychopathology is an intriguing research issue that has generated contrasting results due to methodological differences. Hill and Hruska (1992, p. 1024) justified the efforts devoted to this subject by stating that "if particular disorders in childhood could be found to be associated with later development of alcoholism, then these disorders could be considered as behavioral markers for risk." However, these authors reported that a study of high-risk children aged 8–18 years from families with a multigenerational history of alcoholism had rates of psychopathology similar to those of a control group from families without Axis I disorders of DSM-III-R (American Psychiatric Association, 1987).

Tarter, Laird, and Bukstein (1991) examined the relationship between mental health and psychosocial adjustment among adolescent offspring of substance-abusing parents compared to that of a control group reared by parents who did not have a PSUD. Adolescents who were in inpatient treatment and a community sample were separately studied. The findings indicated that parental substance abuse does not necessarily lead to maladjustment of their offspring.

Other empirical reports based on comparative studies of adolescents with a positive family history of alcoholism (FH+) also report equivocal results (Clair & Genest, 1987; Werner, 1986).

In contrast, Pandina and Johnson (1990) reported that FH+ of a community-based sample of adolescents reported alcohol or drug problems or both at about twice the rate of FH− individuals. These results are supportive of the adult FH+ and FH− literature (Hesselbrock, Stabenau, Hesselbrock, Meyer, & Babor, 1982; Schuckit, 1983).

Earls, Reich, Jung, and Cloninger (1988) conducted a comprehensive controlled family study investigating the frequency and types of psychopathology (DSM-III diagnoses) in children of parents with alcoholism only, children of antisocial parents (usually with alcoholism as a comorbidity), and children of nonalcoholic parents. The subjects were between 6 and 17 years of age, and the assessment of their psychopathology was done without knowledge of the parent's psychiatric status.

Children of alcoholic parents had higher rates of ADHD, oppositional disorder, and CD than did children of nonalcoholic parents. A coexisting ASPD of the father did not increase the rate of psychopathology in the children. A recent progress report of this study added findings based on the full data set (Reich, Earles, Frankel, & Shayka, 1993). Children of alcoholic parents did not have significantly higher rates of depression, but they may be at risk for anxiety. Also, they showed higher rates of oppositional and conduct disorders, but not of ADHD. These findings do not support the opinion that alcoholism and alcoholism with sociopathy are distinct diagnostic categories (Pollock et al., 1990; Schuckit, 1973). Another important finding in this study was that children of two alcoholic parents had an increased probability of a psychiatric disorder compared to children of one alcoholic parent. These results are similar to the findings in adult COAs (McKenna & Pickens, 1981).

No differences between groups regarding rates of alcoholism were found. Anxiety-disorder rates were higher among children of parents with diagnosed psychopathology.

Tarter et al. (1991) try to explain the differences between reports such as the ones cited above by attributing the absence of uniform findings to several factors, including ascertainment source (e.g., clinical or community sample) and family density of substance abuse or alcoholism (i.e., number of affected relatives in proportion to family size). Pollock et al. (1990) ascribe the confusion to biased subject-selection procedures, varied definitions of problematic behaviors and psychiatric disorders among family members and offspring, and sample size. Also, intelligence, psychosocial status, and other protective factors may lead to equivocal findings even when a control group is employed in a study. Moos and Billings (1982) suggested that the extent of the child's exposure to an alcoholic parent was predictive, but they additionally found that the degree of parental functioning in several domains was equally predictive. Also, they found that the emotional well-being of children with alcoholic parents who were in remission was no different than that of children of controls and better than that of children of relapsed parents.

Tarter et al. (1991) assert that being the offspring of parents who have a substance-abuse disorder does not necessarily mean an association with psychopathology. They also caution against uncritical acceptance of the pathologizing effect of parental PSUD on their offspring without referring to the quality and the severity of risk as well as protective factors.

Chapter 5 is devoted to APSUDs and psychiatric comorbidity.

4.5.2.4. Peer Factors

Peer influences play a crucial role in the initiation, development, and maintenance of ASU and the transition to APSUDs. The most consistent and reproducible finding in drug research is the strong relationship between an adolescent's drug behavior and the concurrent drug use of his or her friends (Kandel, 1982). Such similarity results not only from socialization, but also from a process of interpersonal selection (assortative pairing) in which adolescents with similar values and behaviors seek each other out as friends (Kandel, 1978). Girls appear to be more susceptible than boys to the influences of friends, especially in peer-related activities such as dating, and to a degree of attachment and reliance on peers rather than parents (Kandel, 1978).

ASU and especially APSUDs are inversely correlated with conventional behaviors, societal values, and beliefs and positively correlated with various risk-taking behaviors. Jessor and Jessor (1977) introduced a peer-group-dependent developmental psychosocial theory that explains the nature and development of alcohol abuse, drug misuse, and other problem behaviors. Their problem-behavior theory addresses the concept of transition proneness and the interaction between the personality and behavioral characteristics of the individual young drinker, the perceived environment (i.e., the relevant dimension of the larger social environment), and the attributes of the situation in which drinking takes place (Jessor, 1987). The proneness generated by the dynamic interaction of personality, perceived environment, and behavior specifies the likelihood of occurrence of normative development or of problem behavior in multiple domains that may include alcohol abuse, other substance abuse, delinquency, and deviant age-related sexual behaviors. This theory can explain the primary and secondary gains for the deviant adolescents as generated by problem behavior such as using the same preferred drugs or engaging in the same criminal and social activity. Such activities are deeply rooted in the identity-creating process of these groups and are inseparable components of their code of values (e.g., gang activity, satanism).

Oetting and Beauvais (1986) have introduced the peer cluster theory due to their dissatisfaction with theories, such as physiologically oriented disease/addiction models, that emphasize the effects of drugs especially on adolescents, or gateway theories, which focus on the gradual progression from one drug to another. They claim that for youths, the social effects of taking drugs are likely to be more important. This theory is similar to that of Jessor, with one major difference—that is, that it attests to peer relationships and clusters as the most important factors for the initiation and maintenance of APSUDs.

4.6 CONCLUSION

The importance of the interaction between biological and environmental factors for the development of alcoholism and other PSUDs has been recognized. The two are not independent of each other, especially with regard to the expression of the disorders. Although vulnerability may be attributed largely to genetic predisposition, the manifestations and severity of the disorder depend on shared familial environment, cultural, ethnic, and racial factors, and peer-group interactions. It is plausible to conclude that the greater the number and severity of risk factors, the higher the risk for APSUDs.

Further research is needed in all the fields referred to in the introduction to this chapter. Implications for therapeutic interventions (i.e., prevention and treatment) should be targeted whenever possible for the different transitions of ASU and APSUDs.

REFERENCES

Ahmed, S. W., Bush, P. J., Davidson, F. R., & Iannotti, R. J. (1984). Predicting children's use and intentions to use abusable substances. Paper presented at the annual meeting of the American Public Health Association, Anaheim, CA.

Ainsworth, M. D. S., Blehar, M. C., Waters, E., & Wall, S. (1978). *Patterns of Attachment: A Psychological Study of the Strange Situation.* Hillsdale, NJ: Erlbaum Associates.

Alexopoulos, G. S., Lieberman, K. W., & Frances, R. J. (1983). Platelet MAO activity in alcoholic patients and their first-degree relatives. *American Journal of Psychiatry, 140,* 1501–1503.

Allport, G. (1961). *Pattern and Growth in Personality.* New York: Holt, Reinhart, Winston.

American Psychiatric Association (1987). *Diagnostic and Statistical Manual of Mental Disorders,* 3rd ed. Washington, DC: American Psychiatric Association.

American Psychiatric Association (1994). *Diagnostic and Statistical Manual of Mental Disorders,* 4th ed., rev. Washington, DC: American Psychiatric Association.

Bandura, A. (1977). *Social Learning Theory.* Englewood Cliffs, NJ: Prentice-Hall.

Baumrind, D., & Moselle, K. A. (1985). A developmental perspective on adolescent drug abuse. In J. Brook, D. J. Lettieri, D. W. Brook, & B. Stimmel (Eds.), *Alcohol and Substance Abuse in Adolescence* (pp. 41–67). New York: Haworth Press.

Begleiter, H., & Porjesz, B. (1990). Neuroelectric processes in individuals at risk for alcoholism. *Alcohol & Alcoholism, 25,* 251–256.

Begleiter, H., Porjesz, B., Bihari, B., & Kissin, B. (1984). Event-related brain potentials in boys at risk for alcoholism. *Science, 225,* 1493–1496.

Blum, K., Noble, E. P., Sheridan, P. J., Montgomery, A., Ritchie, T., Jagadeeswaran, P., Nogami, H., Briggs, A. H., & Cohn, J. B. (1990). Allelic association of human dopamine D_2 receptor gene in alcoholism. *Journal of the American Medical Association, 263,* 2055–2060.

Bohman, M., Sigvardsson, S., & Cloninger, C. R. (1981). Maternal inheritance of alcohol abuse: Cross-fostering analysis of adopted women. *Archives of General Psychiatry, 38,* 965–969.

Borg, S., Kvande, H., Magnusson, E., & Sjoquist, B. (1980). Salsolinol and solsoline in cerebrospinal lumbar fluid of alcoholic patients. *Acta Psychiatrica Scandinavica Supplement, 286,* 171–177.

Bowlby, J. (1969). *Attachment and loss,* Vol. 1, *Attachment.* New York: Basic Books.

Bowlby, J. (1980). *Attachment and Loss,* Vol. 3, *Loss, Sadness and Depression.* London: Hogarth Press.

Brown, S. A. (1989). Life events of adolescents in relation to personal and parental substance abuse. *American Journal of Psychiatry, 146,* 484–489.

Bry, B. H., McKeon, P., & Pandina, R. J. (1982). Extent of drug use as a function of the number of risk factors. *Journal of Abnormal Psychology, 91,* 273–279.

Buydens-Branchey, L., Branchey, M. H., & Noumair, D. (1989). Age of alcoholism onset. I. Relationship to psychopathology. *Archives of General Psychiatry, 46,* 225–230.

Buydens-Branchey, L., Branchey, M. H., Noumair, D., & Lieber, C. S. (1989). Age of alcoholism onset. II. Relationship to susceptibility to serotonin precursor availability. *Archives of General Psychiatry, 46,* 231–236.

Cadoret, R. J. (1992). Genetic and environmental factors in initiation of drug use and the transition to abuse. In M. Glantz & R. Pickens (Eds.), *Vulnerability to Drug Abuse* (pp. 99–113). Washington, DC: American Psychological Association.

Cadoret, R. J., O'Gorman, T., Troughton, E., & Heywood, E. (1985). Alcoholism and antisocial personality: Interrelationships, genetic and environmental factors. *Archives of General Psychiatry, 42,* 161–167.

Cadoret, R. J., O'Gorman, T., Troughton, E., & Heywood, E. (1986). An adoption study of genetic and environmental factors in drug abuse. *Archives of General Psychiatry, 43,* 1131–1136.

Cantwell, D. (1972). Psychiatric illness in the families of hyperactive children. *Archives of General Psychiatry, 27,* 414–417.

Carmelli, D., Swan, G. E., Robinette, D., & Fabsitz, R. (1992). Genetic influence on smoking—a study of male twins. *New England Journal of Medicine, 327,* 829–833.

Chan, A. W. (1986). Racial differences in alcohol sensitivity. *Alcohol and Alcoholism, 21,* 93–104.

Clair, D., & Genest, M. (1987). Variables associated with the adjustment of offspring of alcoholic fathers. *Journal of Studies on Alcohol, 48,* 345–355.

Clayton, R. R. (1992). Transitions in drug use: Risk and protective factors. In M. Glantz and R. Pickens (Eds.), *Vulnerability to Drug Abuse* (pp. 15–51). Washington, DC: American Psychological Association.

Clifford, C. A., Fulker, D. W., Gurling, H.M.D., & Murray, R. M. (1981). Preliminary findings from a twin study of alcohol use. Twin Research 3 Part c: *Epidemiological and Clinical Studies.* New York: Alan R. Liss.

Cloninger, C. R. (1987). Neurogenetic adaptive mechanisms in alcoholism. *Science, 236,* 410–415.

Cloninger, C. R., Bohman, M., & Sigvardsson, S. (1981). Inheritance of alcohol abuse:

Cross-fostering analysis of adopted men. *Archives of General Psychiatry, 38,* 861–867.

Cloninger, C. R., Christiansen, K. O., Reich, T., & Gottesman, I. I. (1978). Implications of sex differences in the prevalence of antisocial personality, alcoholism, and criminality for familial transmission. *Archives of General Psychiatry, 35,* 941–951.

Cloninger, C. R., Sigvardsson, S., & Bohman, M. (1988). Childhood personality predicts alcohol abuse in young adults. *Alcoholism: Clinical & Experimental Research, 12,* 494–505.

Coccaro, E. F. (1989). Central serotonin and impulsive aggression. *British Journal of Psychiatry, 155,* 52–62.

Cotton, N. S. (1979). The familial incidence of alcoholism: A review. *Journal of Studies on Alcohol, 40,* 89–116.

Davis, V. E., & Walsh, M. J. (1970). Alcohol, amines and alkaloids: A possible biochemical basis for alcohol addiction. *Science, 167,* 1005–1007.

Dembo, R., Dertke, M., LaVoie, L., Border, S., Washburn, M., & Schmeidler, J. (1987). Physical abuse, sexual victimization and illicit drug use: A structural analysis among high risk adolescents. *Journal of Adolescence, 10,* 13–33.

Dinwiddie, S. H. (1992). Patterns of alcoholism inheritance. *Journal of Substance Abuse, 4,* 155–163.

Donovan, J.M. (1986). An etiologic model of alcoholism. *American Journal of Psychiatry, 143,* 1–11.

Earls, F., Reich, W., Jung, K. G., & Cloninger, C. R. (1988). Psychopathology in children of alcoholic and antisocial parents. *Alcoholism: Clinical and Experimental Research, 12,* 481–487.

Erikson, E. H. (1968). *Identity: Youth and Crisis.* New York: Plenum Press.

Famularo, R., Stone, K., Barnum, R., & Wharton, R. (1986). Alcoholism and severe child maltreatment. *American Journal of Orthopsychiatry, 56,* 481–485.

Frezza, M., Di-Padova, C., Pozzatto, G., Terpin, M., Baraona, E., & Lieber, C. S. (1990). High blood alcohol levels in women: The role of decreased gastric alcohol dehydrogenase activity and first pass metabolism. *New England Journal of Medicine, 322,* 95–99.

Glantz, M. D. (1992). A developmental psychopathology model of drug abuse vulnerability. In M. Glantz & R. Pickens (Eds.), *Vulnerability to Drug Abuse* (pp. 389–418). Washington, DC: American Psychological Association.

Goldman, M. S. (1989). Alcohol expectancies as cognitive–behavioral psychology: Theory and practice. In T. Loberg, G. A. Marlatt, P. E. Nathan, & W. R. Miller (Eds.), *Treatment of Addictive Behaviors* (pp. 11–30). Amsterdam: Swets.

Gomberg, E. S. L. (1993). Women and alcohol: Use and abuse. *Journal of Nervous and Mental Disease, 181,* 211–219.

Goodwin, D. W. (1985). Alcoholism and genetics: The sins of the fathers. *Archives of General Psychiatry, 42,* 171–174.

Goodwin, D. W., Schulsinger, F., Hermansen, L., Guze, S. B., & Winokur, G. (1973). Alcohol problems in adoptees raised apart from alcoholic biological parents. *Archives of General Psychiatry, 28,* 238–242.

Gordis, E., Tabakoff, B., Goldman, D., & Berg, K. (1990). Finding the gene(s) for alcoholism. *Journal of the American Medical Association, 263,* 2094–2095.

Hawkins, J. D., & Catalano, R. F. (1989). Risk and protective factors for alcohol and other drug problems: Implications for substance abuse prevention. Unpublished manuscript.

Hawkins, J. D., Lishner, D. M., Catalano, R. F., & Howard, M. O. (1986). Childhood predictors of adolescent substance abuse: Toward an empirically grounded theory. *Journal of Children in Contemporary Society, 18*, 11–49.

Hegedus, A., Alterman, A., & Tarter, R. (1984). Learning achievement in sons of alcoholics. *Alcoholism: Clinical and Experimental Research, 8*, 330.

Hegedus, A., Tarter, R., Hill, S., Jacob, T., & Winsten, N. (1984). Static ataxia: A possible marker for alcoholism. *Alcoholism: Clinical and Experimental Research, 8*, 580–582.

Helzer, J. E., & Pryzbeck, T. R. (1988). The co-occurrence of alcoholism with other psychiatric disorders in the general population and its impact on treatment. *Journal of Studies on Alcohol, 49*, 219–224.

Hesselbrock, V. M., Stabenau, J. R., Hesselbrock, M. N., Meyer, R. E., & Babor, T. F. (1982). The nature of alcoholism in patients with different family histories for alcoholism. *Progressive Neuropsychopharmacology and Biological Psychiatry, 6*, 607–614.

Hill, S. Y., & Hruska, D. R. (1992). Childhood psychopathology in families with multi-generational alcoholism. *Journal of American Academy of Child and Adolescent Psychiatry, 31*, 1024–1030.

Hill, S. Y., Steinhauer, S. R., Smith, T. R., & Locke, J. (1991). Risk markers for alcoholism in high-density families. *Journal of Substance Abuse, 3*, 351–369.

Horrobin, D. F. (1980). A biochemical basis for alcoholism and alcohol-induced damage including the fetal alcohol syndrome and cirrhosis: Interface with essential fatty acid and prostaglandin and alcohol metabolism. *Medical Hypotheses, 6*, 929–942.

Hrubre, Z., & Omenn, G. (1981). Evidence of genetic predisposition to alcoholic cirrhosis and psychosis: Twin concordance for alcoholism and its biological end-points by zygosity among male veterans. *Alcoholism: Clinical and Experimental Research, 5*, 207–235.

Huba, G. J., Wingard, J. A., & Bentler, P. M. (1980). Applications of a theory of drug use to prevention programs. *Journal of Drug Education, 10*, 25–38.

Irwin, M., Schuckit, M., & Smith, T. L. (1990). Clinical importance of age at onset in Type 1 and Type 2 primary alcoholics. *Archives of General Psychiatry, 47*, 320–324.

Jellinek, E. M. (1960). *The Disease Concept of Alcoholism*. New Brunswick: Hillhouse Press.

Jessor, R. (1987). Problem-behavior theory, psychosocial development, and adolescent problem drinking. *British Journal of Addiction, 82*, 331–342.

Jessor, R., & Jessor, S. L. (1977). *Problem Behavior and Psychosocial Development: A Longitudinal Study of Youth*. New York: Academic Press.

Johnson, J. L., Sher, K. J., & Rolf, J. E. (1991). Models of vulnerability to psychopathology in children of alcoholics: An overview. *Alcohol Health & Research World, 15*, 33–42.

Johnston, L. D., O'Malley, P. M., & Bachman, J. G. (1989). *Drug Use, Drinking, and Smoking: National Survey Results from High School, College, and Young Adult Populations 1975–1988*. Rockville, MD: National Institute on Drug Abuse.

Kagan, J., Resnick, J. S., & Snidman, N. (1988). Biological basis of childhood shyness. *Science, 240*, 167–171.

Kaij, L. (1960). *Alcoholism in Twins*. Stockholm: Almquist & Wiksell.

Kandel, D. B. (1975). Stages of adolescent involvement in drug use. *Science, 190*, 912–914.

Kandel, D. B. (1978). *Longitudinal Research on Drug Use: Empirical Findings and Methodological Issues*. New York: Hemisphere-Wiley.

Kandel, D. B. (1982). Epidemiological and psychosocial perspectives on adolescent drug use. *Journal of the American Academy of Child Psychiatry, 20*, 328–347.

Kaplan, H. B. (1980). Self-esteem and self-derogation theory of drug abuse. In D. J. Lettieri, M. Sayers, & H. W. Pearson (Eds.), *Theories on Drug Abuse: Selected Contemporary Perspectives* (pp. 128–131). Rockville, MD: National Institute on Drug Abuse.

Kaprio, J., Koskenvuo, M., Langinvainio, H., Romanov, K., Sarna, S., & Rose, R. J. (1987).

Genetic influences on use and abuse of alcohol: A study of 5638 adult Finnish twin brothers. *Alcoholism: Clinical and Experimental Research, 11,* 349–356.

Kellam, S. G., Simon, M. B., & Ensminger, M. E. (1983). Antecedent of teenage drug use and psychological well-being: A ten year community wide prospective study. In D. Ricks & B. S. Dohrewend (Eds.), *Origins of Psychopathology: Research and Public Policy* (pp. 203–232). Cambridge, MA: Cambridge University Press.

Kendler, K. S., Heath, A. C., Neale, M. C., Kessler, R. C., & Eaves, L. J. (1993). Alcoholism and major depression in women: A twin study of the causes of comorbidity. *Archives of General Psychiatry, 50,* 690–698.

Khantzian, E. J. (1985). The self-medication theory of addictive disorders: Focus on heroin and cocaine dependence. *American Journal of Psychiatry, 142,* 1259–1264.

King, R., Curtis, D., & Knoblich, G. (1992). Biological factors in sociopathy: Relationships to drug abuse behaviors. In M. Glantz & R. Pickens (Eds.), *Vulnerability to Drug Abuse* (pp. 115–136). Washington, DC: American Psychological Association.

Labouvie, E. W., Pandina, R. J., White, H. R., & Johnson, V. (1986). Risk factors of adolescent drug use: A cross sectional study. Unpublished manuscript.

Lee, C., & Bates, J. (1985). Mother–child interaction at age two years and perceived difficult temperament. *Child Development, 56,* 1314–1326.

Lerner, J., & Vicary, J. (1984). Difficult temperament and drug use: Analysis from the New York longitudinal study. *Journal of Drug Education, 14,* 1–8.

Lettieri, D. J., Sayers, M., & Pearson, H. W. (Eds.) (1980). *Theories on Drug Abuse: Selected Contemporary Perspectives.* NIDA Research Monograph 30. Rockville, MD: National Institute on Drug Abuse.

Lex, B. W. (1985). Alcohol problems in special populations. In J. H. Mendelson & N. K. Mello (Eds.), *The Diagnosis and Treatment of Alcoholism,* 2nd ed. (pp. 89–117). New York: McGraw-Hill.

Li, T. Y., Lumeg, L., McBride, W. J., & Murphy, J. M. (1987). Rodents lines selected factors affecting alcohol consumption. *Alcoholism, 11,* 91–96.

Loeber, R. (1985). Patterns of development of antisocial child behavior. *Annals of Child Development, 2,* 77–115.

Loosen, P. T., Wilson, I. C., Dew, B. W., & Tipermas, A. (1983). Thyrotropin releasing hormone (TRH) in abstinent alcoholic men. *American Journal of Psychiatry, 140,* 1145–1149.

Main, M., & Solomon, J. (1986). Discovery of an insecure disorganized/disoriented attachment pattern: Procedures, findings, and implications for the classification of behavior. In M. Yogman & T. B. Brazelton (Eds.), *Affective Development in Infancy* (pp. 95–124). Norwood, NJ: Ablex.

Martin, R., Nagle, R., & Paget, K. (1983). Relationship between temperament and classroom behavior, teacher attitudes, and academic achievement. *Journal of Clinical Psychology, 39,* 1013–1020.

Maziade, M., Caron, C., Cote, R., Boutin, P., & Thiverge, J. (1990). Extreme temperament and diagnosis: A study in a psychiatric sample of consecutive children. *Archives of General Psychiatry, 47,* 477–484.

McKenna, T., & Pickens, R. (1981). Alcoholic children of alcoholics. *Journal of Studies on Alcohol, 42,* 1021–1029.

Merikangas, K. R. (1990). The genetic epidemiology of alcoholism. *Psychological Medicine, 20,* 11–22.

Merikangas, K. R., Leckman, J. F., Prusoff, B. A., Pauls, D. L., & Weissman, M. M. (1985). Familial transmission of depression and alcoholism. *Archives of General Psychiatry, 42,* 367–372.

Miles-Cox, W., & Klinger, E. (1988). A motivational model of alcohol use. *Journal of Abnormal Psychology, 2,* 168–180.

Miller, N. S., Goodwin, D. W., Jones, F. C., Pardo, M. P., Anand, M. M., Gabrielli, W. F., & Hall, T. B. (1987). Histamine receptor antagonism of intolerance to alcohol in oriental population. *Journal of Nervous and Mental Disease, 175,* 661–667.

Moos, R. H., & Billings, A. G. (1982). Children of alcoholics during the recovery process: Alcoholic and matched control families. *Addictive Behaviors, 7,* 155–163.

Morrison, J., & Stewart, M. (1973). The psychiatric status of the legal families of adopted hyperactive children. *Archives of General Psychiatry, 28,* 888–891.

Moss, H. B., Guthrie, S., & Linnoila, M. (1986). Enhanced thyrotropin response to thyrotropin releasing hormone in boys at risk for development of alcoholism: Preliminary report. *Archives of General Psychiatry, 43,* 1137–1142.

Moss, H. B., & Tarter, R. E. (1993). Substance abuse, aggression, and violence: What are the connections? *American Journal on Addictions, 2,* 149–160.

Nathan, P. E. (1988). The addictive personality is the behavior of the addict. *Journal of Consulting and Clinical Psychiatry, 56,* 183–188.

Nathan, P. E. (1990). Integration of biological and psychosocial research on alcoholism. *Alcoholism: Clinical and Experimental Research, 14,* 368–374.

Needle, R. H., Su, S., & Doherty, W. J. (1990). Divorce, remarriage, and adolescent substance use: A prospective longitudinal study. *Journal of Marriage and the Family, 52,* 157–169.

Newcomb, M. D., & Bentler, P. M. (1988). Consequences of adolescent drug use: Impact on the lives of young adults. Beverly Hills, CA: Sage.

Newcomb, M. D., Maddahian, E., & Bentler, P. M. (1986). Risk factors for drug use among adolescents: Concurrent and longitudinal analyses. *American Journal of Public Health, 76,* 525–531.

O'Connor, M. J., Sigman, M., & Brill, N. (1987). Disorganization of attachment in relation to maternal alcohol consumption. *Journal of Consulting and Clinical Psychology, 55,* 831–836.

Oetting, E. R., & Beauvais, F. (1986). Peer cluster theory: Drugs and the adolescent. *Journal of Counseling and Development, 65,* 17–22.

O'Malley, S. S., Jaffe, A. J., Chang, G., Schottenfeld, R. S., Meyer, R. E., & Rounsaville, B. (1992). Naltrexone and coping skills therapy for alcohol dependence. *Archives of General Psychiatry, 49,* 881–887.

Pandina, R. J., & Johnson, V. (1990). Serious alcohol and drug problems among adolescents with a family history of alcoholism. *Journal of Studies on Alcohol, 51,* 278–282.

Partanen, J., Bruun, K., & Markkanen, T. (1966). *Inheritance of Drinking Behavior: A Study on Intelligence, Personality, and Use of Alcohol of Adult Twins,* Vol. 14. Helsinki: The Finnish Foundation for Alcohol Studies.

Piaget, J. (1962). *The Moral Judgment of the Child.* New York: Collier.

Pickens, R. W., Svikis, D. S., McGue, M., Lykken, D. T., Heston, L. L., & Clayton, P. J. (1991). Heterogeneity in the inheritance of alcoholism: A study of male and female twins. *Archives of General Psychiatry, 48,* 19–28.

Pollock, V. E., Briere, J., Schneider, L., Knop, J., Mednick, S. A., & Goodwin, D. W. (1990). Childhood antecedents of antisocial behavior: Parental alcoholism and physical abusiveness. *American Journal of Psychiatry, 147,* 1290–1293.

Pollock, V. E., Volavka, J., Goodwin, D. W., Sarnoff, A. M., Gabrielli, W. F., Knop, J., & Schulsinger, F. (1983). The EEG after school administration in men at risk for alcoholism. *Archives of General Psychiatry, 40,* 854–861.

Reich, W., Earls, F., Frankel, O., & Shayka, J. J. (1993). Psychopathology in children of alcoholics. *Journal of the American Academy of Child and Adolescent Psychiatry, 32,* 995–1002.

Rivinus, T. M. (1991). *Children of Chemically Dependent Parents.* New York: Brunner/Mazel.

Rivinus, T. M. (1992). College age substance abuse as a developmental arrest. *Journal of College Student Psychotherapy, 6,* 141–166.

Robins, L. (1978). Sturdy childhood predictors of adult antisocial behavior: Replications from longitudinal studies. *Psychological Medicine, 8,* 611–622.

Robins, L. N., Helzer, J. E., Weissman, M. M., Orvaschel, H., Gruenberg, E., Burke, J. D., & Regier, D. A. (1984). Life time prevalence of specific psychiatric disorders in three sites. *Archives of General Psychiatry, 41,* 949–958.

Roe, A. (1944). The adult adjustment of children of alcoholic parents raised in foster homes. *Quarterly Journal of Studies on Alcohol, 5,* 378–393.

Sameroff, A. J., & Chandler, M. J. (1975). Reproductive risk and the continuum of caretaking casualty. In F. D. Horowitz (Ed.), *Review of Child Development Research,* Vol. 4 (pp. 187–244). Chicago: University of Chicago Press.

Schenker, S., & Speeg, K. V. (1990). The risk of alcohol intake in men and women: All may not be equal. *New England Journal of Medicine, 322,* 127–129.

Schuckit, M. A. (1973). Alcoholism and sociopathy—diagnostic confusion. *Quarterly Journal of Studies on Alcohol, 34,* 157–164.

Schuckit, M. A. (1983). Alcoholic men with no alcoholic first-degree relatives. *American Journal of Psychiatry, 140,* 439–443.

Schuckit, M. A. (1984). Subjective responses to alcohol in sons of alcoholics and control subjects. *Archives of General Psychiatry, 41,* 879–884.

Schuckit, M. A., Parker, D. C., & Rossman, L. R. (1983). Ethanol-related prolactin responses and risk for alcoholism. *Biological Psychiatry, 18,* 120–126.

Schuckit, M. A., & Irwin, M. D. (1989). An analysis of the clinical relevance of Type 1 and Type 2 alcoholics. *British Journal of Addiction, 84,* 869–876.

Seifer, R., & Sameroff, A. J. (1987). Multiple determinants of risk and invulnerability. In E. J. Anthony & B. J. Cohler (Eds.), *The Invulnerable Child* (pp. 51–69). New York: Guildford Press.

Shedler, J., & Block, J. (1990). Adolescent drug use and psychological health. *American Psychologist, 45,* 612–630.

Sher, K. J., & Levenson, R. W. (1982). Risk for alcoholism and individual differences in the stress-response-dampening effect of alcohol. *Journal of Abnormal Psychology, 19,* 350–367.

Smith, S. S., O'Hara, B. F., Persico, A. M., Gorelick, D. A., Newlin, D. B., Vlahov, D., Solomon, L., Pickens, R., & Uhl, G. R. (1992). Genetic vulnerability to drug abuse: The D_2 dopamine receptor Tag 1 B1 restriction fragment length polymorphism appears more frequently in polysubstance abusers. *Archives of General Psychiatry, 49,* 723–727.

Swaim, R. C., Oetting, E. R., Edwards, R. W., & Beauvais, F. (1989). Links from emotional distress to adolescent drug use: A path model. *Journal of Consulting and Clinical Psychology, 57,* 227–231.

Szatmari, P., Boyle, M., & Offord, D. (1989). ADHD and conduct disorder: Degree of diagnostic overlap and differences among correlates. *Journal of the American Academy of Child and Adolescent Psychiatry, 28,* 865–872.

Tarter, R. (1982). Psychosocial history, minimal brain dysfunction and differential drinking patterns of male alcoholics. *Journal of Clinical Psychology, 38,* 867–873.

Tarter, R. (1991). Developmental behavior–genetic perspective of alcoholism etiology. In M. Galanter (Ed.), *Recent Developments in Alcoholism* (pp. 71–85). New York: Plenum Press.

Tarter, R. E., Blackson, T., Martin, C., Loeber, R., & Moss, H. B. (1993). Characteristics and correlates of child discipline practices in substance abuse and normal families. *American Journal on Addictions, 2,* 18–25.

Tarter, R., & Edwards, K. (1986). Antecedents to alcoholism: Implications for prevention and treatment. *Behavior Therapy, 17,* 346–361.

Tarter, R., Hegedus, A., Goldstein, G., Shelly, C., & Alterman, A. (1984). Adolescent sons of alcoholics: Neuropsychological and personality characteristics. *Alcoholism: Clinical and Experimental Research, 8,* 216–222.

Tarter, R., Laird, S., Kabene, M., Bukstein, O., & Kaminer, Y. (1990). Drug abuse severity in adolescents is associated with magnitude of deviation in temperament traits. *British Journal of Addiction, 85,* 1511–1504.

Tarter, R. E., Laird, S., & Bukstein, O. (1991). Multivariate comparison of adolescent offspring of substance abuse parents: Community and treatment samples. *Journal of Substance Abuse, 3,* 301–306.

Tarter, R. E., & Mezzich, A. C. (1992). Ontogeny of substance abuse: Perspectives and findings. In M. Glantz & R. Pickens (Eds.), *Vulnerability to Drug Abuse* (pp. 149–178). Washington, DC: American Psychological Association.

Thomas, A., & Chess, S. (1984). Genesis and evolution of behavioral disorders: From infancy to early adult life. *American Journal of Psychiatry, 141,* 1–9.

Uhl, G. R., Persico, A. M., & Smith, S. S. (1992). Current excitement with D_2 dopamine receptor gene alleles in substance abuse. *Archives of General Psychiatry, 49,* 157–160.

Virkkunnen, M. (1985). Urinary free cortisol secretion in habitually violent offenders. *Acta Psychiatrica Scandinavica, 72,* 40–44.

Werner, E. (1986). Resilient offspring of alcoholics: A longitudinal study from birth to age 18. *Journal of Studies on Alcohol, 47,* 34–40.

West, M. O., & Prinz, R. J. (1987). Parental alcoholism and childhood psychopathology. *Psychological Bulletin, 102,* 204–218.

Wilson, J. R., & Crowe, L. (1991). Genetics of alcoholism: Can and should youth at risk be identified? *Alcohol Health & Research World, 15,* 11–17.

Zuckerman, M. (1979). *Sensation Seeking: Beyond the Optimal Level of Arousal.* Hillsdale, NJ: Erlbaum.

Dual Diagnosis: Adolescent Psychoactive Substance Use Disorders and Psychiatric Comorbidity

Adolescence is a critical developmental phase for the onset and recognition of psychiatric disorders including psychoactive substance use disorders (PSUDs). The co-occurrence of PSUDs with other psychiatric disorders has been termed a "dual diagnosis" (DD), and the patients so diagnosed have been defined as "dually diagnosed" (DUDI).

The prevalence of DD is high, and the recently increased recognition of the concept of comorbid* disorders has important clinical, public health, and research implications.

From the clinical perspective, subgroups of DUDI individuals may respond differentially to specific therapeutic approaches. Regarding public health interests, subgroups of adolescents with comorbid disorders may be at a higher risk of contracting or manifesting additional disorders and of increased severity of the course of each one of the index disorders. The implications for research on DD are that more homogeneous subgroups within a given diagnostic category can be studied to broaden the knowledge about this diagnostic entity.

This chapter reviews the methodological and nosological issues in diagnosing and understanding the nature of DD, the epidemiology of

---

*The term "comorbidity," introduced by Feinstein (1970), refers to the presence of any additional coexisting ailment in a patient with a particular index disease.

DD, and the specific relationship between a variety of psychiatric disorders and PSUDs of adolescents and their families. Finally, special reference is made to future clinical and research implications concerning prevention and treatment of DD. The literature on comorbidity in adults is used as a departure point in some sections due to the sparsity of data on adolescents.

5.1. NOSOLOGICAL AND METHODOLOGICAL ISSUES

It is generally accepted that comorbidity is the coexistence of two or more distinct disorders in the same individual; however, Achenbach (1990) argued that findings of apparent comorbidity among behavioral and emotional disorders may raise more questions than they answer due to a lack of validated operational definitions for many psychiatric disorders of childhood and adolescence. Achenbach (1990) reviewed five factors that may contribute to the erroneous assumption of comorbidity between disorders: (1) The symptoms used to diagnose the different disorders may result from the same underlying cause. (2) The diagnostic procedures may fail to discriminate accurately between disorders that do not actually occur together with greater than chance incidence. (3) The diagnostic criteria may omit features that would increase the discriminability of a disorder from other disorders. (4) The apparent comorbidity could involve a higher-order pattern of co-occurring problems that should be used to define a single diagnostic entity. (5) By incorrectly placing the border between the normal and the pathological or between two disorders, the categories may not be congruent with the distinctive criteria that define them.

Additional explanations for a perceived comorbidity between disorders include (1) population stratification, (2) chance association, and (3) a treatment-seeking bias known also as "Berkson's fallacy." Berkson (1946) indicated that individuals with more than one disorder are more likely to seek clinical services than are those with only one disorder, leading to an erroneously higher estimate of the prevalence of the association between these disorders than would be the case if each single disorder independently led the sufferer to seek medical care.

Artificial comorbidity may lead to errors in treatment and therefore should be watched for. Caron and Rutter (1991) reviewed the issue of both apparent and real comorbidity, and their monograph is a highly recommended source for understanding concepts and research strategies of comorbidity in child psychopathology.

Achenbach (1990) advocated the separation of conceptual models from diagnostic models in order to improve the clarity of comorbid disorder phenomenology (pp. 272–273):

> Conceptual models are the underlying theoretical concepts of disorders, regardless of the diagnostic procedures used to identify the disorders. Several conceptual models may be used to understand a disorder, and several diagnostic models may be used to identify it. The distinction between the conceptual models for disorders and the diagnostic models for detecting them can be expressed in terms of taxonomy and assessment: "Taxonomy" refers to the conceptual models by which we group cases according to their distinguishing features, whereas "assessment" refers to diagnostic models and procedures for identifying the distinguishing features of individual cases.

It is often unclear whether a patient's symptoms are a consequence of substance abuse per se or are indicative of a comorbid psychiatric disorder. Moreover, in such patients, the sequelae of psychoactive substance intoxication or withdrawal or both are often difficult to distinguish from the signs and symptoms of concurrent psychiatric disorder (Mirin, Weiss, Griffin, & Michael, 1991).

It is important to reemphasize that dual diagnosis is a term limited to the relationship between disorders and is not applicable to symptoms associated with PSUDs, which are considered to be manifestations of the severity of PSUDs.

Rather than accepting reports of DD at face value, one must maintain increased awareness based on an understanding of conceptual and diagnostic models in the practical context delineated above to limit potential pitfalls in a relatively sparsely researched domain.

The diagnostic process of comorbid disorders and the reliability and stability of DD are factors of great importance that as yet have been reported only in research conducted with DUDI adults. Regarding the diagnostic process, information derived from multiple informants is believed to facilitate the process and to enhance the specificity of prevalence estimates of disorders. Also, in the case of DD, a "best estimate" procedure may be helpful in enhancing the accuracy of the diagnostic process. Such a procedure is especially likely to be helpful when data from direct interview either are missing or may be inaccurate if the subject withholds or provides false information. A "best estimate" diagnosis is one made by a clinician on the basis of diagnostic information from a direct interview conducted by another clinician plus information from medical records and from reports of family members (Kosten & Rounsaville, 1992).

It has been reported that current mood disorders and psychotic disorders were less reliably diagnosed in a group with current PSUDs compared to two control groups, one with past PSUDs and the other without a history of PSUD (Bryant, Rounsaville, Spitzer & Williams, 1992). However, the results were adequately reliable to aid in classification. It was also concluded that delaying diagnosis until at least 1–2 weeks after cessation of drug use is likely to improve classification results.

A study of the stability of psychiatric comorbidity in alcoholic men after 1 year revealed that the symptoms are stable over time and therefore constitute a potential target for treatment (Penick, Powell, Liskow, Jackson, & Nickel, 1988). On the other hand, Rounsaville and Kleber (1986) reported good stability of comorbid psychiatric disorders at 6 months of follow-up among opiate addicts, which deteriorated by 2.5 years of follow-up, resulting in a very low rate of stability. Penick et al. (1988) attributed these differences to a threshold effect. Thus, patients over time tend to minimize the number and intensity of symptoms associated with other psychiatric disorders rather than simply to deny all symptoms at one time and acknowledge other symptoms at another. In order to make a reliable and valid psychiatric diagnosis, rating scales are frequently utilized. However, some argue that the assessment of comorbid psychopathology, especially of depression among substance abusers, lacks acceptable specificity. Indeed, the results among adult patients support only limited use of measures (Weiss, Griffin, & Mirin, 1989).

5.2. EPIDEMIOLOGY OF DUAL DIAGNOSIS

Examining the association between disorders in clinical populations alone may generate misleading impressions regarding the magnitude of the comorbidity. Therefore, relationships between disorders are best studied in representative samples of general populations.

5.2.1. Epidemiological Studies in Child and Adolescent Psychiatry

During the 1980s, eight community surveys of the prevalence of psychiatric disorders in children and adolescents generated estimates of moderate to severe disorders that ranged from 14% to 20% (Brandenburg, Friedman, & Silver, 1990). One of these reports also investigated comorbidity of psychiatric disorders in a sample of 792 preadolescents (Anderson, Williams, McGee, & Silva, 1987). Anderson et al. (1987) reported that 17.6% of their cohort were found to have at least one DSM-III psychiatric disorder, and almost 55% of the diagnosed individuals had more than one diagnosis. It can be concluded that psychiatric comorbidity is highly prevalent among children and adolescents in the general population.

5.2.2. Substance-Abuse-Oriented Epidemiological Studies in Adults

A pivotal source for the prevalence of psychiatric disorders, alcohol and substance abuse, and DD in the general population is the Epidemiological Catchment Area (ECA) study. This is a combined NIMH-sponsored household and institutional survey of mental disorders conducted in five metropolitan areas throughout the United States. The analysis is based on data from about 20,000 respondents who were 18 years old and older at the time of entry into the study and included both sexes and multiple racial and ethnic groups (Regier et al., 1988).

The rates of anxiety disorders, major depression, and substance use disorders were high in the age group of 18–24 years (Christie, Burke, Regier, Rae, Boyd, & Locke, 1988). About 22% of the 18- to 30-year-olds had a substance use disorder according to DSM-III, and fewer than one third of them had a comorbid depressive or anxiety disorder manifested before age 20. Moreover, almost 3 of every 4 subjects with psychiatric comorbidity indicated that the substance abuse started later than the other psychiatric disorder(s) (Christie et al., 1988). These findings demonstrate a doubling of risk for subsequent substance use disorders in young adults who have had an earlier depressive or anxiety disorder.

The relationship between major depression and PSUDs in adolescents has recently received increased attention following analysis of the age of onset of psychiatric disorders in the ECA study (Burke, Burke, Rae, & Regier, 1991).

Life-table survival methods were used to examine the hazard rates for major depression as well as for other specific mental disorders. The findings are consistent with a gradual shift to increased rates for major depression between the ages of 15 and 19 years. The report also suggested a similar shift for drug abuse/dependence. Similar but less pronounced changes were found for alcohol abuse/dependence (Burke et al., 1991). For drug abuse/dependence, there has been a shift to a younger age at onset for the most recent cohort as well as an increase in the magnitude of the hazard rate for those respondents born between 1953 and 1966. For alcohol abuse/dependence, there has not been a shift in the peak age of onset.

The evidence of increasing onset from 15 to 19 years of age for major depression, drug abuse/dependence, and possibly alcohol

abuse/dependence raises important questions about the possible association of these conditions. According to Burke et al. (1991, p. 794): "It is
not yet clear whether the earlier occurrence of major depression contributes to an earlier onset of clinical disorders of drug abuse/dependence in
adolescents who may have only experimented with drug use in earlier
cohorts. If so, the shift to an earlier age at onset for major depression
could be one of the factors leading to increased drug abuse/dependence
in the same period of late adolescence."

A study on the degree of association between alcoholism and other
psychiatric disorders in the ECA study population generated a variety of
odds ratios specific to each psychiatric diagnosis (Helzer & Pryzbeck,
1988). The strongest association is with antisocial personality disorder
(ASPD), which has an odds ratio of 21.0, followed by bipolar disorders,
6.2; schizophrenia, 4.0; panic disorder, 2.4; obsessive–compulsive, 2.1;
somatization disorder, 1.8; dysthymia, 1.8; depression, 1.7; phobic disorders, 1.4; anorexia, 1.2; and any core diagnosis, 2.8. Depression and
dysthymia co-occur with alcoholism to a high degree in clinical samples
(Hesselbrock, Meyer, & Keener, 1985); however, their odds ratios here
are relatively weak as compared to those of other categories. It seems
likely that these results are not contradictory, but that depression may
motivate alcoholics to seek treatment (Helzer & Pryzbeck, 1988).

It is important to recognize that the ECA study suffers from several
shortcomings: (1) It is not a representative sample of the entire United
States. (2) It is not a comprehensive survey of the full range of psychiatric disorders. (3) It is based on lifetime rather than cross-sectional
assessment of symptoms and disorders. Also, findings from epidemiological studies in adults that investigate onset of disorders must be interpreted cautiously. Poor recall or reporting or both by older individuals
of either symptoms or onset data, or earlier mortality of those participants with psychiatric disorders in the older cohorts, are of concern in
retrospective analysis of cross-sectional data.

5.2.3. Substance-Abuse-Oriented Epidemiological
Studies in Untreated Adolescents

Little is known about the prevalence of diagnosed PSUDs in adolescents from the community. Early studies conducted in the 1970s with
cohorts of adolescents from the general population usually found a
relationship between substance abuse and psychiatric symptomatology
(Braucht, Brakarsch, Follingstad, & Berry, 1973; McAree, Steffenhagen,
& Zhentlen, 1972; Vener, Stewart, & Hager, 1972). However, these studies suffered from methodological flaws related to their examination of

the participants at only one point in time (Kaminer, 1991). Paton, Kessler, and Kandel (1977) performed a longitudinal study of a representative sample of a large cohort ($N = 8206$) of high school seniors and found a complex relationship between depression and illicit drug use. Lavik and Onstad (1987) reported that in a random sample of 177 adolescents from a junior high school in Norway, users of various psychoactive substances also had higher frequencies of psychiatric symptoms than nonusers. However, no specific symptoms were reported.

Of 275 non-treatment-seeking children and adolescents, 7% received a DSM-III diagnosis of alcohol or substance use disorder (Keller, Lavori, Beardslee, Wunder, & Hasin, 1992). Of the 19 individuals diagnosed with substance use disorder, 89% also received one or more diagnoses.

5.2.4. Dual Diagnosis in Clinical Adolescent Populations

The prevalence of psychiatric disorders among alcoholics and other substance-abusing adults was found to be very high. Ross, Glaser, and Germanson (1988) reported that 78% of their 501 patients with substance use disorders met DSM-III criteria for a lifetime comorbid psychiatric disorder, with 65% suffering from a concurrent psychiatric disorder. A study of opioid addicts by Khantzian and Treece (1985) and a report about 321 alcoholics (Hesselbrock et al., 1985) generated similar results, with 77% receiving a comorbid Axis I diagnosis. Confirming these results is a study that reported that 81% of 339 alcoholics were found to have associated mental disorders (Roy et al., 1991). The most common lifetime disorders were other drug abuse, ASPD, mood disorders, and anxiety disorders.

Studies among treated adolescents with PSUDs also revealed a high prevalence of comorbid disorders, primarily mood or conduct disorders or both. In a study of 459 adolescents seen for psychiatric evaluation in a general hospital emergency room, it was reported that almost half those with elevated blood alcohol levels (17% of the total sample) had at least one additional psychiatric diagnosis, with depression being the most common (Reichler, Clemente, & Dunner, 1983). A study of 41 adolescents admitted to a psychiatric hospital for psychiatric disorders concluded that about 70% were also diagnosed as substance abusers (Roerich & Gold, 1986). However, both studies relied on chart review and on selected patients, circumstances that limit the generalizability of these findings. A report on 100 substance abusers who were interviewed at a youth drop-in counseling center revealed that 16% of the sample were found to suffer from double depression, i.e., a major depression superimposed on a dysthymic disorder (Kashani, Keller, Solomon, Reid, & Mazzola, 1985).

DeMilio (1989) administered a structured clinical interview to evaluate 57 adolescents consecutively admitted for treatment of substance abuse and other concurrent psychiatric disorders. Of those patients, 42% and 35% received a diagnosis of conduct disorder (CD) and major depressive disorder, respectively, according to DSM-III criteria.

The following reports compared the rates of psychopathology in consecutive admissions to inpatient units for adolescent substance abusers with other comorbid psychiatric disorders. The final diagnosis of each patient was made at least 2 weeks after admission and represents a consensus-discharge diagnosis; DSM-III-R diagnostic criteria were used for making the diagnosis in all cases. Kaminer (1991) studied 72 adolescents; 44% and 18% of this cohort were diagnosed with CD and mood disorders, respectively. Another 18% were diagnosed with adjustment disorders with an accompanying mood component, reflecting the difficulty of definitively diagnosing stress-related, short-term-oriented disorders. Begtrup (1989) studied 101 adolescents and reported 28% and 24% as manifesting CD and depressive disorder, respectively. Stowell (1991) reported that among 226 adolescents, 61% were diagnosed with mood disorders and 54% with CD. It is apparent from this report that a considerable percentage of this sample met criteria for a triple diagnosis (TD) of CD–mood disorder–PSUD. Begtrup (1989) and Kaminer (1991) noted 12% and 17%, respectively, of TD composed of the same specific triad reported by Stowell (1991).

Bukstein, Glancy, and Kaminer (1992) examined a sample of 156 inpatient adolescents with DD. CD was diagnosed in 62% and major depression in 30% of this cohort. The rate of TD was 38% and 18% in females vs. males, respectively.

The wide range in prevalence of psychopathology diagnosed in the reports reviewed in this section reflects possible treatment-seeking bias, different referral sources, and various diagnostic models. However, the figures cited underscore the needs of this population for an appropriate treatment for comorbid psychiatric diagnosis including PSUDs.

5.3. RELATIONSHIPS BETWEEN COMORBID DISORDERS

In order to assess the nature of the relationships between PSUDs and other comorbid disorders, it is important to rely on the sparse data available to support or negate the variety of hypotheses on the subject.

Meyer (1986) suggested a list of six possible paradigms:

1. Psychiatric symptoms or disorders developing as a consequence of substance abuse.
2. Psychiatric disorders altering the course of substance abuse.
3. Substance abuse developing as a consequence of psychopathology and dysfunction in the individuals and their families.
4. Substance abuse altering the course of psychiatric disorders.
5. Substance abuse and psychiatric disorders originating from a common vulnerability.
6. Psychiatric disorders and substance abuse being mutually exclusive but coincidentally manifested.

Because the etiology and pathophysiology of PSUDs and other psychiatric disorders are far from being clear, indirect methods such as biological-marker studies, follow-up and follow-back studies, and treatment-response studies are employed to establish the diagnostic validity of disorders. Additional important sources of such data are family and genetic studies (Penick et al., 1988). Since the late 1960s, there has been intensive research activity exploring the genetic and familial transmission of psychiatric disorders. Evidence gathered from adoption, twin, and family studies has suggested familial determinants of numerous conditions, most notably schizophrenia, mood disorders, and alcoholism.

The strongest evidence for a genetic component to substance abuse would come from twin and cross-fostering studies. The main difficulties in conducting such studies are generally low population rates of non-alcohol specific substance abuse and major cross-generational differences in availability of psychoactive substances (Rounsaville, Kosten, et al., 1991). In the absence of twin and cross-fostering studies, family studies represent a useful approach for low-prevalence disorders to identify those that are likely to be influenced by genetically transmitted vulnerabilities. The diagnostic limitations involved in obtaining reliable information from family members regarding PSUDs and other psychiatric disorders need to be considered.

Regardless of the controversy between the disease model and the self-medication model, recent family studies provide information that separating comorbid groups according to the primary–secondary paradigm is not the only way to establish association between comorbid disorders. A bidimensional model, separating individuals with alcohol or other PSUDs from those with comorbid diagnoses, may be more useful in predicting natural history and treatment outcome (Read, Penick, Powell, Nickel, Bingham, & Campbell, 1990). Furthermore, there are reports that focus on family factors related to preference to specific substances.

Many of the studies reviewed in this section were done with adult co-horts; however, they carry great importance for prevention among children and siblings of patients with PSUDs or with DD.

5.4. SPECIFIC SUBSTANCES OF CHOICE AND COMORBID PSYCHOPATHOLOGY

This self-medication theory of substance abuse suggests that individuals are predisposed to addiction because they suffer from painful affective states or related psychiatric disorders or both (Khantzian, 1985). Moreover, it has been hypothesized that specific expectations for the effects of use of psychoactive substances may lead to substance preference or avoidance.

Generalization of this concept to empirical research can be found in substance-specific family studies. Studies designed to explore for evidence of two or more familial transmitted subtypes of PSUDs with and without accompanying psychiatric disorders are reviewed in this section.

5.4.1. Alcohol

Findings from families of alcoholics suggest that two familial transmitted subtypes of alcoholism can be defined on the basis of the presence or absence of coexistent anxiety or depression or both (Merikangas, Leckman, Prusoff, Pauls, & Weissman, 1985). High rates of ASPD, depression, and alcoholism among relatives of alcoholics was not related to a common pathway of genetic transmission. It is probable that there is familial clustering of social risk factors that are related to the development of these disorders. This clustering of sociocultural factors would explain the frequently observed association of these disorders (Merikangas, Leckman, et al., 1985).

Strong associations were identified between offspring psychopathology and alcoholism in fathers, particularly among black families (Luthar, Merikangas, & Rounsaville, 1993).

In a review of the genetic and clinical implications of alcoholism and affective disorders, Schuckit (1985) estimated that 20–30% of adult alcoholics develop secondary affective disorder. In a clinical cohort of inpatient adolescents with PSUDs, secondary depressive disorder was more common than its primary form in a 3.5:1 ratio. Nonremission of the depression in the secondary-depression group within a 3-week period of abstinence was the rule rather than the exception (Bukstein et al., 1992). It was also concluded that utilizing the primary–secondary paradigm could not aid in showing differential prediction of a mood-disorder remission among adolescents with comorbid PSUDs, major depressive disorder (MDD), and in some cases also CD. In examining parental psychopathology, the same study revealed that secondary MDD did not appear to predict an increased number of parents with substance abuse. Keller, Lavori, Beardslee, Wunder, and Hasin (1992) speculated that the comorbidity of substance use disorders and affective disorders in adolescents and their parents may be a manifestation of a single illness. This study, which was reviewed in Section 5.2.3, draws its strength from a non-treatment-seeking cohort, although the sample was small. Mirin et al. (1991) found no significant differences in the rate of alcoholism between brothers and fathers of DUDI abusers of substances other than alcohol. However, mothers had a significantly higher prevalence rate of alcoholism than sisters, regardless of whether the proband was an alcoholic or not. They attributed these results to sex-related age of onset of alcoholism (Cloninger, 1987). A study among 424 college students that examined the cause–effect dilemma indicated that while anxiety appeared to antedate alcoholism, depression appeared to be a consequence of both heavy drinking and drug abuse (Deykin, Levy, & Wells, 1987).

5.4.2. Sedatives–Hypnotics

Many patients with a preference for sedatives–hypnotics meet criteria for anxiety and mood disorders (Mirin et al., 1991). Other studies show that abuse of benzodiazepines is relatively low among patients with anxiety disorders (Garvey & Tollefson, 1986). A recent study reported on a differential response to the benzodiazepine Alprazolam on the basis of the presence of a family history of alcoholism (Ciraulo, Barnhill, & Ciraulo, 1989). Another study investigating mental disorders among alcoholics focused on alcoholism typology and cerebrospinal fluid (CSF) neuropeptides (Roy et al., 1991). Elevation of CSF concentrations of diazepam-binding inhibitor and somatostatin in alcoholics with late onset compared to early onset was reported. It has been postulated that anxious personality traits, and the rapid development of tolerance and dependence on the antianxiety effects of alcohol, are associated with the diazepam-binding inhibitor, which has a role in the pathophysiological state of anxiety and depression. It is noteworthy that such a profile suits the description of the Type 1 alcoholism of Cloninger (1987).

In contrast, it has been shown by King, Curtis, and Knoblich (1992) that minor tranquilizers such as benzodiazepines act as antiaggression agents and may be the drugs of choice among aggressive polysubstance abusers characterized by low levels of phenylacetic acid, a metabolite of phenylethylamine. These findings suggest that further research is needed on the interaction between psychopathology and the use of and response to specific sedative–hypnotic substances in families of substance abusers, especially alcoholics.

5.4.3. Cocaine

The very few studies of the role of family psychiatric disorders in the vulnerability to different types of substance use disorders and to coexistent psychiatric disorders in different substance-specific abusing groups have not, as of now, generated conclusive data regarding cocaine. A very recent family study suggests that a higher incidence of drug abuse and alcoholism occurs among relatives of cocaine abusers than among those of opioid addicts (Luthar et al., 1993).

A study of 298 cocaine abusers seeking treatment reported a higher rate of a history of childhood attention deficit disorder, mania, and alcoholism compared with opioid addicts (Rounsaville, Anton, Carroll, Budde, Prusoff, & Gawin, 1991). Also, compared with opioid addicts, cocaine abusers had substantially lower rates of major depression and ASPD. Mirin et al. (1991) reported in their study of 120 cocaine addicts that about 40% had concurrent nondrug psychopathology, including patients with major depression, some of whom may have used cocaine in an attempt to self-medicate depressed affects. An interesting phenomenon regarding patients with bipolar/cyclothymic disorder is that few of these patients used cocaine primarily during periods of hypomania or mania. Their use of cocaine appears to be an effort to enhance an endogenously produced "high," not an effort to self-medicate.

King et al. (1992) suggested a cocaine–dopamine–histrionic triad as an expression of the reward-centered incentive–motivation system. Psychostimulants including cocaine enhance dopamine activity, and it has been hypothesized that histrionic personality traits may lead to preferring cocaine in order to increase low basal dopaminergic activity (Cloninger, 1987).

5.4.4. Opioids

The relationships between opioid abuse and comorbid psychiatric disorders generated great interest, especially with regard to anxiety and depressive symptomatology (e.g., acute vs. chronic effects, cause vs. effect). A high rate of affective disorders according to DSM-III criteria was diagnosed among opioid abusers (Mirin et al., 1991; Rounsaville, Weissman, Wilber, Crits-Christoph, & Kleber, 1982). These findings considered together with the results of the recent study by Luthar et al. (1993) suggest that the presence or absence of depression could be of value as a criterion in subtyping opiate addicts.

The one adoption study that has addressed determinants of drug abuse found a high rate of ASPD among substance abusers; however, the relevance of this work to opiate addiction is limited by the heterogenous nature of drug abuse and the low incidence of opiate addiction in that sample (Cadoret, Troughton, O'Gorman, & Heywood, 1986).

Rounsaville, Kosten, et al. (1991) studied a sample of 877 first-degree relatives of 201 opiate addicts with normal controls and came to the following conclusions: (1) Compared with relatives of normal subjects, opiate addicts' relatives had substantially higher rates of alcoholism, drug abuse, depression, and ASPD. (2) Relatives of depressed opiate-addicted probands had elevated rates of major depression and anxiety disorders, but not of other disorders, suggesting the validity of subtyping opiate addicts by the presence or absence of major depression. (3) In contrast, relatives of antisocial opiate addicts had rates of disorders that were not significantly different from those of relatives of opiate addicts without ASPD.

Age and sex had a significant influence on rates of disorders. Younger relatives and males had higher rates of drug abuse, ASPD, and alcoholism, while female subjects had higher rates of depression and anxiety disorders. Finally, this important study did not support the validity of a familially transmitted subtype of ASPD in opiate addicts in contrast to depression.

The vulnerability to substance abuse and psychopathology among siblings of opioid abusers was the focus of another important study by the Yale University group (Luthar, Anton, Merikangas, & Rounsaville, 1992). This study enrolled 476 siblings of 201 opioid abusers. The results gave the following indications: (1) The siblings had substantially higher rates of drug abuse, alcoholism, major depression, ASPD, and general anxiety as compared to rates in the community. (2) Rates of drug abuse and ASPD were higher among siblings than among parents; also, rates of major depression were higher among male siblings than among fathers, while alcoholism occurred more frequently among addicts' sisters than among mothers. (3) The presence of a major psychiatric disorder significantly increased the risk of developing substance abuse among siblings, although no specificity of transmission of comorbid disorders was indicated. (4) Psychopathology appeared to precede drug abuse in terms of age of onset in this group.

5.5. PSYCHIATRIC COMORBIDITY

After the preceding review of the comorbidity dilemma from the standpoint of the preferred substance of abuse, this section explores the subject from the orientation of psychiatric disorders. The following disorders are reviewed: mood disorder, anxiety disorders, dissociative disorders, CD–ASPD continuum (CD-ASPDC), attention deficit hyperactivity disorder (ADHD), eating disorders, cluster B of personality disorders (PDs), schizophrenia, and pathological gambling (PG) according to DSM-IV (American Psychiatric Association, 1994). As noted before, the relative scarcity of adolescent-oriented research is clear, and the literature on comorbidity in adults is utilized as appropriate in reviewing various disorders. DSM-III-R terminology is used unless studies that predate the DSM-III-R era are cited.

5.5.1. Mood Disorders

5.5.1.1. Unipolar Depressive Disorder

It has been established that maternal mood disorder and offspring depression are associated; similarly, there is evidence that as compared to controls, children of depressed parents show elevated rates of substance abuse (Luthar et al., 1993).

Familial aggregation of both major depression and alcoholism has been frequently noted and established by twin and cross-fostering studies. The clustering of depression, alcoholism, and ASPD within individuals and families has also been frequently observed (Merikangas, Leckman, et al., 1985). Despite this clustering, the independence of transmission of these disorders has been demonstrated in several studies (Merikangas, Weissman, Prusoff, Pauls, & Leckman, 1985). Specificity of transmission for depression and anxiety disorders in the children aged 6–17 of probands with these disorders has been reported (Weissman, Leckman, Merikangas, Gammon, & Prusoff, 1984).

Merikangas, Weissman, et al. (1985) utilized the primary–secondary paradigm in assessing psychiatric disorders of offspring of parents with primary depression and secondary alcoholism. This controlled study also compared children and adolescent offspring vs. adult offspring (the cutoff point was 18 years of age). The results of this study indicated that the rates of major depression, anxiety disorders, and ASPD are higher among offspring over the age of 18 of probands with depression alone than among offspring of controls. The rates of alcoholism were similar in the two groups, suggesting that the probands with depression only were no more likely to transmit alcoholism to their offspring than were the control probands. Similar results emerged for the offspring aged 6–17 (who were designated as manifesting CD rather than ASPD).

Offspring of the secondary alcoholics had a 3-fold greater risk of alcoholism than did offspring of controls and of probands with depression only, and a 5-fold and 20-fold greater risk of ASPD compared with offspring of probands with depression only and of controls, respectively. Risks of CD-ASPD were significantly increased among offspring of probands with depression alone and were further increased among offspring of secondary alcoholics. The CD-ASPDC and its association with PSUDs and other disorders is further discussed in Section 5.5.4.

Higher rates of alcoholism in the families of depressed women, but not in the families of depressed men, were reported by Winokur and Coryell (1991). This large controlled study sample of 723 directly interviewed adult relatives of 326 probands with primary unipolar depression is the first to report such findings. According to the authors, it is simply because other investigators (Merikangas, Weissman, et al., 1985; Weissman et al., 1984) did not separate their sample by gender. Regarding the sex distribution of severity and type of psychiatric disorders experienced by adolescents involved in substance use, it is suggested that the distribution is similar for males and females for anxiety as well as for depression (Boyle & Offord, 1991; Deykin et al., 1987).

The influence of alcoholism on the course of primary major depression was examined by Hirschfeld, Kosier, Keller, Lavori, and Endicott (1989). Contrary to expectations, during a 2-year period of follow-up, two groups of depressive patients with and without concurrent alcoholism did not differ in time to recovery or time to relapse into a subsequent major depression. Alcoholism was related in this study only to worse functioning in social relationships. On the other hand, a study of the effect of depression on alcoholism did not find characteristics of depression useful in predicting remission from alcoholism (Hasin, Endicott, & Keller, 1989). In another study of adult alcoholics, the severity of the accompanying depression was inversely correlated with the level of improvement of alcoholism, suggesting that severity and not hierarchy or chronology of the psychopathology is an important factor for course and treatment outcome of substance abuse (Rounsaville, Kosten, Weissman, & Kleber, 1986). Additional concurrent family problems exacerbated the outcome.

Finally, Dilsaver (1987) hypothesized an integrative model for affective disorders and substance abuse based on symptomatic overlap. He claimed that disturbances of mood and affect can be treated by prescribed medications or by substances of abuse and that they all interact with cholinergic and aminergic neurotransmitter systems. Self-medication of psychiatric symptoms may be the common denominator in explaining this model (Bukstein, Brent, & Kaminer, 1989).

5.5.1.2. Bipolar Disorder

The prevalence of bipolar disorder in the United States population is 1.1%; the percentage of adult patients with bipolar disorders in populations seeking treatment for substance abuse exceeds this prevalence in all nine studies reported to date. The range varies from 1.9% to 30.0% and is attributed to diagnostic criteria that include the bipolar spectrum disorders in less restrictive studies (Brady & Lydiard, 1992). Kaminer (1991) reported that 5 inpatients were diagnosed with a DSM-III-R consensus diagnosis of bipolar disorder among 72 consecutive admissions of DUDI adolescents (6.9% of the sample).

According to the ECA study, bipolar disorder had an odds ratio of 6.2 and 6.6 respectively, for co-occurrence with alcoholism (Helzer & Pryzbeck, 1988) and with drug or alcohol abuse (Regier et al., 1990). The rates of substance abuse among adult bipolar patients according to the studies reviewed by Brady and Lydiard (1992) vary between 21% and 58%.

The data concerning a family–genetic link between bipolar disorder and PSUDs are as yet inconclusive. A family study of bipolar patients revealed high rates of alcoholism (Helzer & Winokur, 1974). Other studies found no higher risk in these families than in families of control subjects (Dunner, Hensel, & Fieve, 1979; Morrison, 1974).

Cocaine appeared to be overrepresented among psychoactive substances preferred by patients with bipolar disorder. Mirin et al. (1991) found that 5.4% of opiate abusers, 6.8% of depressant abusers, and 17.5% of stimulant abusers met DSM-III-R criteria for bipolar spectrum disorder.

The course of bipolar disorder accompanied with alcohol or other substance of abuse is unclear due to different measures of remission of the mood disorder vs. that of the PSUD. There is a need to further clarify the relationship between bipolar disorder and PSUD with an additional special emphasis on offspring of patients with the bipolar-disorder spectrum with or without comorbid PSUD.

5.5.2. Anxiety Disorders

Studies of the magnitude of alcohol abuse among patients with anxiety disorders revealed a high prevalence of comorbidity (Bibb & Chambless, 1986; Smail, Stockwell, Canter, & Hodgson, 1984).

Another group of studies has also indicated a relatively high prevalence of anxiety disorders among alcoholics (Hesselbrock et al., 1985; Mullaney & Trippett, 1979). Schuckit (1985) reported that anxiety symptoms followed symptoms of alcoholism; other studies suggest the opposite (Hesselbrock et al., 1985) or consider these findings equivocal (Bibb & Chambless, 1986).

A review of the literature on the relationship between alcoholism and anxiety disorders in adults (Kushner, Sher, & Beitman, 1990) concluded that a majority of studies agree on the following conclusions: (1) In agoraphobia and social phobia, alcohol abuse appears more likely to be secondary to the anxiety disorder (i.e., in accord with the self-medication theory). (2) Panic disorder without agoraphobia and generalized anxiety disorder tend to follow alcohol abuse (i.e., in accord with the disease model). (3) Simple phobia does not appear to be related to alcohol abuse.

Hill, Steinhauer, Smith, and Locke (1991) studied children and adolescents of families with three generations of alcoholic adults and reported the results of comparing members of high- and low-risk groups for alcoholism. They found that children who were at high risk for developing alcoholism were 2.2 times as likely to have a psychiatric diagnosis, most likely an anxiety or phobic disorder.

Bradley and Hood (1993) studied 28 adolescents referred for the treatment of panic attacks. Of these subjects, 27 had at least one comorbid psychiatric disorder but no PSUD.

A high prevalence of panic attacks and panic-related disorders was reported among alcoholics (Pollard, Detrick, Flynn, & Frank, 1990), but comparable prevalence rates can be found in depressed patients as well. The relationship between anxiety and mood symptomatology/disorders and their association with PSUDs is intriguing. Studies of the clinical phenomenology and natural history of depressive syndromes suggest a close phenotypic relationship between symptoms of anxiety and depression in many patients, and indeed an anxious subgroup of depressed patients has been identified (Leckman, Weissman, Merikangas, Pauls, & Prusoff, 1983).

Pure panic disorder diagnosed at age 21 showed a strong tendency to develop into pure depression or mixed panic and depression at 7-year follow-up (Vollrath & Angst, 1989). Also, the natural history of anxiety disorders is frequently complicated with depression (Angst & Vollrath, 1991). Leckman et al. (1983) reported that depression plus panic disorder in probands was associated with a markedly increased incidence among relatives of any one or more of major depression, panic disorder, phobia, and alcoholism than in the relatives of probands with major depression only. In another family study, Weissman et al. (1984) found that the rate of substance abuse and agoraphobia among children of probands with depression and anxiety was higher than it was among children of either a control group or of the probands with depression only.

Merikangas, Leckman, et al. (1985) found an increased risk of anxiety disorders and depression in relatives of probands with alcoholism, which could be attributed specifically to the presence of alcoholism in addition to an anxiety disorder in the proband. This finding suggested that the alcoholism in these probands may result from self-medication of anxiety symptoms.

That some forms of anxiety disorders in childhood (such as separation anxiety disorder) as well as various adult anxiety disorders respond to treatment with antidepressants might be construed as suggesting a link between anxiety and depression disorders (Gittleman-Klein & Klein, 1973). It is noteworthy that the 10th revision of the *International Classification of Diseases* (ICD-10) contains an entity of anxiety–depression disorder. Except for the family studies described, no other studies involving adolescents have been reported to explore the comorbidity of anxiety disorders with PSUDs. Follow-up studies are warranted, especially with regard to the continuity between the anxiety disorders of childhood and adolescence and the anxiety or mood disorders, or both, of adulthood. Exploration of the relationship of anxiety and mood disorders of childhood and adolescence to PSUDs is needed.

5.5.3. Dissociative Disorders

Until recently, dissociative disorders were thought to be rare. There is increasing evidence that they are more common than once believed (Ross, 1991). Research on the relationship between dissociative disorders and PSUDs is sparse, although it has been suggested that PSUDs may conceal dissociative states. An increased interest in the psychological consequences of child physical and sexual abuse and posttraumatic stress disorder (PTSD) revealed that they co-occur with dissociative disorders (Saxe et al., 1993). A study of 100 adult subjects diagnosed as substance abusers concluded that 34% had a dissociative disorder and that 43% reported childhood abuse (Ross, Kronson, Koensgen, Barkman, Clark, & Rockman, 1992). It has been reported that two thirds of the patients with dissociative disorders also received a diagnosis of PSUD and also a DSM-III-R Axis II diagnosis of borderline personality disorder, a disorder that has a high prevalence of comorbid PSUD (Saxe et al., 1993). Another recent study of 265 male inpatient substance abusers revealed that 41% scored within the clinical range on a screening instrument for dissociative disorders (Dunn, Paolo, Ryan, & Van Fleet, 1993).

Further studies on the magnitude and nature of the comorbidity between dissociative disorders and PSUD are warranted, with special attention to minority groups and adolescents. Follow-up controlled studies of children and adolescents with PTSD are recommended to ensure proper methodology.

5.5.4. Conduct Disorder–Antisocial Personality Disorder Continuum

CD-ASPDC has long been strongly associated with PSUD. This disorder has the highest odds ratio of comorbidity with alcoholism: >21 according to the ECA study (Helzer & Pryzbeck, 1988). This association may be due, in part, to the fact that substance abuse is one of the diagnostic criteria for ASPD. Additionally, intoxication with various substances leads to behavioral disinhibition, thus lowering the threshold for antisocial behavior (Bukstein et al., 1989). Association between the use of illicit substances and violent behavior, and between alcohol use and homicide, suggests a direct causative relationship between substance use and antisocial behavior.

The relationship between ASPD and PSUD is complex and not yet fully understood. The nosological confusion regarding this relationship is being addressed in the early 1990s by reintroduction of the term "psychopathy." It has been suggested that the nosological entity of ASPD will be divided into two terms: a "true" psychopathy (a term characterized by lack of empathy, secondary gain-oriented behavior, and lack of remorse) and a "neurotic" psychopathy (Gerstley, Alterman, McLellan, & Woody, 1990). Such a differentiation will also favor a differential treatment response of behavioral–cognitive intervention in a structured setting for true psychopathy and medication and psychotherapy for neurotic psychopathy (Alterman & Cacciola, 1991).

To receive the diagnosis of ASPD according to DSM-III-R criteria, an individual must show antisocial behaviors before the age of 15 and must manifest 3 of a possible 12 antisocial behaviors. Indeed, CD is usually manifested at least 2–3 years before substance abuse is diagnosed. Even in subjects reporting very high rates of conduct symptoms, the ages of the first episode of drunkenness and of drug use were 12 and 14.5, respectively (Robins & McEvoy, 1990). In a prospective follow-up study, it was found that 23–55% of children with CD developed ASPD as adults (Robins & Ratcliff, 1979). However, follow-up of adolescents to adulthood showed that the prevalence of ASPD dropped, suggesting a maturation process (Mannuzza, Klein, Bessler, Malloy, & LaPadula, 1993).

The comorbidity and clinical course of children with CD were investigated in a cohort of 51 children diagnosed with disruptive behavior disorders (Keller, Lavori, Beardslee, Wunder, Schwartz, et al., 1992). These disorders include ADHD, CD, and oppositional defiant disorder (ODD) and may carry some or all of the following sequelae: poor psychopathological prognosis, legal difficulties, academic deficits, and abuse of alcohol or other substances or both. ODD is believed to be either an early manifestation or a mild form of CD. CD may also be a complication experienced by about 25% of children with ADHD (Klein & Mannuzza, 1991). The disruptive behavior disorder could at times pose a difficulty for interviewers to completely differentiate between the courses of the two disorders. Of the children studied by Keller, Lavori, Beardslee, Wunder, Schwartz, et al. (1992), 84% received at least one other psychiatric diagnosis and 39% received a diagnosis of DSM-III affective disorder. High rates of alcoholism and alcoholism with additional diagnosis of MDD were diagnosed among the patients.

Depressive and anxiety symptom clusters co-occur with CD-ASPDC far more than expected by chance in general population studies. Most females develop a depressive or anxiety disorder by early adulthood. For males with CD, the trend is opposite, with the highest prevalence of depression or anxiety disorder diagnosed in preadolescence and decreasing into adulthood (Zoccolillo, 1992). The study by Merikangas, Weissman, et al. (1985) was discussed in Section 5.5.1.1 with regard to secondary alcoholism with major depression in probands and the psychiatric disorders in their offspring. The risk of CD-ASPD was significantly increased among offspring of probands with depression alone and was further increased among offspring of secondary alcoholics. There was a highly significant linear change in the rate of alcoholism and CD-ASPD according to whether one or both parents were alcoholic. There was a 2-fold greater risk of alcoholism and a 3-fold greater risk of CD-ASPD among offspring when both parents were affected than when only one parent was affected. This specificity in the effects of assortative mating on children's behavior could be related to modeling of parental behavior, genetic factors, or both.

It has been hypothesized that a subtype of CD may be an early nonspecific manifestation of mood–anxiety disorders or alcoholism–substance abuse or both (Merikangas, Weissman, et al., 1985). The independence of alcoholism and ASPD on one hand and the suggested role of CD as a common underlying pathology on the other hand are important questions waiting to be pursued.

5.5.5. Attention-Deficit Hyperactivity Disorder

There has been frequent expectation for ADHD and PSUD to be associated with each other in the adult-oriented literature (Khantzian, Bean-Bayog, & Blumenthal, 1991). However, there are two conflictual approaches attempting to specify the nature of the relationship between ADHD and PSUDs (Kaminer, 1992). The adult-psychiatry-oriented approach emphasizes the direct path between ADHD and PSUDs based on a conceptual model of the self-medication theory and on a diagnostic model of retrospective studies (Achenbach, 1990). The other school is child- and adolescent-psychiatry-oriented, and it argues that only about one fourth of ADHD children who are at high risk for developing CD may develop PSUDs during the course of CD-ASPDC.

Longitudinal, prospective, controlled, and blind studies support the latter approach (Klein & Mannuzza, 1991; Mannuzza et al., 1993; Weiss, Hechtman, Milroy, & Perlman, 1985), as does a large-sample Canadian epidemiological study that posited that "ADHD is not related to PSUD in any meaningful way" (Boyle & Offord, 1991, p. 699). It is noteworthy that Szatmari, Boyle, and Offord (1989) also concluded that children with ADDH and CD appear to represent a true hybrid disorder rather than one diagnosis or the other. This hybrid is what the British literature termed "hyperkinetic conduct disorder" (Werry, 1992). Biderman, Newcorn, and Sprich (1991) studied comorbidity of ADHD with other disorders such as CD, major depression, and anxiety disorders and concluded that subtyping of these children might be delineated on the basis of the co-occurring disorder. In conclusion, ADHD plus CD may be a distinct subtype.

A prospective long-term follow-up study, with blind systematic clinical assessments, investigated the psychiatric status of 91 white males. This was a 13-year evaluation of subjects who were diagnosed with DSM-II hyperkinetic reaction of childhood (an equivalent of the present ADHD) before 1975 (Mannuzza et al., 1993). Probands had significantly higher rates than the control group of ADHD symptoms (11% vs. 1%), ASPD (18% vs. 2%), and drug abuse disorders (16% vs. 4%). Significant comorbidity occurred between antisocial and drug disorders. In fact, 59% of subjects with CD progressed to PSUD.

Childhood ADHD predicted antisocial and drug abuse disorders if at least one of the primary symptoms of ADHD (attentional difficulty, impulsivity, and hyperactivity) had been retained into adulthood. In contrast, probands without symptoms in adolescence and early adulthood did not differ significantly from controls in the rates of antisocial and substance use disorders. Self-medication by cocaine of adults diagnosed with attention deficit disorder–residual type (ADD-RT) according to DSM-III criteria was not substantiated. The simplistic relationship between ADHD and PSUDs should be viewed in a critical fashion, and it is noteworthy that there is a considerable risk in identifying future drug abusers on the basis of early behavior problems (Kaminer, 1992).

Future research efforts are essential to improve diagnostic procedures and classification among children and adolescents with ADHD and comorbid psychiatric disorders and of adults diagnosed with ADD-RT or ADHD, with special emphasis on differentiating age-appropriate symptoms from the full syndrome, and lifetime diagnosis of ADHD versus residual ADHD (Caroll & Rounsaville, 1993). Such research is important in order to avoid merely creating a mirror image of the childhood clinical picture of this disorder in adults. Also, it is imperative to develop prevention–intervention techniques for children with ADHD alone or with a comorbid CD.

5.5.6. Personality Disorders—Cluster B

Cluster B of DSM-III-R personality disorders includes ASPD, borderline PD, histrionic PD, and narcissistic PD. It is not expected to diagnose PD before the patient reaches 18 years of age. The rationale behind this rule is that adolescence is an age of emotional–psychological growth and repair and diagnosis of PD might therefore be premature and merely define a temporary state. This argument may not hold, for more than strict nosological reasons. It is evident that characteristics or profiles of specific personality disorder(s) are recognizable early in adolescence. Furthermore, continuity from adolescence to adulthood has been predicted, although not yet validated.

Borderline PD is characterized by a pervasive pattern of instability of mood, interpersonal relationships, and self-image. Impulsiveness that is potentially self-damaging, chronic emptiness, and boredom are common. Substance abuse is extremely common in borderline PD, with reported prevalences ranging from 11% to 69% (Dulit, Fyer, Haas, Sullivan, & Frances, 1990). However, the criteria for substance use disorders in these studies were generally not well defined. Kaminer (1991) reported that 11% of adolescents admitted to an inpatient unit for DUDI adolescents received a DSM-III-R diagnosis of borderline PD. Dulit et al. (1990) reported that when substance abuse was not used as a diagnostic criterion, 23% of the cohort no longer met DSM-III borderline PD criteria. These data suggest that there might be a subgroup of borderline patients for whom substance use plays a primary role in the development of psychopathology. Borderline patients were reported to prefer sedative–hypnotics or alcohol and to suffer from a concurrent major depression at higher rates than those with other PDs (Mirin & Weiss, 1991). The tendency of borderline patients to exhibit serious self-injurious behavior, bulimia, and suicidal behavior increases the chance that a psychoactive substance will be used for self-destructive behavior or accidental overdose. Such events can take place following an impulsive reaction to mood changes, perception of rejection, or boredom.

Other PDs from cluster B also appear to be represented among substance abusers; however, they have been researched less than ASPD and borderline PD. More than one disorder from cluster B may be diagnosed concomitantly. Also, PDs from other clusters may be associated with PSUD, although this relationship has not been researched as yet.

It is timely to refer here to the commonly used term "addictive personality." Although there is no data base to support this definition, personality traits and disorders as discussed in this chapter do influence risk-taking.

It is noteworthy that the incentive–motivation system in the brain has been postulated to be neuromodulated by the neurotransmitter dopamine. It has also been hypothesized that histrionic personality and individuals with ASPD may crave excitement, including psychoactive substance use, due to a low basal dopaminergic activity (Cloninger, 1987).

The role of PD in the development of PSUDs and vice versa awaits further study, especially among adolescents and young adults.

5.5.7. Schizophrenia

No studies on the comorbidity of PSUD and schizophrenia among adolescents have yet been reported. Schizophrenia was second only to mania in its association with alcoholism in the ECA study (Helzer & Pryzbeck, 1988). Between 25% and 50% of schizophrenic patients use psychoactive substances during their lifetimes. However, clinical experience suggests that adult patients diagnosed with schizophrenia tend to refrain from use of hallucinogens and stimulants, which may exacerbate psychotic symptomatology.

5.5.8. Eating Disorders

An accumulating body of data suggests a high prevalence of PSUDs in patients with eating disorders as well as among first-degree relatives.

A high incidence of substance abuse can be found among bulimic patients compared to those with restrictive anorexia nervosa, with rates ranging from 6% to 31% (Hatsukami, Mitchell, Eckert, & Pyle, 1986). Bulimic patients were reported to have a high prevalence of comorbid affective disorders, between 35% and 88%, and family studies concluded that at least one first-degree relative received the DSM-III diagnosis of an affective disorder (Hatsukami et al., 1986).

Eating disorders are more prevalent among females. Bulik (1987) suggested that this phenomenon represents an alternative expression for behaviors that are culturally restrictive for women, such as aggressive behavior and addiction. Biopsychosocial factors are responsible for shaping the individual's anorexic or bulimic behavior and neurophysiological adaptation. The personal experience of reduction of tension and anxiety, the feeling of loss of control, and the accompanying changes of mood after binge eating were compared to intoxication. Bulimic or anorexic behavior is then continued to maintain a dependency rather than to get high (Bukstein et al., 1989). Bulimia nervosa is associated with alcohol abuse among female high school students (Timmerman, Wells, & Chen,1990). Abuse of diuretics, laxatives, and diet pills is common among patients with eating disorders. Bulik (1992) reviewed 10 studies examining drugs commonly abused with eating disorders. Even cocaine was reported to be used for the purpose of dieting, on the basis of information from the National Cocaine Hotline (Jonas, Gold, Sweeney, & Pottash, 1987). However, it is important to understand the purpose of using medications or drugs in the "service" of the disorder as compared to abuse of a psychoactive substance. Anorexia nervosa (AN) is uncommon among adults with PSUD. Also, AN is a rare disorder among males. However, the rate of the disorder among male body builders who had used anabolic steroids was reported to be more than ten times more prevalent than among nonuser controls (Pope, Katz, & Hudson, 1993). In addition, a rare syndrome termed "reverse anorexia" was described in male anabolic steroid users. This disorder of body image is characterized by the belief that a person appears small and weak even though he is actually large and muscular.

It is safe to conclude that eating disorders are not common among patients with PSUDs, although PSUD is common among bulimic patients. Continued studies of individuals and families regarding the aforementioned comorbidity are important.

5.5.9. Pathological Gambling

The criteria for PG disorder in DSM-IV are almost identical to those for the substance-related disorders category (American Psychiatric

Association, 1994). These criteria show that the problem is similar to other forms of addiction. A family study indicated that 50% of children of pathological gamblers were pathological gamblers themselves (Lesieur & Heineman, 1988). Evidence is mounting that PG overlaps with other addictions, especially PSUDs, and presents a difficulty for treatment. Multiple addictions in the family of the gambler put the offspring of a gambling parent or parents at a risk identical to that of children of alcoholics or substance abusers. Increased stress, deception of spouse, fiscal and legal problems, and high rate of divorce characterize such a family.

Very little research on PG among adolescents has been reported. However, 57% of students in a southern New Jersey sample showed clear signs of pathological gambling. Of these gamblers, 32% gambled at least once a week during the past year and 86% gambled in the past year (Lesieur & Klein, 1987).

Further research is warranted to explore the magnitude of PG among adolescents. Also, it is imperative to clarify the relationship between PG, PSUDs, and other psychiatric disorders in the adolescent and among family members.

5.6. CLINICAL AND RESEARCH IMPLICATIONS

There is growing recognition that the population of substance abusers is not a unitary, homogeneous one. The pursuit of knowledge concerning the nosology, magnitude, and nature of DD in various DUDI subpopulations has critical implications for the advancement of prevention and treatment strategies.

Given the high rates of psychiatric disorders among adults with PSUDs, it is likely that their offspring are at high risk for PSUDs and other psychiatric disorders. Also, siblings of adolescents with PSUDs or other psychopathology or both constitute high-risk groups. Continued research on the relationship and course of PSUDs and other psychiatric disorders and the development of prevention and treatment approaches in these families are urgent priorities for the health system.

The relationship between the most prevalent comorbid psychiatric disorders (i.e., mood disorders, CD-ASPDC) and APSUDs should be thoroughly researched. Special emphasis on gender differences is imperative due to changes in secular trends. An intriguing new phenomenon that has not been explored is the emergence of adolescent female gangs. The members of these groups typically abuse drugs and are involved in aggressive–violent behaviors toward both sexes.

In terms of policy implications, it should be noted that more than

45% of the estimated 31 million Americans with no health insurance coverage (1987 figures) are 24 years old or younger (Burke et al., 1991). The need to ensure adequate services and access to these programs is imperative and must include services for DUDI adolescents.

Increased awareness and recognition of DD and improved diagnostic assessment and treatment skills of clinicians should be emphasized in medical and health teaching and training facilities.

REFERENCES

Achenbach, T. M. (1990). Comorbidity in child and adolescent psychiatry: Categorical and quantitative perspectives. *Journal of Child and Adolescent Psychopharmacology, 1,* 271–278.

Alterman, A. I., & Cacciola, J. S. (1991). The antisocial personality disorder diagnosis in substance abusers: Problems and issues. *Journal of Nervous and Mental Disease, 179,* 401–409.

American Psychiatric Association (1994). *Diagnostic and Statistical Manual of Mental Disorders,* 4th ed. Washington, DC: American Psychiatric Association.

Anderson, J. C., Williams, S., McGee, R., & Silva, P. A. (1987). DSM-III disorders in preadolescent children. *Archives of General Psychiatry, 44,* 69–76.

Angst, J., & Vollrath, M. (1991). The natural history of anxiety disorders. *Acta Psychiatrica Scandinavica, 84,* 446–452.

Begtrup, R. O. (1989). Dual diagnosis in adolescents: Co-existing substance abuse disorders and other psychiatric illnesses. Presented at East Tennessee State University Grand Rounds, August.

Berkson, J. (1946). Limitations of the application of four fold table analysis to hospital data. *Biometry Bulletin, 2,* 47–53.

Bibb, J. L., & Chambless, D. L. (1986). Alcohol use and abuse among diagnosed agoraphobics. *Behavior Research Therapy, 24,* 49–58.

Biderman, J., Newcorn, J., & Sprich, S. (1991). Comorbidity of attention deficit hyperactivity disorder with conduct, depressive, anxiety, and other disorders. *American Journal of Psychiatry, 148,* 564–577.

Boyle, M. H., & Offord, D. R. (1991). Psychiatric disorder and substance use in adolescence. *Canadian Journal of Psychiatry, 36,* 699–705.

Bradley, S. J., & Hood, J. (1993). Psychiatrically referred adolescents with panic attacks: Presenting symptoms, stressors, and comorbidity. *Journal of the American Academy of Child and Adolescent Psychiatry, 32,* 826–829.

Brady, K. T., & Lydiard, R. B. (1992). Bipolar affective disorder and substance abuse. *Journal of Clinical Psychopharmacology, 12,* 17S–22S.

Brandenburg, N. A., Friedman, R. M., & Silver, S. E. (1990). The epidemiology of childhood psychiatric disorders: Prevalence findings from recent studies. *Journal of the American Academy of Child and Adolescent Psychiatry, 29,* 76–83.

Braucht, G. N., Brakarsch, D., Follingstad, D., & Berry, K. L. (1973). Deviant drug use in adolescence: A review of psychological correlates. *Psychology Bulletin, 79,* 92–106.

Bryant, K. J., Rounsaville, B., Spitzer, R. L., & Williams, J. (1992). Reliability of dual diagnosis, substance dependence and psychiatric disorders. *Journal of Nervous and Mental Disease, 180,* 251–257.

Bukstein, O. G., Brent, D. A., & Kaminer, Y. (1989). Comorbidity of substance abuse and other psychiatric disorders in adolescents. *American Journal of Psychiatry, 146,* 1131–1141.

Bukstein, O. G., Glancy, L. J., & Kaminer, Y. (1992). Patterns of affective comorbidity in a clinical population of dually-diagnosed adolescent substance abusers. *Journal of the American Academy of Child and Adolescent Psychiatry, 31,* 1041–1045.

Bulik, C. M. (1987). Drug and alcohol abuse by bulimic women and their families. *American Journal of Psychiatry, 144,* 1604–1606.

Bulik, C. M. (1992). Abuse of drugs associated with eating disorders. *Journal of Substance Abuse, 4,* 69–90.

Burke, K. C., Burke, J. D., Rae, D. S., & Regier, D. A. (1991). Comparing age at onset of major depression and other psychiatric disorders by birth cohorts in five U.S. community populations. *Archives of General Psychiatry, 48,* 789–795.

Cadoret, R. J., Troughton, E., O'Gorman, T. W., & Heywood, E. (1986). An adoption study of genetic and environmental factors in drug abuse. *Archives of General Psychiatry, 43,* 1131–1136.

Caroll, K. M., & Rounsaville, B. J. (1993). History and significance of childhood attention deficit disorders in treatment-seeking cocaine abusers. *Comprehensive Psychiatry, 34,* 75–82.

Caron, C., & Rutter, M. (1991). Comorbidity in child psychopathology: Concepts, issues, and research strategies. *Journal of Child Psychology and Psychiatry, 132,* 1063–1080.

Christie, K. A., Burke, J. D., Regier, D. A., Rae, D. S., Boyd, J. H., & Locke, B. Z. (1988). Epidemiologic evidence for early onset of mental disorders and higher risk of drug abuse in young adults. *American Journal of Psychiatry, 145,* 971–975.

Ciraulo, D. A., Barnhill, J. G., & Ciraulo, A. M. (1989). Parental alcoholism as a risk factor in benzodiazepine abuse: A pilot study. *American Journal of Psychiatry, 146,* 1333–1335.

Cloninger, D. R. (1987). Neurogenetic adaptive mechanisms in alcoholism. *Science, 236,* 410–416.

DeMilio, L. (1989). Psychiatric syndromes in adolescent substance abusers. *American Journal of Psychiatry, 146,* 1212–1214.

Deykin, E. Y., Levy, J. C., & Wells, V. (1987). Adolescent depression, alcohol and drug abuse. *American Journal of Public Health, 77,* 178–182.

Dilsaver, S. C. (1987). The psychopathologies of substance abuse and affective disorders: An integrative model. *Journal of Clinical Psychopharmacology, 7,* 1–10.

Dulit, R. A., Fyer, M. R., Haas, G. L., Sullivan, T., & Frances, A. J. (1990). Substance use in borderline personality disorder. *American Journal of Psychiatry, 147,* 1002–1007.

Dunn, G. E., Paolo, A. M., Ryan, J. J., & Van Fleet, J. (1993). Dissociative symptoms in a substance abuse population. *American Journal of Psychiatry, 150,* 1043–1047.

Dunner, D. L., Hensel, B. M., & Fieve, R. R. (1979). Bipolar illness: Factors in drinking behavior. *American Journal of Psychiatry, 136,* 583–585.

Feinstein, A. R. (1970). The pre-therapeutic classification of comorbidity in chronic disease. *Journal of Chronic Disease, 23,* 455–468.

Garvey, M. J., & Tollefson, G. D. (1986). Prevalence of misuse of prescribed benzodiazepines in patients with primary anxiety disorder or major depression. *American Journal of Psychiatry, 143,* 1601–1603.

Gerstley, L. J., Alterman, A. I., McLellan, A. T., & Woody, G. E. (1990). Antisocial personality disorder in patients with substance abuse disorders: A problematic diagnosis. *American Journal of Psychiatry, 147,* 173–178.

Gittleman-Klein, R., & Klein, D. F. (1973). School phobia diagnostic considerations in the light of imipramine effects. *Journal of Nervous and Mental Disease, 156,* 199–215.

Hasin, D. S., Endicott, J. E., & Keller, M. B. (1989). RDC alcoholism in patients with major affective syndromes: 2-Year course. *American Journal of Psychiatry, 146,* 318–328.

Hatsukami, D., Mitchell, J. E., Eckert, E. D., & Pyle, R. (1986). Characteristics of patients with bulimia only, bulimia with affective disorders, and bulimia with substance abuse problems. *Addictive Behaviors, 11,* 399–406.

Helzer, J. E., & Pryzbeck, T. R. (1988). The co-occurrence of alcoholism with other psychiatric disorders in the general population and its impact on treatment. *Journal of Studies on Alcohol, 49,* 219–224.

Helzer, J. E., & Winokur G. (1974). A family interview study of male manic depressives. *Archives of General Psychiatry, 31,* 73–77.

Hesselbrock, M. N., Meyer, R. E., & Keener, J. J. (1985). Psychopathology in hospitalized alcoholics. *Archives of General Psychiatry, 42,* 1050–1055.

Hill, S. Y., Steinhauer, S. R., Smith, T. R., & Locke, J. (1991). Risk markers for alcoholism in high density families. *Journal of Substance Abuse, 3,* 351–369.

Hirschfeld, R., Kosier, T., Keller, M. B., Lavori, P. W., & Endicott, J. (1989). The influence of alcoholism on the course of depression. *Journal of Affective Disorders, 16,* 151–158.

Jonas, J. M., Gold, M. S., Sweeney, D., & Pottash, A. (1987). Eating disorders and cocaine abuse: A survey of 259 cocaine abusers. *Journal of Clinical Psychiatry, 48,* 47–50.

Kaminer, Y. (1991). The magnitude of concurrent psychiatric disorders in hospitalized substance abusing adolescents. *Child Psychiatry and Human Development, 22,* 89–95.

Kaminer, Y. (1992). Clinical implications of the relationship between attention deficit hyperactivity disorder and psychoactive substance use disorders. *The American Journal on Addictions, 1,* 257–264.

Kashani, J. H., Keller, M. B., Solomon, N., Reid, J. C., & Mazzola, D. (1985). Double depression in adolescent substance abuse. *Journal of Affective Disorders, 8,* 153–157.

Keller, M. B., Lavori, P. W., Beardslee, W., Wunder, J., & Hasin, D. (1992). The clinical course and outcome of substance abuse disorders in adolescents. *Journal of Substance Abuse Treatment, 9,* 9–14.

Keller, M. B., Lavori, P. W., Beardslee, W. R., Wunder, J., Schwartz, C. E., Roth, J., & Biederman, J. (1992). The disruptive behavioral disorder in children and adolescents: Comorbidity and clinical course. *Journal of the American Academy of Child and Adolescent Psychiatry, 31,* 204–209.

Khantzian, E. J. (1985). The self-medication hypothesis of addictive disorders: Focus on heroin and cocaine dependence. *American Journal of Psychiatry, 142,* 1259–1264.

Khantzian, E. J., Bean-Bayog, M., & Blumenthal, S. (1991). Substance abuse disorders: A psychiatric priority. *American Journal of Psychiatry, 148,* 1291–1300.

Khantzian, E. J., & Treece, C. (1985). DSM-III psychiatric diagnosis in narcotic addicts: Recent findings. *Archives of General Psychiatry, 42,* 1067–1077.

King, R., Curtis, D., & Knoblich, G. (1992). Biological factors in sociopathy: Relationships to drug abuse behaviors. In M. Glantz & R. Pickens (Eds.), *Vulnerability to Drug Abuse* (pp. 115–135). Washington, DC: American Psychological Association.

Klein, R. G., & Mannuzza, S. (1991). Accuracy of retrospective self-reports of childhood separation anxiety and ADHD. Presented at the American Academy of Child and Adolescent Psychiatry Annual Meeting, San Francisco.

Kosten, T. A., & Rounsaville, B. J. (1992). Sensitivity of psychiatric diagnosis based on the best estimate procedure. *American Journal of Psychiatry, 149,* 1225–1227.

Kushner, M. G., Sher, K. J., & Beitman, B. D. (1990). The relation between alcohol problems and the anxiety disorders. *American Journal of Psychiatry, 147,* 685–695.

Lavik, N. J., & Onstad, S. (1987). Drug use and psychiatric symptoms in adolescents. *Acta Psychiatrica Scandinavica, 73,* 437–440.

Leckman, J. F., Weissman, M. M., Merikangas, K. R., Pauls, D. L., & Prusoff, B. A. (1983). Panic disorder and major depression. *Archives of General Psychiatry, 40,* 1055–1060.

Lesieur, H. R., & Heineman, M. (1988). Pathological gambling among youthful multiple substance abusers in a therapeutic community. *British Journal of Addiction, 83,* 765–771.

Lesieur, H. R., & Klein, R. (1987). Pathological gambling among high school students. *Addictive Behaviors, 12,* 129–145.

Luthar, S. S., Anton, S. F., Merikangas, K. R., & Rounsaville, B. J. (1992). Vulnerability to substance abuse and psychopathology among siblings of opioid abusers. *Journal of Nervous and Mental Disease, 180,* 153–161.

Luthar, S. S., Merikangas, K. R., & Rounsaville, B. J. (1993). Parental psychopathology and disorders in offspring: A study of relatives of drug abusers. *Journal of Nervous and Mental Disease, 181,* 351–357.

Mannuzza, S., Klein, R. G., Bessler, A., Malloy, P., & LaPadula, M. (1993). Adult outcome of hyperactive boys. *Archives of General Psychiatry, 50,* 565–576.

McAree, C. P., Steffenhagen, R. A., & Zhentlen, L. S. (1972). Personality factors and patterns of drug usage in college students. *American Journal of Psychiatry, 128,* 890–893.

Merikangas, K. R., Leckman, J. F., Prusoff, B. A., Pauls, D. L., & Weissman, M. M. (1985). Familial transmission of depression and alcoholism. *Archives of General Psychiatry, 42,* 367–372.

Merikangas, K. R., Weissman, M. M., Prusoff, B. A., Pauls, D. L., & Leckman, J. F. (1985). Deppressives with secondary alcoholism: Psychiatric disorders in offspring. *Journal of Studies on Alcohol, 46,* 199–204.

Meyer, R. E. (1986). *Psychopathology and Addictive Disorders.* New York: Guilford Press.

Mirin, S. M., & Weiss, R. D. (1991). Substance abuse and mental illness. In R. J. Frances & S. I. Miller (Eds.), *Clinical Textbook of Addictive Disorders* (pp. 271–298). New York: Guilford Press.

Mirin, S. M., Weiss, R. D., Griffin, M. L., & Michael, J. L. (1991). Psychopathology in drug abusers and their families. *Comprehensive Psychiatry, 32,* 36–51.

Morrison, J. R. (1974). Bipolar affective disorder and alcoholism. *American Journal of Psychiatry, 131,* 1130–1133.

Mullaney, J. A., & Trippett, C. J. (1979). Alcohol dependence and phobias: Clinical description and relevance. *British Journal of Psychiatry, 135,* 656–673.

Paton, S., Kessler, R., & Kandel, D. (1977). Depressive mood and adolescent illicit drug use: A longitudinal analysis. *Journal of General Psychology, 131,* 267–289.

Penick, E. C., Powell, B. J., Liskow, B. I., Jackson, J. O., & Nickel, E. J. (1988). The stability of coexisting psychiatric syndromes in alcoholic men after 1 year. *Journal of Studies on Alcohol, 49,* 395–405.

Pollard, C. A., Detrick, P., Flynn, T., & Frank, M. (1990). Panic attacks and related disorders in alcohol dependent, depressed and nonclinical samples. *Journal of Nervous and Mental Disease, 178,* 180–185.

Pope, H. G., Katz, D. L., & Hudson, J. I. (1993). Anorexia nervosa and reverse anorexia among 108 male body builders. *Comprehensive Psychiatry, 34,* 406–409.

Read, M. R., Penick, E. C., Powell, B., Nickel, E. J., Bingham, S. F., & Campbell, J. (1990). Subtyping male alcoholics by family history of alcohol abuse and co-occurring psychiatric disorders: A bi-dimensional model. *British Journal of Addiction, 85,* 367–378.

Regier, D. A., Boyd, J. H., Burke, J. D., Rae, D. S., Myers, J. K., Kramer, M., Robins, L. N., George, L. K., Karno, M., & Locke, B. Z. (1988). One-month prevalence of mental disorders in the U.S. based on five epidemiologic catchment sites. *Archives of General Psychiatry, 45,* 977–986.

Regier, D. A., Farmer, M. E., Rae, D. S., Locke, B. Z., Keith, S. J., Judd, L. L., & Goodwin, F. K. (1990). Comorbidity of mental disorders with alcohol and other drug abuse: Results from the Epidemiologic Catchment Area (ECA) study. *Journal of the American Medical Association, 264,* 2511–2518.

Reichler, B. D., Clemente, J. L., & Dunner, D. L. (1983). Chart review of alcohol problems in adolescent psychiatric patients in an emergency room. *Journal of Clinical Psychiatry, 44,* 338–339.

Robins, L. N., & McEvoy, L. (1990). Conduct problems as predictors of substance abuse. In L. N. Robins & M. Rutter (Eds.), *Straight and Devious Pathways from Childhood to Adulthood* (pp. 182–204). Cambridge, England: Cambridge University Press.

Robins, L. N., & Ratcliff, K. S. (1979). Risk factors in the continuation of childhood antisocial behavior into adulthood. *International Journal of Mental Health, 7,* 96–111.

Roerich, H., & Gold, M. S. (1986). Diagnosis of substance abuse in an adolescent psychiatric population. *International Journal of Psychiatric Medicine, 16,* 137–143.

Ross, C. A. (1991). Epidemiology of multiple personality disorder and dissociation. *Psychiatric Clinics of North America, 14,* 503–517.

Ross, C. A., Kronson, J., Koensgen, S., Barkman, K., Clark, P., & Rockman, G. (1992). Dissociative comorbidity in 100 chemically dependent patients. *Hospital and Community Psychiatry, 48,* 860–862.

Ross, H. E., Glaser, F. B., & Germanson, T. (1988). The prevalence of psychiatric disorders in patients with alcohol and other drug problems. *Archives of General Psychiatry, 45,* 1023–1031.

Rounsaville, B. J., Kosten, T. R., Weissman, M. M., & Kleber, H. D. (1986). Prognostic significance of psychiatric disorders in treated opiate addicts. *Archives of General Psychiatry, 43,* 739–745.

Rounsaville, B. J., Kosten, T. R., Weissman M. M., Prusoff, B., Pauls, D., Anton, S. F., & Merikangas, K. (1991). Psychiatric disorders in relatives of probands with opiate addiction. *Archives of General Psychiatry, 48,* 33–42.

Rounsaville, B. J., & Kleber, H. D. (1986). Psychiatric disorders in opiate addicts: Preliminary findings on the course and interaction with program type. In R. E. Meyer (Ed.), *Psychopathology and Addictive Disorders* (pp. 140–168). New York: Guilford Press.

Rounsaville, B. J., Anton, S. F., Carroll, K., Budde, D., Prusoff, B., & Gawin, F. (1991). Psychiatric diagnoses of treatment-seeking cocaine abusers. *Archives of General Psychiatry, 48,* 43–51.

Rounsaville, B. J., Weissman, M. M. Wilber, C. A., Crits-Cristoph, K., & Kleber, H. D. (1982). Diagnosis and symptoms of depression in opiate addicts: Course and relationship to treatment outcome. *Archives of General Psychiatry, 39,* 151–156.

Roy, A., DeJong, J., Lamparski, D., Adinoff, B., George, T., Moore, V., Garnett, D., Kerisch, M., & Linnoila, M. (1991). Mental disorders among alcoholics. *Archives of General Psychiatry, 48,* 423–427.

Saxe, G. N., Van der Kolk, B. A., Berkowitz, R., Chinman, G., Hall, K., Lieberg, G., & Schwartz, J. (1993). Dissociative disorders in psychiatric inpatients. *American Journal of Psychiatry, 150,* 1037–1042.

Schuckit, M. A. (1985). The clinical implications of primary diagnostic groups among alcoholics. *Archives of General Psychiatry, 42,* 1043–1044.

Smail, P., Stockwell, T., Canter, S., & Hodgson, R. (1984). Alcohol dependence and phobic states I: A prevalence study. *British Journal of Psychiatry, 144,* 53–57.

Stowell, R. J. (1991). Dual diagnosis issues. *Psychiatric Annals, 21,* 98–104.

Szatmari, P., Boyle, M., & Offord, D. R. (1989). ADDH and conduct disorder: Degree of diagnostic overlap and differences among correlates. *Journal of the American Academy of Child and Adolescent Psychiatry, 28,* 865–872.

Timmerman, B. A., Wells, L. A., & Chen, S. (1990). Bulimia nervosa and associated alcohol abuse among secondary school students. *Journal of the American Academy of Child and Adolescent Psychiatry, 29,* 118–122.

Vener, A. M., Stewart, C. S., & Hager, D. L. (1972). Depression and the adolescent in middle America. Paper presented at the 67th annual meeting of the American Sociological Association in New Orleans, LA.

Vollrath, M., & Angst, J. (1989). Outcome of panic and depression in a seven-year follow-up: Results of the Zurich study. *Acta Psychiatrica Scandinavica, 80,* 591–596.

Weiss, G., Hechtman, L., Milroy, T., & Perlman, L. (1985). Psychiatric status of hyperactives as adults: A controlled prospective 15-year follow up of 63 hyperactive children. *Journal of the American Academy of Child Psychiatry, 24,* 211–220.

Weiss, R. D., Griffin, M. C., & Mirin, S. M. (1989). Diagnosing major depression in cocaine abusers: The use of depression rating scales. *Psychiatry Research, 28,* 335–343.

Weissman, M. M., Leckman, J. F., Merikangas, K. R., Gammon, G. D., & Prusoff, B. A. (1984). Depression and anxiety disorders in parents and children: Results from the Yale family study. *Archives of General Psychiatry, 41,* 845–852.

Werry, J. S. (1992). Child psychiatric disorders: Are they classifiable? *British Journal of Psychiatry, 161,* 472–480.

Winokur, G., & Coryell, W. (1991). Familial alcoholism in primary unipolar major depressive disorder. *American Journal of Psychiatry, 148,* 184–188.

Zoccolillo, M. (1992). Co-occurrence of conduct disorders and its outcomes with depressive and anxiety disorders: A review. *Journal of the American Academy of Child and Adolescent Psychiatry, 31,* 547–556.

Adolescent Substance Use and Adolescent Psychoactive Substance Use Disorders: Relation to Suicidal Behavior

The leading external causes of adolescent morbidity and mortality are motor vehicle accidents, homicide, and suicide, in declining order. Adolescent psychoactive substance use disorders (APSUDs) and unprotected sex leading to teenage pregnancies, abortions, and communicable diseases including acquired immunodeficiency syndrome (AIDS) are also major problems of epidemic proportion. In the United States, homicide represents the second-leading cause of death, accounting for 11.7 deaths/100,000 in the 15- to 19-year age group. However, among black adolescent males, homicide is the leading cause of death (Bearinger & Blum, 1987). Substance abuse, availability of arms, social stressors, low socioeconomic status, and increased interpersonal violence contribute to the problem.

This chapter primarily reviews the association between APSUDs and suicidal behavior. Additional high-risk behaviors/activities that are presumed to be associated with PSUDs and suicide, such as the occult—particularly satanism and music preferences—are also illuminated.

6.1. SUICIDAL BEHAVIOR

Many studies have reported an elevated risk ratio for suicidal behavior in adults diagnosed with PSUDs (Galanter & Castaneda, 1985; Goodwin, 1979; Miles, 1977; Roy & Linnoila, 1986). The sparsity of literature on the relationship between suicidal behavior and adolescent substance use (ASU) or APSUDs causes concern for the following reasons:

1. Suicide rates for the 15- to 24-year age group have almost tripled since the late 1950s, and suicide is now the second leading cause of death for this age group (Holinger, 1987).
2. Adolescents display the highest involvement with psychoactive substances.
3. Concomitant psychopathologies, especially conduct and mood disorders, have been identified as risk factors for adolescent suicide and are frequently diagnosed in adolescents with PSUDs (Bukstein, Brent, & Kaminer, 1989).

Retrospective studies and psychological autopsy investigations of adolescent suicides provide most of the data about the relationship between suicidal behavior and APSUDs, although methodological constraints limit the generalization of conclusions derived from such studies (Shafii, Steltz-Lenarsky, Derrick, Beckner, & Whittinghill, 1988; Tunvig, 1988).

This section assesses the nosology and epidemiology of suicidal behavior, examines the nature of the association between APSUDs and suicidal behavior, and discusses clinical and research implications.

6.1.1. Nosology and Epidemiology

The association between suicidal behavior and PSUDs has been hypothesized and studied since the dawn of modern psychiatry. Menninger (1938) formulated addiction as a protracted form of chronic suicide. This conception of self-destructive behavior is represented almost 50 years later in the DSM-III-R criteria for PSUD, which require the continued use of a psychoactive substance despite the individual's knowledge of the deleterious effects of the substance on functioning in various life domains.

Suicidal behavior comprises a spectrum ranging from suicidal ideas and suicidal threats to suicidal attempts and completed suicides (Kaminer, 1992). Suicidal ideation is a common phenomenon among adolescents and college students, with a lifetime prevalence between 54% and 62% (Garland & Zigler, 1993). It is of great importance to specify which behavior within the suicidal behavior spectrum is being studied.

The rate of suicide among 15- to 19-year-olds increased from 5.2/100,000 in 1970 to 9.0/100,000 in 1984 (Centers for Disease Control, 1986) and to 11.3/100,000 in 1988 (National Center for Health Statistics, 1968–1991). The age group of 15–24 years displayed a suicide rate of 12.5/100,000 per year (Holinger, 1987). Between 6% and 13% of adolescents have reported at least one suicide attempt in their lives (Shaffer, 1988). Among completed suicides, males outnumber females by 4:1; among suicide attempters, the ratio is inverted (Levy & Deykin, 1989). In reviewing 12 studies of gender distribution among adult alcohol suicides, it was reported that men outnumbered women by 10:1 (Roy & Linnoila, 1986). It is estimated that suicidal behavior is underreported; however, attempted suicides by adolescents with PSUDs range from 11% to 23% (Kaminer, 1992). There are differences in suicide rates and suicide reports among various races, religions, and ethnic groups, mainly because of religious implications, concerns for the family, and other factors. Hispanics and African Americans traditionally have had a lower suicide rate than whites, but the gap has been narrowing. Native Americans have the highest suicide rate of any ethnic group in the United States. Perhaps the high incidence of ASU and APSUDs among this group may help explain the recent upward trend in overall adolescent suicide rates (Marzuk, Tardiff, Leon, Stagic, Morgan, & Mann, 1992).

6.1.2 Range between Suicidal Ideations and Attempts

An excellent study by Levy and Deykin (1989) examined the occurrence of suicidal ideations, suicide attempts, major depression, and substance abuse in a sample of 424 apparently healthy college students 16–19 years old. The data from this study indicate a high rate of suicidal thoughts experienced by more than a quarter of the cohort at one time or another in their lives. The authors concluded that these findings highlight both the lack of specificity of such thoughts as predictors of more serious behavior and their transitory nature. Students with a DSM-III diagnosis of substance abuse had a higher risk of suicidal ideation or behavior than did students without this diagnosis. A diagnosis of substance abuse was also associated with a prolonged desire to be dead (a factor considered to be a more specific risk factor for a suicide attempt), thus elevating the risk among this group compared to non-substance-abusers (Levy & Deykin, 1989). It is noteworthy that APSUD has not only been related to seriousness of suicide attempts as measured by the desire to be dead but also has been associated with medical seriousness and lethality of suicide attempts (Brent, 1987; Robbins & Alessi, 1985).

6.1.3. Completed Suicides

For every adolescent suicide, there are between 20 and 200 attempts, compared to an adult ratio of 1:6 (Shaffer, 1988). Yet the data regarding the association of attempted and completed suicides and AP-SUDs are limited. Benson and Holmberg (1984) reported in a Scandinavian prospective study that after 10-year follow-up of 9th grade students, the rate of suicide was higher among substance abusers than among non-substance-abusers. Hoberman and Garfinkel (1988) concluded that of 229 adolescent suicides, 13% were alcohol abusers and 15% were substance abusers. In a Canadian study of 190 adolescent suicides, 33% were diagnosed with alcohol abuse and 17% were diagnosed with substance abuse (Thompson, 1987). The San Diego suicide study concluded that substance abuse is the most important single factor contributing to the increase in suicide rates among youths in the United States (Rich, Young, & Fowler, 1986). A psychological postmortem study reported that 70% of adolescent suicides were drug or alcohol abusers (Shafii et al., 1988), and Sturner (1986) found that at least 15 of 70 adolescent suicides had a history of substance abuse.

The wide range of results cited (from 13% to 70%) points to the differences between the methods used to establish a diagnosis of PSUD. Sturner (1986) and Rich et al. (1986) utilized information obtained from extensive toxicological techniques. Other studies relied on data received from psychological autopsies. It is important to illuminate problems associated with data generated by psychological autopsies: (1) The information obtained is often incomplete, and (2) bias may be introduced when the examiner knows that the patient committed suicide (Shafii et al., 1988). A common problem in retrospective studies such as most of the reports noted in this section is the inclusion of subjects whose suicide occurred several years before their charts were reviewed or other methods of data collection were utilized. This delay raises the possibility of relying on incomplete data and potential cohort differences.

6.1.4. Specificity of Substance of Abuse

Studies indicate that there are different opinions regarding the relationship between type of substance abused and likelihood of suicidal behavior. In a clinical and demographic study of 413 adults hospitalized for suicide attempts, only a diagnosis of alcoholism predicted eventual suicide (Beck & Steer, 1989). The risk of alcoholics eventually committing suicide was over 5 times greater than that of nonalcoholics. Cocaine use may play a role in youth suicide either because of concomitant depression or personality disorder, or because psychostimulants may enhance suicide risk directly by changing brain neurochemistry, or because of both factors (Marzuk et al., 1992). In a report of 33 adolescents 11–20 years old who completed suicide, 7 (21%) had used cocaine prior to death. Hispanics were 3.3 times and African Americans were 1.9 times more likely to have used cocaine before suicide than whites. Both cocaine and alcohol had been used in 12% of the cases (Marzuk et al., 1992). Multiple substance abuse was the norm among youth suicides (Fowler, Rich, & Young, 1986; Rydelius, 1984; Sturner, 1986). Schwartz, Comerci, and Meeks (1987) reported that 21% of 107 adolescent LSD users revealed that they or a close friend had been involved in an accident or had made a serious suicide attempt while under the influence of LSD. Tunvig (1988) suggested that suicide was not related to any specific substance of abuse. It appears that the data on this issue are not yet conclusive.

6.1.5. Suicidal Behavior and Other Variables

Other variables that affect investigation of the relationship between APSUDs and suicidal behavior include suicide methods, parental substance use, family dysfunction, duration of PSUD, and history of treatment for PSUD or for dual diagnosis (DD).

There is growing evidence that adolescents with PSUDs are more likely to commit suicide with firearms than are nonabusers; this tendency is especially prominent among males (Brent, Perper, & Allman, 1987; Marzuk et al., 1992). Females prefer ingestion or overdose of drugs. Firearm-related suicide among African-American teenage males aged 15 to 19 doubled from 1982 to 1987. The rate for white males was nearly twice as high. This is not surprising following reports that firearms caused more than 36,000 deaths among Americans in 1990, including about 19,000 suicides and 16,000 homicides (McGinnis & Foege, 1993). Comparison data indicate that firearm-related suicide and homicide rates for young males in the United States are many times greater than the rates in other industrialized nations (e.g., homicide rates 12 to 273 times greater).

Parental substance abuse has not been found to be associated with offspring suicide among adolescents with PSUDs; however, further research on this issue and other parental factors is warranted (McKenry, Tishler, & Kelley, 1983; Murphy & Wetzel, 1982). A recent study on suicidality in girls predicted that the risk for suicidal behavior increases with family dysfunction that is also associated with alcohol abuse (King, Hill, Naylor, Evans, & Shain, 1993).

The history of APSUDs before suicides of young adults was studied by Fowler et al. (1986). They reported that substance abuse was typically present for at least 9 years before suicide was committed. Tunvig (1988) reported that chronicity of substance abuse increased the suicide rate among adolescents.

Treatment history appears to be of prominent importance. Adult substance abusers who have not sought treatment were reported to be at special risk for suicide (Hasin, Grant, & Endicott, 1988). Fowler et al. (1986) reported that lack of accessibility to mental health facilities among young substance abusers may have had an impact on their suicide rate.

6.1.6. Role of Psychiatric Comorbidity

Recent publications have emphasized the importance of investigating suicide in a growing number of adolescents with no apparent psychopathology (Apter et al., 1993; Brent, Perper, Moritz, Baugher, & Allman, 1993). However, psychiatric comorbidity accompanies PSUDs in a majority of adolescent suicides. Mood disorders, especially major depressive disorder (MDD), are the most frequently diagnosed disorders among adolescents manifesting suicidal behavior. Crumley (1990) reported that the majority of suicide victims (82%) had a primary mood disorder. In a recent study of psychiatric risk factors for adolescent suicide, Brent, Perper, Moritz, Allman, et al. (1993) reported the following results: The most significant disorders according to a declining odds ratio (OR) were major depression (OR = 27), bipolar mixed state (OR = 9), substance abuse (OR = 8.5), and conduct disorder (OR = 6). Substance abuse combined with mood disorder carried twice the risk factor of substance abuse alone (OR = 17), a finding consistent with the report by Shafii et al. (1988). These findings support the DD concept (Deykin, Buka, & Zeena, 1992). However, in a study by Levy and Deykin (1989), about half the adolescents who admitted having made a suicide attempt did not meet diagnostic criteria for major depression at any time in their lives. These authors suggest that the strong association found in psychiatric samples could be partly explained by Berkson's fallacy (Berkson, 1946). Levy and Deykin (1989) also concluded that MDD and substance abuse were independent albeit interactive risk factors for suicidal ideations and for suicide attempts. King et al. (1993) reported that depression severity has been associated with personal thoughts about suicide or self-reported suicidal ideations; however, depression severity was not related to the severity of clinician-documented suicidal behavior.

A high level of measured hopelessness is a common finding among depressed individuals. The role of hopelessness in predicting suicide by attempters is equivocal; however, an association between feelings of hopelessness and subsequent suicide attempts among adults has been found (Beck, Steer, Kovacs, & Garrison, 1985). Carlson and Cantwell (1982) reported similar findings among children and adolescents. In a more recent study, Beck and Steer (1989) reported that application of a hopelessness scale was not useful as a predictive instrument for suicide among alcoholic adults.

Impulsive rather than planned suicides by adolescents have been reported in large numbers (Shaffer, 1988). Many adolescents manifest suicidal behavior shortly after an acute crisis such as perceived rejection or interpersonal conflict; an acute disciplinary act; sexual assault, especially for females; or immediate loss. It has been suggested that intoxication for the purpose of self-medication, which often follows a crisis, may trigger suicide in an adolescent who feels shame, humiliation, or frustration. There is an ongoing debate whether homosexuality in adolescence is a risk factor for suicide (Garland & Zigler, 1993).

Conduct disorder (CD), antisocial personality disorder (ASPD), and borderline personality disorder have long been associated with PSUDs. These disorders are characterized by a tendency toward life-threatening and impulsive or aggressive acts or both.

The relationship between suicide, aggression, and alcoholism was supported by the report that Type 2 alcoholics were 4 times more likely to have attempted suicide than were Type 1 alcoholics (Buydens-Branchey, Branchey, & Noumair, 1989). Low levels of the neurotransmitter serotonin in alcoholism, depression, suicide, and aggression have been hypothesized as the biological etiological correlate of these disorders/behaviors (Coccaro, 1989). An additional specific link between violent behavior and suicide in adolescents was demonstrated by a study in which a substantial number of suicide victims had significant homicidal ideation with a homicidal plan within a week of their death (Brent, Perper, Moritz, Allman, et al., 1993).

Other comorbid psychiatric disorders have not yet been reported to be related to suicidal behavior among adolescents with PSUDs. However, there are increasing data about suicide attempts in adults suffering from panic disorder with and without comorbid PSUDs (Lepine, Chignon, & Teherani, 1993; Weissman, Klerman, Markowitz, & Ouellette, 1989).

The question of whether adolescents diagnosed with panic disorder and other anxiety disorders may have increased vulnerability to suicidal behavior merits further study. Finally, Brent, Perper, Moritz, Allman, et al. (1993) reported the association of overanxious disorder and suicide as increased but almost always in the context of MDD.

6.1.7. Relationship between Suicidal Behavior, Intoxication, Overdosing, and the Single-Car Accident

For any age group, intoxication often precedes suicide attempts. In a study of 197 adolescent suicides, 46% had detectable blood alcohol levels, yet many of these individuals were not diagnosed as substance abusers or substance dependent (Brent et al., 1987). Patel, Roy, and Wilson (1972) studied 352 admissions of adolescents who attempted suicide; 41% of the boys and 19% of the girls had been drinking immediately before they made the attempt.

It has been suggested that adolescents may use psychoactive substances, especially alcohol, as a means of bolstering their courage to carry out a suicide attempt (Patel et al., 1972). Another common explanation ties intoxication either to impaired judgment or to a decrease in inhibitions that may lead to impulsive, self-destructive acts. No systematic research has substantiated these speculations.

The interplay between suicidal behavior and psychoactive substance overdose (OD) is intriguing. Parker (1981) compared low-intent with high-intent overdosing adolescents. He found that the low-intent group perceived overdosing as similar to "getting drunk" and viewed it almost exclusively as an escape from tension. The high-intent group perceived overdosing and suicide in quite similar terms. Tunvig (1988) reported a high rate of OD fatalities among adolescents with PSUDs. It is generally accepted that the so-called "accidental" and intentional OD of psychoactive substances with or without other pharmacological agents accounts for the majority of unsuccessful suicide attempts, mainly among females. Victims of completed suicide usually tend to use more violent means such as firearms and often get intoxicated before the act.

About half of all teenage traffic accident fatalities involve an intoxicated adolescent driver (Bearinger & Blum, 1987). There are conflicting reports regarding the dilemma as to whether some road accidents resulting in death are disguised suicides, especially those involving a lone intoxicated driver in a single-car accident (Jenkins & Salisbury, 1980). The main difficulty in these cases lies in ascertaining the suicide intent. Anecdotal information and clinical reports elicited from patients suggest that such an interpretation is occasionally valid.

6.2. MUSIC PREFERENCE AND SATANISM

The relationship between the increasing rates of APSUDs and suicidal behavior during the last 30 years has been well established (Rich et al., 1986). Also, the late 1960s and the early 1970s saw the emergence of interest in the occult and cults including satanism. Related literature emerged, such as *The Satanic Bible* (Lavey, 1969) and *The Satanic Rituals* (Lavey, 1972). Part of midstream pop music also went through various mutations that led to the birth of alternative (psychedelic and underground) music, which was followed by the development of heavy metal music. The relationship between these phenomena (satanism, heavy metal music) and behaviors/disorders (suicidal behavior, APSUDs) has received widespread attention following highly publicized homicides and suicides, as reviewed by King (1988). This discovery led to the implication of heavy metal music and interest in the occult as contributing factors. On the other hand, some critics claim that these phenomena are being inappropriately blamed for the failure of American society to provide its high-risk youth with resources, alternatives, and guidance that will limit the development of deviant behaviors and problematic life-styles.

6.2.1. Music Preference

There are at present about 20 different definitions and "buzzwords" for popular music streams ("New Buzzwords," 1993). Some of them have quickly become widespread through massive exposure on music television (MTV), others are played on specific radio stations such as college networks, and some single or few streams are particularly identified with certain subcultures, with only minimal overlapping.

The 1990s have recycled 1970s alternative music and thrust it into the mainstream through vast exposure. Heavy metal and thrash music are related streams that originated in the late 1960s in England and then invaded the United States and the rest of the world. This music is characterized by high-volume fast guitar riffs and a thundering percussion section. Themes such as violence, female sexual abuse, and satanic worshipping have been common. Profane and offensive lyrics have upset parents and educators and have contributed to the increased appeal of this music, particularly among white adolescent males. Two heavy metal acts, Judas Priest and Ozzy Osbourne, were sued by parents of adolescents who committed suicide while listening to songs of these bands that contain lyrics related to hopelessness and suicide. The cases were dismissed.

Only two studies have been reported on the possible link between music preference and substance abuse in hospitalized adolescents (King, 1988; Weidinger & Demi, 1991). They suggested that significantly higher percentages of disturbed or drug-abusing adolescents prefer heavy metal music.

A recent study on a community population of adolescents examined the relationship between suicidal behavior and music preference (Martin, Clarke, & Pearce, 1993). A marked gender bias was shown to exist, with 74% of girls preferring pop music compared with 70.7% of boys preferring rock or heavy metal music. Feeling sadder after listening to any type of preferred music appeared to distinguish the most disturbed group, which was more vulnerable to suicidal thoughts and actions. Also, girls' preference for rock or heavy metal music was linked with a history of more suicidal behavior, depression, and delinquency and more difficult family background as compared with the majority of females, who indicated no interest in this category of music (Martin et al., 1993).

With regard to the message of the music, the cohort admitted that heavy metal music contains messages of violence, substance abuse, death, and satanism and few messages about love, happiness, and the environment. However, only 33% agreed with the predominant message.

Since 1985, there have been public efforts in the United States to deal with music that is perceived as offensive and that promotes violence at large and especially against women and policemen. The Parents' Music Resource Center is an example of an organization that was formed to educate and put pressure on record companies to be more selective about lyrics of songs and to rate music according to its potential harmfulness for youngsters. The critics view the acts of this center as censorship and as a violation of the First Amendment. King (1988, p. 301) expressed a view that has been shared at some national conferences on drug abuse that "heavy metal music represents a public health problem."

6.2.2. Satanism in Adolescence

The word "Satan" is derived from the Hebrew word for adversary and first appears in the Old Testament. This was translated to the Greek as "diabolos" ("accuser"), which is the origin of the English word "devil" (Nurcombe & Unutzer, 1991). In Christianity, the devil developed into the supernatural enemy of God and mankind. Satan demands sacrifices in order to increase his powers and satanic worshipers frequently offer human and animal blood and flesh, pain, and sexual rituals. A detailed history of satanism can be found in *The Black Arts* by Cavendish (1967).

There is formal satanic church worship in the United States, as exemplified by the Church of Satan and the Temple of Set. They have a formal membership and distribute newsletters (Nurcombe & Unutzer, 1991). These churches have considerable influence on adolescent "dabblers." Adolescents have always been curious about the dark side of religion, culture, and cults. It is commonly accepted that a superficial interest in mysticism, magic, witchcraft, and satanism is a developmental phase of adolescence (Russell, 1988). Adolescents typically rely on relevant available books, play heavy metal and thrash music, display occult jewelry, wear black clothing and makeup, or have tattoos of popular satanic signs, such as the pentagram, 666, upside-down cross, and the like. However, they do not join in any organized activity, rituals of animal sacrifice, or a formal group.

There have been several disturbing reports in the media about adolescents who were involved in ritualistic animal mutilations or sacrifices or who broke into graveyards and violated graves. There has been at least one detailed case study of ritualistic child abuse in the medical literature (Nurcombe & Unutzer, 1991). This case study, a report by Gould (1987), and a review of 36 cases of sexual abuse in which investigators detected bizzare ritualistic elements (Finkelhor, Williams, Burns, & Kalinowski, 1988) are in contrast to a 1989 report of the FBI stating that "serious satanic cult crimes were entirely unsubstantiated" (Komrad, 1992, p. 55). Komrad (1992) suggests that they are most probably cases of multigenerational abuse, especially of females, in families with ASPDs and criminal activity, or, as in the first known description of an adult survivor who as a child and/or an adolescent was victimized physically and/or sexually in Satanic rituals, it is a case of multiple personality disorder (Smith & Pazder, 1980).

A review and discussion of cults is beyond the scope of this section; the interested reader is referred to Galanter (1989). Briefly, however, a satanic group may organize in a charismatic cult format. Adolescents who join cults may be sucked into deeper involvement and may find it difficult to get out. Galanter (1990, p. 543) explained that cults operate according to the model of a charismatic group, characterized by

> a high level of cohesiveness, an intensely held belief system, and a profound influence on its members' behavior. It is charismatic because of the commitment of the member to a . . . transcendent goal as frequently articulated by a charismatic leader or ascribed to the progenitor of the group.

Although most cults renounce the use of psychoactive substances, cult leaders may be users or abusers, and in the name of cult leadership they may victimize other members, particularly young or female victims.

Multiple cases of homicides, suicides, sexual abuse, and other antisocial activity were reported in two well-known cults led by Jim Jones in Guiana in 1979 and David Koresh in Texas in 1993.

In my clinical experience, I have seen sporadic cases, and received first-hand reports, of a small number of adolescents who had participated in ceremonies of sacrificing animals or drinking their blood or both. Most of these youngsters were loners, unhappy with their family life, reported powerlessness and low self-esteem, and were frequently engaged in daydreaming and fantasies about the death of other people. Satanism had strong appeal to these adolescents as an escape and as a soothing experience (Wheeler, Wood, & Hatch, 1988). A more sophisticated minority of adolescents practicing satanism were charismatic individuals who were diagnosed with ASPD and PSUD that followed CD of childhood. They were leaders in their class or among their peers and enjoyed the fear reported by adults and peers with regard to satanism. They gained power and thrived on the excitement of satanic activity and the satisfaction generated by their ability to recruit other adolescents who, in order to belong to the group, had to fulfill such missions as stealing small pets and providing alcohol for ceremonies.

In summary, the small number of cases of adolescents expected to arrive for diagnosis and treatment following alleged satanic activity should go through assessment for psychopathology and family dysfunction. Secrecy and denial should be expected. However, the same therapeutic approach as that for the assessment of any deviant behavior/problem is applicable. It is recommended that the therapist be knowledgeable concerning satanic symbols and rituals. Nurcombe and Unutzer (1991) suggest that even though the evidence of ritual abuse is sketchy, a high index of suspicion is appropriate.

6.3. CONCLUSION

There is an unfortunate mental and conceptual gap that precludes adults from acknowledging and accepting adolescent behaviors in the context of normal adolescent development. Behaviors such as adolescent substance use, early sexual experimentation, risky driving, musical preference, and even an occasional interest in the occult are components of the adolescent life-style. Jessor (1991, p. 600) defined a life-style as "an organized pattern of interrelated behaviors" and emphasized the expressiveness and function of the concept.

A behavior should be considered risky when it can compromise physical health and psychosocial aspects of successful adolescent development. PSUDs, unprotected sex, violent behavior, driving while intoxicated, school dropout, and immersion in the occult are some obvious examples.

The clinical utility of life-style as a useful concept is measured by its focus on the adolescent as a whole rather than on each potentially risky behavior.

PSUD is a high-risk factor for suicidal behavior. An adolescent male who is likely to be intoxicated and to have access to a firearm is at the highest risk for suicide. An additional diagnosis of conduct disorder, mood disorder, or personality disorder, and lack of intervention by a mental health professional, especially after a precipitating stressful event, previous suicide attempts, and homicidal ideations, add to the risk. Although there has been a clear association between depression and suicidal behavior among adolescents (Pfeffer, 1986), the clinician should exercise caution in assuming that suicide risk declines significantly following an adolescent's response to treatment for depressive symptomatology. The existence of other high-risk factors such as substance abuse and other environmental factors is still a threat.

It is difficult to predict who will commit suicide, even among high-risk adolescents. However, decreased availability of firearms and treatment of PSUD and other accompanying psychopathology are important.

Research on adolescents with PSUDs and the suicidal behavior spectrum is particularly valuable when the methodological design is solid, the studies provide a longitudinal perspective, and a random double-blind design is utilized. Finally, biological factors and markers should be explored in these adolescents and first-degree relatives. Only comprehensive and sound research will be able to provide us with extended understanding of the subject.

Adolescent suicide prevention is discussed in conjunction with PSUD prevention in Chapter 9.

REFERENCES

Apter, A., Bleich, A., King, R. A., Kron, S., Fluch, A., Kotler, M., & Cohen, D. J. (1993). Death without warning? A clinical postmortem study of suicide in 43 Israeli adolescent males. *Archives of General Psychiatry, 50,* 138–143.

Bearinger, L., & Blum, R. W. (1987). Adolescent medicine and psychiatry: Trends, issues and needs. *Psychiatric Annals, 17,* 775–779.

Beck, A. T., & Steer, R. A. (1989). Clinical predictors of eventual suicide: A 5-to-10-year prospective study of suicide attempters. *Journal of Affective Disorders, 17,* 203–209.

Beck, A. T., Steer, R. A., Kovacs, M., & Garrison, B. (1985). Hopelessness and eventual suicide: A 10 year prospective study of patients hospitalized with suicidal ideation. *American Journal of Psychiatry, 142,* 559–563.

Benson, G., & Holmberg, M. B. (1984). Drug-related mortality in young people. *Acta Psychiatrica Scandinavica, 70*, 525–534.

Berkson, J. (1946). Limitations of the application of fourfold table analysis to hospital data. *Biomedical Bulletin, 2*, 47–53.

Brent, D. A. (1987). Correlates of the medical lethality of suicide attempts in children and adolescents. *Journal of the American Academy of Child and Adolescent Psychiatry, 26*, 87–89.

Brent, D. A., Perper, J. A., & Allman, C. J. (1987). Alcohol, firearms and suicide among youth. *Journal of the American Medical Association, 257*, 3369–3372.

Brent, D. A., Perper, J., Moritz, G., Allman, C., Friend, A., Roth, C., Schweers, J., Balach, L., & Baugher, M. (1993). Psychiatric risk factors for adolescent suicide: A case–control study. *Journal of the American Academy of Child and Adolescent Psychiatry, 32*, 521–529.

Brent, D. A., Perper, J., Moritz, G., Baugher, M., & Allman, C. (1993). Suicide in adolescents with no apparent psychopathology. *Journal of the American Academy of Child and Adolescent Psychiatry, 32*, 494–500.

Bukstein, O. G., Brent, D. A., & Kaminer, Y. (1989). Comorbidity of substance abuse and other psychiatric disorders in adolescents. *American Journal of Psychiatry, 146*, 1131–1141.

Buydens-Branchey, L., Branchey, M. H., & Noumair, D. (1989). Age of alcoholism onset: Relationship to psychopathology. *Archives of General Psychiatry, 46*, 225–230.

Carlson, G. A., & Cantwell, D. P. (1982). Suicidal behavior and depression in children and adolescents. *Journal of the American Academy of Child Psychiatry, 21*, 361–368.

Cavendish, Y. (1967). *The Black Arts*. New York: Putnam.

Centers for Disease Control (1986). *Youth Suicide in the United States, 1970–1980*. Atlanta: Centers for Disease Control.

Coccaro, E. F. (1989). Central serotonin and impulsive aggression. *British Journal of Psychiatry, 155*, 52–62.

Crumley, F. E. (1990). Substance abuse and adolescent suicidal behavior. *Journal of the American Medical Association, 263*, 3051–3056.

Deykin, E. Y., Buka, S. L., & Zeena, T. H. (1992). Depressive illness among chemically dependent adolescents. *American Journal of Psychiatry, 149*, 1341–1347.

Finkelhor, D., Williams, L. M., Burns, N., & Kalinowski, M. (1988). *Sexual Abuse in Daycare: A National Study Final Report:* Durham, NH: University of New Hampshire.

Fowler, R. C., Rich, C. L., & Young, D. (1986). San Diego suicide study II: Substance abuse in young cases. *Archives of General Psychiatry, 43*, 962–965.

Galanter, M. (1989). *Cults: Faith, Healing, and Coercion*. New York: Oxford University Press.

Galanter, M. (1990). Cults and zealous self-help movements: A psychiatric perspective. *American Journal of Psychiatry, 147*, 543–551.

Galanter, M., & Castaneda, R. (1985). Self-destructive behavior in the substance abuser. *Psychiatric Clinics of North America, 8*, 251–261.

Garland, A. F., & Zigler, E. (1993). Adolescent suicide prevention: Current research and social policy implications. *American Psychologist, 48*, 169–182.

Goodwin, D. W. (1979). Alcoholism and heredity: A review and hypothesis. *Archives of General Psychiatry, 36*, 57–61.

Gould, C. (1987). Satanic ritual abuse: Child victims, adult survivors, system response. *California Psychologist, 1*, 1–5.

Hasin, D., Grant, B., & Endicott, J. (1988). Treated and untreated suicide attempts in substance abuse patients. *Journal of Nervous and Mental Disease, 176*, 289–294.

Hoberman, H. M., & Garfinkel, B. D. (1988). Completed suicide in youth. *Canadian Journal of Psychiatry, 33*, 494–502.

Holinger, P. D. (1987). *Violent Deaths in the US: An Epidemiological Study of Suicide, Homicide, and Accidents.* New York: Guilford Press.

Jenkins, J., & Salisbury, P. (1980). Single car road deaths—disguised suicides? *British Medical Journal, 281,* 1041.

Jessor, R. (1991). Risk behavior in adolescence: A psychosocial framework for understanding and action. *Journal of Adolescent Health, 12,* 597–605.

Kaminer, Y. (1992). Psychoactive substance abuse and dependence as a risk factor in adolescent attempted and completed suicide. *The American Journal on Addictions, 1,* 21–29.

King, C. A., Hill, E. M., Naylor, M., Evans, T., & Shain, B. (1993). Alcohol consumption in relation to other predictors of suicidality among adolescent inpatient girls. *Journal of the American Academy of Child and Adolescent Psychiatry, 32,* 82–88.

King, P. (1988). Heavy metal music and drug abuse in adolescents. *Postgraduate Medicine, 83,* 295–304.

Komrad, M. S. (1992). Should we believe patients' claims of satanic cult abuse? *Psychiatric Times, April,* 54–55.

Lavey, A. (1969). *The Satanic Bible.* New York: Avon.

Lavey, A. (1972). *The Satanic Rituals.* New York: Avon.

Lepine, J. P., Chignon, J. M., & Teherani, M. (1993). Suicide attempts in patients with panic disorders. *Archives of General Psychiatry, 50,* 144–149.

Levy, J. C., & Deykin, E. Y. (1989). Suicidality, depression, and substance abuse in adolescence. *American Journal of Psychiatry, 146,* 1462–1467.

Martin, G., Clarke, M., & Pearce, C. (1993). Adolescent suicide: Music preference as an indicator of vulnerability. *Journal of the American Academy of Child and Adolescent Psychiatry, 32,* 530–535.

Marzuk, P. M., Tardiff, K., Leon, A. C., Stagic, M., Morgan, E. R., & Mann, J. J. (1992). Prevalence of cocaine use among residents of New York City who committed suicide during a one-year period. *American Journal of Psychiatry, 149,* 371–375.

McGinnis, J. M., & Foege, W. H. (1993). Actual causes of death in the United States. *Journal of the American Medical Association, 270,* 2207–2212.

McKenry, P. C., Tishler, C. L., & Kelley, C. (1983). The role of drugs in adolescent suicide attempts. *Suicide and Life Threatening Behaviors, 13,* 166–175.

Menninger, K. (1938). *Man Against Himself.* New York: Harcourt Brace Jovanovich.

Miles, C. P. (1977). Conditions predisposing to suicide: A review. *Journal of Nervous and Mental Disease, 164,* 231–246.

Murphy, G. E., & Wetzel, R. D. (1982). Family history of suicidal behavior among suicide attempters. *Journal of Nervous and Mental Disease, 170,* 86–90.

National Center for Health Statistics (1968–1991). *Vital Statistics of the U.S.,* Vol. 2, *Mortality—Part A* (for the years 1966–1988). Washington, DC: U.S. Government Printing Office.

The new buzzwords for new-music fans. (1993, July 23). *The New York Times.*

Nurcombe, B., & Unutzer, J. (1991). The ritual abuse of children: Clinical features and diagnostic reasoning. *Journal of the American Academy of Child and Adolescent Psychiatry, 30,* 272–276.

Parker, A. (1981). The meaning of attempted suicide to young parasuicides. *British Journal of Psychiatry, 139,* 306–312.

Patel, A. R., Roy, M., & Wilson, G. M. (1972). Self-poisoning and alcohol. *Lancet, 2,* 1099–1102.

Pfeffer, C. R. (1986). *The Suicidal Child.* New York: Guilford Press.

Rich, C. L., Young, D., & Fowler, R. C. (1986). San Diego suicide study I: Young versus old subjects. *Archives of General Psychiatry, 43,* 577–582.

Robbins, D. R., & Alessi, N. E. (1985). Depressive symptoms and suicidal behavior in adolescence. *American Journal of Psychiatry, 142,* 588–592.

Roy, A., & Linnoila, M. (1986). Alcoholism and suicide. *Suicide and Life Threatening Behaviors, 16,* 162–191.

Russell, A. (1988). *The Prince of Darkness.* New York: Cornell University Press.

Rydelius, P. A. (1984). Deaths among child and adolescent psychiatric patients. *Acta Psychiatrica Scandinavica, 70,* 119–126.

Schwartz, R. H., Comerci, G. D., & Meeks, J. E. (1987). Patterns of use by chemically dependent adolescents. *Journal of Pediatrics, 111,* 936–938.

Shaffer, D. (1988). The epidemiology of teen suicide: An examination of use factors. *Journal of Clinical Psychiatry (Supplement), 49,* 36–41.

Shafii, M., Steltz-Lenarsky, J., Derrick, A. M., Beckner, C., & Whittinghill, J. R. (1988). Comorbidity of mental disorders in the post-mortem diagnosis of completed suicide in children and adolescents. *Journal of Affective Disorders, 15,* 227–233.

Smith, M., & Pazder, L. (1980). *Michelle Remembers.* New York: Congdon & Lattes.

Sturner, W. Q. (1986). Adolescent suicide fatalities. *Rhode Island Medical Journal, 69,* 471–474.

Thompson, T. R. (1987). Childhood and adolescent suicide in Manitoba: A demographic study. *Canadian Journal of Psychiatry, 32,* 264–269.

Tunvig, K. (1988). Fatal outcome in drug addiction. *Acta Psychiatrica Scandinavica, 77,* 551–566.

Weidinger, C. K., & Demi, A. S. (1991). Music listening preferences and preadmission dysfunctional psychosocial behaviors of adolescents hospitalized on an inpatient psychiatric unit. *Journal of Child and Adolescent Psychiatry and Mental Health Nursing, 4,* 3–8.

Weissman, M. M., Klerman, G. L., Markowitz, J. S., & Ouellette, R. (1989). Suicidal ideation and suicide attempts in panic disorder and attacks. *New England Journal of Medicine, 321,* 1209–1214.

Wheeler, B. R., Wood, S., & Hatch, R. J. (1988). Assessment and intervention with adolescents involved in satanism. *Social Work, Nov.–Dec.,* 547–550.

CHAPTER 7

Human Immunodeficiency Virus/Acquired Immunodeficiency Syndrome and Psychoactive Substance Use Disorders in Children and Adolescents

The acquired immunodeficiency syndrome (AIDS) represents the end-stage manifestation of a prolonged infection with the human immunodeficiency virus (HIV). Children and adolescents may contract AIDS from sexual contact with any infected person, following injection with contaminated blood, or from pre- or perinatal transmission.

This chapter reviews various aspects of HIV and AIDS in relation to psychoactive substance use disorders (PSUD) in parents and their children as well as among adolescents.

7.1. EPIDEMIOLOGY

Females and children with HIV infection currently represent two of the fastest-growing populations in the HIV/AIDS epidemic in the United States (Etemad & Ponton, 1991). According to the report of the CDC (1991), there are an estimated 10,000 children (under 13 years of age) with HIV infection and about 3,100 with AIDS. The vast majority of pediatric AIDS victims (84%) contracted the disease from their mothers in the perinatal period. Of the mothers, 49% were intravenous drug users (IVDUs) and 21% were sex partners of IVDUs, and 16% of these children were born either to mothers with HIV infection, risk not specified, or to sex partners of males with HIV, risk unspecified (AACAP HIV Issues Committee, 1991). Infection by blood products accounts for fewer than 3% of children with AIDS, and sexual molestation by infected adults is rarely a documented source of HIV infection in children.

Some obstetric services have reported HIV-seropositive rates of 1–3% among their pregnant patients (Nanda, 1990). National figures in the United States of HIV-positive women giving live birth are 0.08–0.66% (Ellerbrock & Rogers, 1990). A study in the United Kingdom reported a seroprevalence of 0.04–0.49% (Peckham et al., 1990). The large range of seroprevalence in epidemiological reports reflects differences, especially between states (e.g., 50% of HIV/AIDS cases in the United States come from only 6 states). Also, significant differences exist between rates reported in the inner city vs. rural areas.

The most recognized adolescent risk group consists of disenfranchised inner city youngsters using psychoactive substances and engaging in unprotected sex. Also, homeless youths and male or female prostitutes of adolescent age are at high risk for AIDS and HIV transmission to others. The prevalence of teenage pregnancy in the United States is the highest in the industrialized world, and teenage females who are IVDUs or engage in unprotected sex, or both, may infect their fetuses.

The proportion of HIV-positive females to males is less favorable (1:7) for adolescents than for adults (1:15) according to the CDC (1991) report. A survey of over 1 million serum specimens from applicants for United States military service (age under 20 years) revealed that the prevalence for HIV-seropositivity was 0.34/1000 (Burke et al., 1990). The ratio between males and females was 35:32, and the prevalence among black recruits was 3.5 times and almost 6 times higher than among Hispanics and whites, respectively (Burke et al., 1990).

A Congressional report issued in April 1992 revealed that more than 5000 individuals under 24 years of age have died of AIDS, which is now the sixth leading cause of death among the age group of 15- to 24-year-olds. The number of teenagers who are HIV-positive is not known, but during the years 1989–1991, the cumulative number of 13- to 24-year-olds diagnosed with AIDS increased by 77%.

7.2. PATHOGENESIS AND CLINICAL FEATURES OF HUMAN IMMUNODEFICIENCY VIRUS INFECTION

Pregnancy is considered a mildly immunosuppressive state; however, infections may be more difficult to treat in pregnant women because of decreased lymphocyte function and levels of T4 lymphocytes. T-cells are involved in the regulation of both cell-mediated and humoral responses. In these responses, T-helper cells are required for effective augmentation of responses to antigenic challenge, and they are often referred to as T4 cells. HIV has a particular predilection for these cells, and the infection and destruction of T4 cells is believed to constitute the primary source of morbidity in AIDS (Schleifer, Delaney, Tross, & Keller, 1991).

There is no conclusive evidence that pregnancy accelerates the course of early asymptomatic HIV disease or that HIV disease significantly affects pregnancy outcome in asymptomatic women.

The exact route of perinatal transmission is unclear. The virus has been identified in fetuses at 15 weeks, in the amniotic fluid, and in breast milk of infected women (AACAP HIV Issues Committee, 1991). The infant could be infected during labor and delivery, although the results are conflicting regarding the role of cesarean section as a technique to reduce the risk of HIV transmission.

The risk of perinatal transmission is estimated as between 20% and 35% (Ellerbrock & Rogers, 1990; European Collaborative Study, 1988). Incubation periods (i.e., the phase between fetal/infant infection and diagnosis of AIDS) have been described as following either a short course (median 4.1 months) or a long course (median 6.1 years).

Many infants will test positive for HIV antibody at birth, but this result may reflect maternal antibodies. A definitive diagnosis can be better made after maternal antibodies for HIV disappear by 12–17 months after birth.

It is important to distinguish between pediatric and adult AIDS. Serious bacterial sepsis and lymphoid interstitial pneumonitis are major problems in children. HIV can directly infect cells in the central nervous system, producing both neoplastic involvement and an encephalopathy. Neurological findings include motor dysfunction, developmental delay, and progressive loss of developmental milestones and cognitive functioning. Microephaly, chronic encephalopathy, and seizure disorders have also been reported (AACAP HIV Issues Committee, 1991). Children are less likely than adults to develop Kaposi's sarcoma and B-cell lymphoma.

The lives of these children are frequently complicated by the death or the progressive complications of the AIDS-infected parent, who may be unable to provide appropriate care. Also, the same circumstances that have led the mother to become an IVDU or HIV-positive or both could undermine her caregiving capacity, thus leaving the child "at risk" emotionally (Belfer, Krener, & Miller, 1988).

Adolescents are a group at growing risk for HIV infection and AIDS. Many are misinformed about the disease. The frequency of AIDS in adolescents rises with age; the long incubation period indicates that many 20- to 29-year olds were infected as adolescents (AACAP HIV Issues Committee, 1991).

The course of AIDS in adolescents resembles that in adults more than that in children. Also, the risk of suicidal behavior among adolescents with HIV seropositivity or AIDS is higher than in the general population. This rate is likely to be similar to suicidal behavior rates among individuals with debilitating and potentially fatal illnesses (Cote, Biggar, & Dannenberg, 1992; Gala et al., 1992). HIV infection has been associated with high prevalence rates of psychiatric and organic–mental disorders including mood, anxiety, adjustment, and substance abuse disorders (Gala et al., 1992).

7.3. PSYCHOACTIVE SUBSTANCE USE DISORDERS AND THE RISK OF HUMAN IMMUNODEFICIENCY VIRUS INFECTION

Psychoactive substances may impair judgment and reduce inhibition, thus leading to risky sexual behavior; condoms also were less likely to be used if use of alcohol or other psychoactive substance was combined with sex (CDC, 1991).

The relationship between the use of specific psychoactive substances and increased risk factors for AIDS has been investigated.

7.3.1. Opioids

Compromised immune function as a result of exposure to opiates may add to the risk of infection and disease progression. This increased risk results from more than simply the use of shared needles (Schleifer et al., 1991). In addition to decreased lymphocyte functional responses, a significant reduction in numbers of T-cells has been reported among opiate users. Incubation of heroin addicts' cells with the opiate antagonist naloxone reversed some of the immune effects (MacGregor, 1988).

Impairment in cell-mediated immunity related to heroin use has also been suggested. Further investigations are needed to shed more light on this matter.

7.3.2. Alcohol

Acute alcohol consumption has been implicated experimentally in the impairment of both cellular and humoral immunity (MacGregor, 1988). It is difficult, however, to extrapolate these experimental results to naturalistic settings in humans. Natural killer cell activity, which plays a role in resistance to viral infection and neoplasia and may be involved in progression of HIV infection, is also inhibited by alcohol use. Alterations in immune function are thought to play a role in the increased susceptibility to infection found in alcoholics (Adams & Jordan, 1984).

7.3.3. Other Substances

Studies of the effects of cocaine and marijuana on human immunity have been conflicting (MacGregor, 1988). The relationship between polysubstance abuse and the function of the immune system has been examined. Opiates have been found to depress immune function and cocaine may reverse this depression when used in combination; however, alcohol attenuates the effect of cocaine (Donahoe & Falek, 1988).

Other factors may further compromise the immune system and increase the risk of HIV infection and disease. These factors include malnutrition, life stress, and depression, which are highly prevalent in substance abusers. Interventions to treat these factors may therefore have important benefits (Schleifer et al., 1991).

7.4. PREVENTION

Women with positive HIV status [tested by the enzyme-linked immunosorbent assay (ELISA) and confirmed by the Western blot] may wish to avoid pregnancy, since there is a substantial risk (50%) of transmission to the fetus *in utero*. It has been reported that 38% of women terminated their pregnancies after learning they were seropositive (Schleifer et al., 1991).

By law, partner notification must be carried out, but to be effective it should be complemented with other outreach and educational interventions (AACAP HIV Issues Committee, 1991). Primary prevention among adolescents is increasing, although it is noteworthy that education for safer sex needs to stress the 5–15% failure rate of condoms in protecting against HIV transmission (Krener, 1991).

7.5. GUIDELINES FOR TREATMENT

A confidential pre- and post-HIV test counseling session is important, and HIV infection control and treatment need to be implemented following a seropositive result. Anti-HIV drug therapy with zidovudine (AZT) reduces morbidity, especially in children with AIDS dementia and encephalopathy. Assessment of neuropsychological functioning and psychiatric needs is important. Access to health and social care is crucial, especially for children with infected parents or who are orphaned (AACAP HIV Issues Committee, 1991).

7.6. CONCLUSION

The increased number of children and adolescents afflicted with HIV/AIDS and the association of maternal addiction and unsafe sex with perinatal transmission are major reasons for concern. Additional resources for prevention, treatment, and research of this epidemic are needed.

Additional information about other aspects of maternal and infancy addiction is delineated in Chapter 8.

REFERENCES

AACAP (American Academy of Child and Adolescent Psychiatry) HIV Issues Committee (1991). Information sheet, annual meeting, San Francisco.

Adams, H., & Jordan, C. (1984). Infections in the alcoholic. *Medical Clinics of North America, 68,* 179–200.

Belfer, M. L., Krener, P. K., & Miller, F. B. (1988). AIDS in children and adolescents. *Journal of the American Academy of Child and Adolescent Psychiatry, 27,* 147–151.

Burke, D. S., Brundage, J. F., Goldenbaum, M., Gardner, L. I., Peterson, M., Visintine, R., & Redfield, R. R. (1990). Human immunodeficiency virus infections in teenagers. *Journal of the American Medical Association, 263,* 2074–2077.

CDC (Centers for Disease Control) (1991). *HIV/AIDS Surveillance Reports.* Atlanta: Centers for Disease Control.

Cote, T. R., Biggar, R. J., & Dannenberg, A. L. (1992). Risk of suicide among persons with AIDS: A national assessment. *Journal of the American Medical Association, 268,* 2066–2068.

Donahoe, R. M., & Falek, A. (1988). Neuroimmunomodulation by opiates and other drugs of abuse: Relationship to HIV infection and AIDS. *Advances in Biochemical Psychopharmacology, 44,* 145–158.

Ellerbrock, T. V., & Rogers, M. F. (1990). Epidemiology of human immunodeficiency virus infection in women in the United States. *Obstetrics and Gynecology Clinics of North America, 17,* 523–543.

Etemad, J., & Ponton, L. (1991). Impact of HIV on child and adolescent psychiatry. *Journal of the American Academy of Child and Adolescent Psychiatry, 30,* 721–722.

European Collaborative Study (1988). Mother-to-child transmission of HIV infection. *Lancet, 2,* 1039–1042.

Gala, C., Pergami, A., Catalan, J., Riccio, M., Durbano, F., Musicco, M., Baldeweg, T., & Invernizzi, G. (1992). Risk of deliberate self-harm and factors associated with suicidal behavior among asymptomatic individuals with human immunodeficiency virus infection. *Acta Psychiatrica Scandinavica, 86,* 70–75.

Krener, P. (1991). HIV spectrum disease. In M. Lewis (Ed.), *Child and Adolescent Psychiatry* (pp. 994–1003). Baltimore: Williams & Wilkins.

MacGregor, R. (1988). Alcohol and drugs as co-factors for AIDS. *Advances in Alcohol and Substance Abuse, 7,* 47–71.

Nanda, D. (1990) Human immunodeficiency virus infection in pregnancy. *Obstetrics and Gynecology Clinics of North America, 17,* 617–625.

Peckham, C. S., Tedder, R. S., Briggs, M., Ades, A. E., Hjelm, M., Wilcox, A. H., Parra-Mejia, N., & O'Connor, C. (1990). Prevalence of maternal HIV infection based on unlinked anonymous testing of newborn babies. *Lancet, 335,* 516–519.

Schleifer, S. J., Delaney, B. R., Tross, S., & Keller, S. E. (1991). AIDS and addictions. In R. J. Frances & S. I. Millder (Eds.), *Clinical Textbook of Addictive Disorders* (pp. 299–319). New York: Guilford Press.

CHAPTER 8

Maternal and Infancy Addiction: Adolescent Mothers and Their Offspring

Adolescent psychoactive substance use disorders (APSUDs) and un-planned pregnancy are two of the most prevalent public health prob-lems in the United States. Pregnancy and parenting during adolescence place adolescent females and their infants at increased risk for present and future medical, economic, and psychosocial problems. Concurrent PSUD adds to the severity of these problems (Zuckerman, Amaro, & Beardslee, 1987). This chapter reviews and discusses APSUDs in adoles-cent females who are pregnant or mothers, or both, and their offspring. It provides an update of the relatively limited information available on the prevalence, patterns, and outcomes of APSUDs among pregnant adolescents and adolescent mothers with their infants.

8.1. PSYCHOACTIVE SUBSTANCE USE, PSYCHOACTIVE SUBSTANCE USE DISORDERS, AND SEXUAL ACTIVITY IN ADOLESCENCE

As reviewed at length in Chapter 3, adolescent substance use (ASU) and APSUDs are more common among adolescent males as compared to females; however, the gender gap appears to be narrowing. It has also been reported that about 70% of adolescent females under 18 years of age were engaged in full sexual activity (Blum, 1991). It is generally accepted that there is a positive correlation between ASU and sexual behavior for both male and female adolescents (Newcomb & Bentler,

1988; Yamaguchi & Kandel, 1987). It is expected that a longitudinal study addressing the subject in a national sample of adolescents will reveal positive relationships between prevalence and incidence of intercourse and extent of drug use and delinquency.

Sexually active adolescent females were assessed for their tobacco smoking in a controlled study (Zabin, 1984). Not only was a higher rate of smoking reported among the sexually active group, but also smoking has been found to be negatively associated with age of first intercourse and with consistent contraceptive behaviors. Additionally, smoking has been reported to correlate positively with rates of unplanned pregnancy.

These findings are in accord with the problem-behavior theory (Jessor & Jessor, 1977). This theory suggests that adolescents who engage in one problem behavior are also prone to experience a variety of problem behaviors that constitute a behavioral syndrome. These problem behaviors are considered to be stable from adolescence to young adulthood. Measures of problem behaviors such as delinquency, sexual intercourse, and ASU were correlated positively with each other and negatively with several measures of conventional behavior, thus confirming the generalizability of the theory (Farrell, Danish, & Howard, 1992).

8.1.1. Adolescent Pregnancy

Among sexually active adolescent females in the United States, about 24% will experience at least one pregnancy before age 18 (Hayes, 1987). Approximately 60% of the 1 million annual unintended adolescent pregnancies will be carried to term. About 40% of adolescent pregnancies in the United States account for 26.2% of all induced abortions. Many of the reported correlates of early pregnancy and adolescent motherhood are similar to correlates reported for early ASU (Gilchrist, Gillmore, & Lohr, 1990).

A comparison of adolescents who carry their pregnancies to term vs. those who choose to abort reveals that females from the first group are more likely to be younger at first intercourse and at first pregnancy, to come from a lower socioeconomic status, to drop out of school or to have lower academic aspirations and achievements, to come from conflictual family situations, and to be at high risk for APSUDs (Gilchrist et al., 1990).

Adolescent pregnancy, delivery, and parenthood are characterized by more obstetrical, medical, and psychosocial problems, as well as more severe difficulties, compared with other age groups (Blum, 1991). Common obstetrical complications include toxemia and premature delivery.

Low birth weight for gestational age and increased risk of perinatal morbidity are characteristic of the neonate. Adolescent mothers' medical problems during pregnancy and delivery, complications during abortions (the rate of which is highest in the adolescent age group), postpartum depression and anxiety, and impaired parenthood are a few of the issues that characterize morbidities related to adolescent pregnancy.

8.1.2. Adolescent Pregnancy and Psychoactive Substance Use Disorders

Any psychoactive substance use in pregnancy may be considered abuse due to the potential damage to the fetus and mother and according to DSM-IV criteria (American Psychiatric Association, 1994).

The overall incidence of substance abuse during pregnancy was found to be 11% (Chasnoff, 1989). Adolescents constitute about 20% of pregnant females who abuse psychoactive substances (Marques & McKnight, 1991). Alcohol consumption among pregnant females was found to decrease from 32% to 20% between the years 1985 and 1988 (Serdula, Williamson, Kendrick, Anda, & Byers, 1991). The study, conducted in 21 states and surveying pregnant women over 18 years of age, concluded that no decline was observed among women under 25 years of age.

It has been estimated that approximately 400,000 newborns are delivered every year to mothers who abused psychoactive substances during pregnancy (Chasnoff, 1988). Gomby and Shiono (1991) estimated that in the late 1980s, about 4.5% of babies born in the United States were exposed to cocaine, more than 17% were exposed to marijuana, 73% were exposed to alcohol, and perhaps 2–3% were exposed to opiates. They concluded that between 550,000 and 740,000 infants annually may have been exposed *in utero* to illegal psychoactive substances (alcohol and nicotine not included).

Hagan (1987) found that 83% of addicted women had one or more parents with PSUDs, 67% of them had been sexually abused, and 60% had been physically abused. Also, many of them had a partner who qualified for a diagnosis of PSUD. Amaro and Zuckerman (1990) investigated the psychosocial profile of pregnant adolescents with PSUDs and found that such disorders were associated with a characteristic profile of risk factors. Compared to non-drug-users, pregnant adolescents with PSUDs were more likely to have a history of elective abortion and venereal diseases, report more negative life events in the previous year, experience violence during pregnancy, and have a male partner with PSUD. Siblings, friends, and partners of adolescent mothers who use psychoactive substances provide a social context of support for use (Amaro & Zuckerman, 1990). Also, a report of having been high while at school was a significant risk factor for continued psychoactive substance use during pregnancy (Kokotailo, Adger, Duggan, Repke, & Joffe, 1992). These findings have implications for prevention and intervention.

8.1.3. Maternal Medical Sequelae of Psychoactive Substance Use Disorders

Pregnant females with PSUDs have an increased incidence of medical and obstetrical complications, the majority of which appear to be related to the use of psychoactive substances, their high-risk life-style, and their tendency to neglect health care (Silver, Wapner, Loriz-Vega, & Finnegan, 1987). Most of the frequent obstetrical complications of females with PSUDs may be listed in one of two categories: (1) infection [e.g., chorioamnionitis, septic thromophlebitis, acquired immunodeficiency syndrome (AIDS)] and (2) vasospasm or contraction of blood vessels [e.g., abruptio placentae, premature labor, intrauterine growth retardation (IUGR)] (Miller & Hyatt, 1992). However, deficient nutrition, toxic adulterants that are mixed with specific drugs, physical abuse, and maternal depression may affect the pregnant female pre- and postpartum and could have an impact on the outcome of the pregnancy.

8.1.4. Neonatal Complications of Maternal Substance Abuse

All known psychoactive substances cross the placenta. There are three major areas in which the neonatal effects of PSUDs in pregnancy are manifested: congenital anomalies, neonatal and infant medical complications, and neurobehavioral changes (Miller & Hyatt, 1992). Zuckerman and Bresnahan (1991, p. 1388) suggest that

> the development of an infant affected by exposure to psychoactive substances is best understood through a multifactorial model consisting of interrelated prenatal and postnatal factors. The prenatal effects of drugs on the central nervous system (CNS) are seen as creating biological vulnerability, that is, dysfunction that may be completely or in part compensated by the brain itself and by competent caretaking, but that renders the child more vulnerable to the effects of poor caretaking.

Prenatal influences of psychoactive substances are associated with a smaller head circumference; however, it is not yet known whether a structural effect on the brain is indicated. The relative weights of the severity, duration, and dosage of abused psychoactive substances and of other possible associated life circumstances of these females relative to the insult to the fetus are unclear. Discontinuation of substance use during pregnancy and satisfactory postnatal caretaking of the child reduce and may even eliminate the effects.

The brain of a newborn has a significant capacity for adaptation. It appears that perinatal factors exert their influence primarily in early infancy, whereas social or environmental factors become predominant in subsequent development (Zuckerman & Bresnahan, 1991). Unfortunately, maternal addiction is associated with prenatal and postnatal impaired self-caring, child abuse, and neglect.

Fetal abuse in the form of PSUD by the mother and, additionally, physical assault by the mother or her partner or both are not uncommon (Condon, 1986). Violence within the maternal–paternal–fetal child triad has been explained by hypotheses ranging from the psychobiology of pregnancy to the psychology of aggression. Abdominal trauma, although unlikely to seriously damage the fetus, may precipitate labor, with resultant prematurity and low birth weight. Fetal abuse has also been suggested as an antecedent of child abuse. One of the explanations for subsequent child abuse is associated with low birth weight of infants born to mothers with PSUDs. Children small for age and infants with poor arousal may either not elicit sufficient caretaking from their parents or be the victims of parental violence (Smith & Hanson, 1974; Zuckerman & Bresnahan, 1991). These children may develop post-traumatic stress disorder (PTSD) later in childhood or adolescence, and they are also prone to become child-abusing parents.

Maternal depression is more prevalent among mothers with PSUDs. This comorbidity, like other medical and mental health comorbidities, has been shown to be associated with impaired mother–infant interactions, psychosomatic symptoms of preschoolers, injuries, and learning disabilities and psychiatric disorders among school-aged children (Zuckerman & Beardslee, 1987). An assessment of pregnant substance-abusing teenagers by the Beck Depression Inventory (Beck, 1976) suggested that they obtained a mean score comparable to that of the general adolescent population (Burns, Melamed, Burns, Chasnoff, & Hatcher, 1985). This report confirmed findings from a similar study of adolescents (Teri, 1982). The results of both studies also indicated that pregnant teenage addicts were less depressed than older pregnant women with PSUDs.

Infants born to mothers who have used various psychoactive substances during pregnancy are known to have a 5- to 10-times-greater risk of dying from sudden infant death syndrome (SIDS), as compared to a control group. The use of opiates, cocaine, PCP, and polysubstances was recorded among the women who participated in the study (Davidson-Ward et al., 1986).

8.2. RELATIONSHIP BETWEEN MATERNAL ABUSE OF SPECIFIC PSYCHOACTIVE SUBSTANCES AND NEONATAL AND FURTHER CHILDHOOD MORBIDITY

8.2.1. Tobacco

Most studies reveal that 25–35% of pregnant women smoke throughout pregnancy. There is also a strong association between alcohol and cigarette consumption during pregnancy (Kwok, Correy, Newman, & Curran,1983; Streissguth, Darby, Barr, & Smith, 1983). An extensive body of literature has documented quite conclusively that smoking during pregnancy is associated with a number of negative outcomes. These ill effects include increased complications during pregnancy, reduced fetal growth, and an increased risk of perinatal mortality (Fried & Watkinson, 1990). Fried and Watkinson (1990) reported in a longitudinal follow-up of 36- and 48-month-old children that a negative dose–response association was observed between the children's cognitive scores (particularly a verbal subscale) and maternal smoking.

Maternal smoking postpartum has been associated with behavior problems among children (Weitzman, Gortmaker, & Sobol, 1992). Smokers' children were found to have an increased rate of conflicts with peers and various psychopathologies. Abstaining from smoking during pregnancy but then resuming the habit did not make a difference. Weitzman et al. (1992) hypothesized that smoking during and after pregnancy might alter the children's brain structure or function or might affect either the mother's behavior or her tolerance toward the children.

8.2.2. Alcohol

The fetal alcohol syndrome (FAS) was first described by Jones, Smith, Ulleland, and Streissguth (1973). In the 1980s, a set of minimal criteria for the diagnosis of FAS was developed: (1) prenatal and/or postnatal growth retardation; (2) CNS involvement (signs of neurological abnormality, developmental delay, or intellectual impairment); (3) characteristic facial dysmorphology, with at least two of three signs (microcephaly; microophthalmia and/or short palpebral fissures; poorly developed philtrum, thin upper lip, or flattening of the maxillary area (Rosett & Weiner, 1985).

FAS has become the third most common known cause of mental retardation in the United States, affecting about 1 in 750 live births (Little & Streissguth, 1981). A diagnosis of partial FAS may be given to a child with fewer than the three criteria noted above, and of 1,000 alcoholic women, 5–9 will bear children affected by FAS (Abel & Sokol, 1987). Alcohol has a dose–teratogenic effect relation, and the synergistic effect of poor nutrition and smoking may have an additional impact on outcome.

The precise mechanism of alcohol's effect on the fetus is unknown as yet; however, it appears that the first trimester is the critical period for teratogenic effects (Kuzma & Sokol, 1982). There appears to be a subset of FAS children who show a pattern of improvement over time; however, hyperactivity, distractibility, and short attention span have been associated with FAS later in life at ages 4 and 7 years for the vast majority of children. Also, exposure of the fetus to 8 or more drinks per day has been associated with a decrement of 5 IQ points (Streissguth, Sampson, & Barr, 1989). These effects are referred to as "fetal alcohol effects." However, these studies have been criticized for a deficiency in control groups.

8.2.3. Marijuana

Marijuana abuse during pregnancy was found to be correlated with lower birth weight and shorter length; this impaired fetal growth is similar to that seen in infants exposed to the hypoxic effects of maternal cigarette smoking (Zuckerman & Bresnahan, 1991). Findings that heavy marijuana smoking may affect the neurophysiological integrity of the newborn have been reported, mainly regarding sleep and arousal states. A 4-year follow-up of children born to mothers abusing marijuana (more than 6 joints per week) found significantly lower scores in verbal and memory domains (Fried & Watkinson, 1990).

8.2.4. Cocaine and Amphetamines

Cocaine and amphetamines have a comparable impact on pregnancy and similar physiological effects. There is a large body of information regarding the effects of maternal cocaine use on pregnancy outcome. Cocaine's vasoactive properties have been implicated in the following maternal complications: abruptio placentae, spontaneous abortion, preterm labor, and risk for fetal/neonatal problems including IUGR, rare congenital abnormalities such as urogenital anomalies and distal limb deformities, reduced head circumference, hemorrhagic lesions, congenital abnormalities, prematurity, increased perinatal mortality, seizures, infarction, and necrotizing enterocolitis (Chasnoff, Griffith, Freier, & James, 1992).

It may be difficult to ascertain the relative weight of prenatal exposure to cocaine vs. the postnatal environment in causation of the behavioral syndrome noted in Section 8.2.1. Also, there is no scientific support for the mythical description of "crack kids" popularized in the media, which predicts a generation of brain-damaged kids. This label is damaging due to its potential as a self-fulfilling prophecy and should be eradicated.

8.2.5. Opioids

In the United States, as many as 10,000 infants a year may be born to women who used opioids, usually heroin or methadone (Hans, 1989). Low birth weight is associated with maternal opioid abuse; however, it is also associated with poor maternal nutrition during pregnancy. Participation in a methadone maintenance (MM) program during pregnancy has been associated with reduced fetal mortality and normal fetal growth (Finnegan, 1986). By 3 years of age, no difference in head circumference between opioid-exposed infants and controls was reported (Zuckerman & Bresnahan, 1991).

Applicants for MM must be above 18 years of age by Federal regulations; therefore, MM for adolescents is a legally sensitive issue. However, most states have accepted either or both parental consent and careful monitoring and reporting to the health and legal authorities as a solution.

Neonatal abstinence syndrome (NAS) is seen when the neonate experiences withdrawal symptoms, usually within 72 hours after delivery. A subacute form may continue up to 6 months (Finnegan, 1991).

8.2.6. Phencyclidine (PCP)

PCP studies in pregnant females are scarce; however, a high risk for teratogenic effects in the skeletal system was reported. Also, a high rate of spontaneous abortions, decreased fertility, and broken chromosomes has been noted, as reviewed by Kaminer and Feingold (1991).

8.2.7. Breast-feeding

It has been noted recently that psychoactive substances are excreted in small amounts in breast milk and may cause and even continue the infant's dependency on these substances, thus affecting the infant's development (Frank, Bauchner, Zuckerman, & Fried, 1992). The substances detected in breast milk are alcohol, nicotine, sedatives, opiates, cocaine, caffeine, and marijuana.

It is noteworthy that the AIDS virus is transmitted in maternal milk; therefore, women with HIV-positive status or AIDS should not breast feed.

8.3. PREVENTION AND INTERVENTION

Substance abuse among pregnant adolescents has declined voluntarily and substantially (Gilchrist et al., 1990). Also, Moss and Hensleigh (1988) reported that most substance abuse was terminated after 12–16 weeks of pregnancy among Hispanic and white pregnant adolescents. These studies suggest that secondary prevention among pregnant adolescents with PSUDs is effective for certain subgroups. However, it is not possible as yet to predict remission in PSUDs during pregnancy.

If prevention of continued PSUD during pregnancy fails, there is an intensified need for continued follow-up of the mother and child after delivery. Mothers who did not attend prenatal clinics and who are diagnosed with PSUDs during their hospitalization for delivery are also at high risk for dropout from follow-up. Neither the age, ethnicity, marital status, and type of psychoactive substance use by the female during pregnancy nor the duration, type, and number of addiction problems are significantly different between dropouts and active participants in treatment (Chan, Wingert, & Wachsman, 1986). The dropouts' newborns were found to have lower birth weight and shorter gestation.

It is important to note that most dysfunctional mothers may fail to return for follow-up, leading to a bias toward retaining children with more favorable outcomes. As delineated in Section 8.1.4, the quality of the postnatal environment appears to be of great importance in compensating for prenatal insults due to PSUDs (Chasnoff et al., 1992).

Children born to adolescent mothers are at higher risk than those born to adult mothers. Therefore, provision of services in a model of "one-stop shopping" is recommended. This plan provides multidimensional treatment for pregnant females and also incentives for compliance with appointments (e.g., food, clothing, laundry services).

A successful behavioral–cognitive therapy for the reduction and elimination of smoking among pregnant adolescents was reported (Duffy & Coates, 1989). Such a program may be generalized for other psychoactive substances.

A special emphasis on psychopharmacological treatment for the mother and child dyad is needed, especially to prevent or treat opiate-induced NAS. When pharmacological intervention is recommended, the treatment of choice is paregoric or phenobarbital. Finnegan (1986) developed an NAS scoring system of neonatal behavior.

No studies have shown a specific developmental dysfunction attributable to a specific PSUD, and it is important to remember that polysubstance abuse in pregnancy is the rule rather than the exception.

Follow-up studies extended into late childhood and beyond combined with improved design of controlled prospective studies may increase the knowledge of those who need to design effective intervention programs. Finally, the legal status of the dilemma, i.e., what to do with a pregnant female who abuses psychoactive substances, is unclear. However, there is a growing trend toward treating these mothers and away from sending them to jail as had been the case in the recent past.

8.4. CONCLUSION

More treatment programs, especially for pregnant adolescents with PSUDs, are needed. Medical, psychiatric, education or employment, and legal problems of the mother should be attended to, as well as the needs of the newborn and other first-degree relatives, including other children in the family.

REFERENCES

Abel, E. L., & Sokol, R. J. (1987). Incidence of fetal alcohol syndrome and economic impact of FAS-related anomalies. *Alcohol and Drug Dependence, 19*, 51–70.

Amaro, H., & Zuckerman, B. (1990). Psychoactive substance use and adolescent pregnancy: Compounded risk among inner city adolescent mothers. In M. E. Colten & S. Gore (Eds.), *Adolescent Stress: Causes and Consequences* (pp. 223–236). New York: Aldine de Gruyter.

American Psychiatric Association (1994). *Diagnostic and Statistical Manual of Mental Disorders*, 4th ed. Washington, DC: American Psychiatric Association.

Beck, A. (1976). *Cognitive Therapy and the Emotional Disorders*. New York: International Universities Press.

Blum, R. W. (1991). Global trends in adolescent health. *Journal of the American Medical Association, 265*, 2711–2719.

Burns, K. I., Melamed, J., Burns, W., Chasnoff, I., & Hatcher, R. (1985). Chemical dependence and clinical depression in pregnancy. *Journal of Clinical Psychology, 41*, 851–854.

Chan, L. S., Wingert, W. A., & Wachsman, L. (1986). Differences between dropouts and active participants in a pediatric clinic for substance abuse mothers. *American Journal of Drug and Alcohol Abuse, 12*, 89–99.

Chasnoff, I. J. (1988). Drug use in pregnancy: Parameters of risk. *Pediatric Clinics of North America, 35,* 1403–1412.

Chasnoff, I. J. (1989). Drug use and women: Establishing a standard of care. *Annals of the New York Academy of Sciences, 68,* 208–210.

Chasnoff, I. J., Griffith, D. R., Freier, C., & James, M. (1992). Cocaine/polydrug use in pregnancy: Two-year follow-up. *Pediatrics, 89,* 284–289.

Condon, J. T. (1986). The spectrum of fetal abuse in pregnant women. *Journal of Nervous and Mental Disease, 174,* 509–516.

Davidson-Ward, S. L., Schuetz, S., Krishna, V., Bean, X., Wingert, W., Wachsman, L., & Keens, T. G. (1986). Abnormal sleeping ventilatory pattern in infants of substance-abusing mothers. *American Journal of Diseases of Children, 140,* 1015–1020.

Duffy, J., & Coates, T. J. (1989). Reducing smoking among pregnant adolescents. *Adolescence, 93,* 29–37.

Farrell, A. D., Danish, S. J., & Howard, C. W. (1992). Relationship between drug use and other problem behaviors in urban adolescents. *Journal of Consulting and Clinical Psychiatry, 60,* 705–712.

Finnegan, L. P. (1986). Neonatal abstinence syndrome: Assessment and pharmacotherapy. In F. F. Rubaltelli & B. Granati (Eds.), *Neonatal Therapy: An Update* (pp. 182–204). New York: Elsevier Science Publishers.

Finnegan, L. P. (1991). Perinatal substance abuse: Comments and perspectives. *Seminars in Perinatology, 15,* 331–339.

Frank, D. A., Bauchner, H., Zuckerman, B. S., & Fried, L. (1992). *Journal of the American Dietetic Association, 92,* 215–217.

Fried, P. A., & Watkinson, B. (1990). 36- and 48-month neurobehavioral follow-up of children prenatally exposed to marijuana, cigarettes, and alcohol. *Developmental and Behavioral Pediatrics, 11,* 49–58.

Gilchrist, L. D., Gillmore, M. R., & Lohr, M. J. (1990). Drug use among pregnant adolescents. *Journal of Consulting Psychology, 58,* 402–407.

Gomby, D. S., & Shiono, P. H. (1991). Estimating the number of substance-exposed infants: The future of children. *Center for the Future of Children, 1,* 17.

Hagan, T. A. (1987). *A Retrospective Search for the Etiology of Drug Abuse: A Background Comparison of a Drug-Addicted Population of Women and a Control Group of Non-Addicted Women.* NIDA Research Monograph Series of Health and Human Services. Washington, DC: Department of Health and Human Services.

Hans, S. L. (1989). Developmental consequences of prenatal exposure to methadone. *Annals of the New York Academy of Sciences, 68,* 195–207.

Hayes, C. D. (1987). *Risking the Future: Adolescent Sexuality, Pregnancy and Childbearing,* Vol 1. Washington DC: National Academy Press.

Jessor, R., & Jessor, S. L. (1977). *Problem Behavior and Psychosocial Development: A Longitudinal Study of Youth.* New York: Academic Press.

Jones, K. L., Smith, D. W., Ulleland, C. N., & Streissguth, A. P. (1973). Pattern of malformation in offspring of chronic alcoholic mothers. *Lancet, 1,* 1267–1271.

Kaminer, Y., & Feingold, M. (1991). Abuse of illegal psychoactive substances in pregnancy. *Harefuah, 121,* 524–526.

Kokotailo, P. K., Adger, H., Duggan, A. K., Repke, J., & Joffe, A. (1992). Cigarette, alcohol, and other drug use by school-age pregnant adolescents: Prevalence, detection, and associated risk factors. *Pediatrics, 90,* 328–334.

Kuzma, J., & Sokol, R. (1982). Maternal drinking behavior and decreased intrauterine growth. *Alcoholism, Clinical and Experimental Research, 6,* 396–402.

Kwok, P., Correy, J. F., Newman, N. M., & Curran, J. T. (1983). Smoking and alcohol consumption during pregnancy. *Medical Journal of Australia, 1,* 220–223.

Little, R., & Streissguth, A., (1981). Effects of alcohol on the fetus: Impact and prevention. *Canadian Medical Association Journal, 125,* 159–164.

Marques, P. R., & McKnight, A. J. (1991). Drug abuse risk among pregnant adolescents attending public health clinics. *American Journal of Drug and Alcohol Abuse, 17,* 399–414.

Miller, W. H., & Hyatt, M. C. (1992). Perinatal substance abuse. *American Journal of Drug and Alcohol Abuse, 18,* 247–261.

Moss, N., & Hensleigh, P. A. (1988). Substance use by Hispanic and white non-Hispanic pregnant adolescents: A preliminary survey. *Journal of Youth and Adolescence, 17,* 531–541.

Newcomb, M. D., & Bentler, P. M. (1988). *Consequences of Adolescent Drug Use: Impact on the Lives of Young Adults.* Newbury Park, CA: Sage.

Rosett, H. L., & Weiner, L. (1985). Alcohol and pregnancy: A clinical perspective. *Annual Review of Medicine, 36,* 73–80.

Serdula, M., Williamson, D. F., Kendrick, J. S., Anda, R. F., & Byers, T. (1991). Trends in alcohol consumption by pregnant women. *Journal of the American Medical Association, 265,* 876–879.

Silver, H., Wapner, R., Loriz-Vega, M., & Finnegan, L. P. (1987). Addiction in pregnancy: High risk intrapartum management and outcome. *Journal of Perinatology, 3,* 178–184.

Smith, S., & Hanson, R. (1974). 134 Battered children: A medical and psychological study. *British Medical Journal, 3,* 666–670.

Streissguth, A. P., Darby, B. L., Barr, H. M., & Smith, J. R. (1983). Comparison of drinking and smoking patterns during pregnancy over a six-year interval. *American Journal of Obstetrics and Gynecology, 145,* 716–724.

Streissguth, A. P., Sampson, P. D., Barr, H. M. (1989). IQ at age 4 in relation to maternal alcohol use and smoking during pregnancy. *Developmental Psychology, 25,* 3–11.

Teri, L. (1982). The use of the Beck Depression Inventory with adolescents. *Journal of Abnormal Child Psychology, 10,* 277–284.

Weitzman, M., Gortmaker, S., & Sobol, A. (1992). Maternal smoking and behavior problems in children. *Pediatrics, 90,* 342–349.

Yamaguchi, K., & Kandel, D. (1987). Drug use and other determinants of premarital pregnancy and its outcomes: A dynamic analysis of competing life events. *Journal of Marriage and the Family, 49,* 257–270.

Zabin, L. S. (1984). The association between smoking and sexual behavior among teens in U.S. contraceptive clinics. *American Journal of Public Health, 74,* 261–263.

Zuckerman, B. S., Amaro, M., & Beardslee, W. R. (1987). Mental health of adolescent mothers: The implications of depression and drug use. *Journal of Developmental and Behavioral Pediatrics, 8,* 111–116.

Zuckerman, B. S., & Beardslee, W. R. (1987). Maternal depression: A concern for pediatricians. *Pediatrics, 79,* 110–117.

Zuckerman, B. S., & Bresnahan, K. (1991). Developmental and behavioral consequences of prenatal drug and alcohol exposure. *Pediatric Clinics of North America, 38,* 1387–1406.

PART II

Interventions: Prevention of Adolescent Substance Use and Assessment and Treatment of Psychoactive Substance Use Disorders

CHAPTER 9

Prevention of High-Risk Behaviors: Adolescent Substance Use, Adolescent Psychoactive Substance Use Disorders, and Suicide

Efforts to prevent use and abuse of psychoactive substances by children and adolescents focus on interventions designed to reduce substance supply and demand. According to a report by the Board of Trustees of the AMA (1991), law enforcement and health authorities curtail the supply aspects by closing gaps in the drug control system, eradicating illicit drugs at the point of production, achieving balance between the demand for and supply of drugs manufactured for medical use and the control of diversion of such drugs to the illicit market, and obstructing or intercepting the trafficking in illicit drugs. According to the same report, reducing the demand involves deferring or precluding initiation of use by nonusers, reducing all use of illicit drugs and inappropriate use of licit drugs, and engaging in programs of prevention, treatment, and rehabilitation.

Understanding early predictors of adolescent substance use (ASU) and the transitions involved in the progression to adolescent psychoactive substance use disorders (APSUDs) is critical for effective prevention. Defining target populations, outcome goals, and measurements for effective prevention strategies and programs is also necessary. The resources and participants to be enlisted in the prevention endeavors need to be defined and may be drawn from many sources, including immediate families, schools, community organizations, policy makers, and the media.

This chapter utilizes data reviewed earlier in this book regarding the onset and development of ASU and APSUDs to address the present state of and future perspective for effective prevention. The chapter also reviews adolescent suicide prevention because of the high incidence of suicidal behavior among adolescents with PSUDs. Successful efforts to reduce the prevalence of substance abuse can be utilized to introduce prevention–intervention in suicidal and other high-risk behaviors.

9.1. ETIOLOGICAL DETERMINANTS

A considerable body of literature concerning the etiological determinants of substance use, abuse, and dependence has been published, although most of the publications failed to discriminate among the levels of involvement. Most users to not make the transition to become abusers; therefore, it is crucial to understand the roles and the mechanisms of the factors responsible for the development of ASU vs. APSUDs. A detailed discussion of these factors is beyond the purpose of this chapter and is presented in other chapters. However, it is worthwhile to briefly review the pivotal factors and conceptual framework responsible for this transition.

Genetic markers and twin and adoption studies provide evidence for the heritability of the liability for alcoholism and to a lesser extent for other PSUDs. The individual at risk is exposed immediately after birth and throughout life to environmental risk and protective factors. Among the most influential environmental factors are family, school, and peers. Psychopathology such as PSUDs may be the result of interactions of temperamental predisposition (e.g., difficult temperament) with environmental factors. However, there is a bidirectional "threshold effect" that may expose the child to the results of increased risk or corrective experiences that from the standpoint of intervention may, respectively, enable or cause the individual to return to the "under-the-threshold" range or to remain in/progress to the "beyond-the-threshold" range (Tarter & Mezzich, 1992).

As the child matures, flexibility of behavioral repertoire diminishes, because habitual patterns of behavior become more and more firmly established. This crystallization of responses to environmental stimuli and interaction style makes interventions increasingly difficult to apply (Tarter, 1992). If this stabilization of deviance happens "under the threshold," it demands intervention in the form of prevention. However, if it occurs "beyond the threshold," treatment is the intervention of choice. Thus, from a pragmatic perspective, it appears that prevention and treatment are two subsets of intervention curricula that are to be applied at different chronological and severity points on the continuum of the subclinical phenomenon and the clinical disorder.

9.1.1. Individual Attributes as Risk Factors

The 1986 Anti-Drug Abuse Act defined high-risk youth (Clayton, 1992, p. 16) as

> children and teenagers under age 18 who, because of the presence of certain characteristics and conditions, are especially likely to use illegal drugs and/or alcohol.

This definition recognizes "characteristics" (i.e., constitutional traits) and "conditions" (i.e., environmental circumstances) as instrumental for the development of PSUDs. The nine risk factors included in the 1986 Act are as follows: (1) the economically disadvantaged; (2) children of substance-abusing parents; victims of (3) physical, (4) sexual, or (5) psychological abuse; (6) runaways or homeless youth; (7) school dropouts; (8) pregnant adolescents; and (9) adolescents who have attempted suicide. As Clayton (1992) noted, these are the "types" of children and adolescents for whom services are rendered in the communities. There is also a certain level of confusion in these risk factors, however, because most of them could serve as effects as well as causes of PSUDs, depending on the temporal ordering and direction of the relationship. These risk factors are in accord with the conceptual framework presented in the problem-behavior theory (Jessor & Jessor, 1977) and with the increasingly recognized reality that adolescents at high risk for PSUDs or who have already developed PSUDs have multiple problems or deviant behaviors such as delinquency, suicidal behavior, unplanned pregnancy, and more.

9.2. A CRITICAL REVIEW OF CURRENT PREVENTION APPROACHES FOR ADOLESCENT SUBSTANCE USE AND ADOLESCENT PSYCHOACTIVE SUBSTANCE USE DISORDERS

There is a growing recognition that the present prevention approaches to ASU and APSUDs are deficient. The greatest concern is that the multifactorial determinants that contribute to the manifestation of the disorders are not fully recognized or acknowledged (Tarter, 1992). Furthermore, the paucity of studies that carefully define the target population and the outcome goals for prevention by addressing specific behaviors, and the lack of control groups, leave the arena to simplistic and mostly untested prevention strategies that do not serve the most needy youth at risk for APSUDs.

The most common approaches to primary or early prevention are media campaigns and education programs. The goal of primary prevention among children and adolescents is to defer or preclude initiation of drug use, especially cigarettes, alcohol, and marijuana. These targeted "gateway" drugs (Kandel, 1982) serve as "villains" based on the fear-arousal model of prevention (Goodstadt, 1980). Even experimental use of these drugs is portrayed as dangerous, especially in mass media campaigns. Films and videos that dramatize the risks associated with drug use are usually utilized. The traditional education program is a prevention strategy used mainly in the form of information dissemination. An approach making use of informative materials to increase knowledge of the consequences of drug use, and promotion of an antidrug attitude in a classroom setting accompanied by displays of substances and relevant literature, is common.

These approaches to prevention among children and adolescents were found to be ineffective by empirical studies, as reviewed by Schinke, Botvin, and Orlani (1991). The assumption that increased knowledge will decrease drug use was found to be invalid. In fact, there were reports that this approach may serve to increase adolescents' curiosity, which may initiate substance use (Swisher, 1979).

Media campaigns may tackle prevention by aiming at reducing harmful behaviors related to drinking. Success in the decrease of injuries related to drunk driving suggests that media intervention with motivated individuals is effective (Nathan, 1990). At the same time, however, the media indirectly provoke the adolescent to seek out cigarettes and alcohol by portraying the products as harmless and "cool" to use (e.g., Joe Camel, beer commercials). Coate and Grossman (1987) reported that use of alcohol by youths declines when either the price of alcoholic beverages or the legal drinking age increases. This finding should encourage community efforts to influence appropriate legislation.

Affective education, designed to increase self-esteem and enhance responsible decision-making and personal growth, was another approach to prevention in the 1970s. No information on drugs was included in the program, yet the expectation was that the youngsters would be able to make the right decision regarding drug use (Swisher,

1979). Also, the idea that alternative activities offered to adolescents would substitute for drug use was presented in the early 1980s (Swisher & Hu, 1983). Athletic, academic, and vocational programs were the most commonly offered alternatives.

Both approaches, i.e., affective education and alternative activities, were found to be ineffective in the prevention of drug use. In fact, in the quest for a "natural high," as experienced in wilderness programs and in some entertainment and vocational programs, there were reports of increased substance abuse (Schinke et al., 1991). Reports regarding the ineffectuality of these approaches to primary prevention were supported by two recent publications (Pentz, Dwyer, & MacKinnon, 1989; Tobler, 1986). It was concluded that a unidimensional approach to prevention in an extremely heterogeneous population is likely to be ineffective for a large percentage of participants (Tarter, 1992).

A more advanced strategy for prevention is based on a psychosocial approach. These prevention programs are aimed at enhancing self-esteem (Schaps, Moskowitz, & Malvin, 1986) and social skills (Botvin, Baker, & Filazzola, 1990). These strategies are employed as part of primary, secondary, and tertiary prevention strategies and usually utilize manuals in group settings. Such strategies are rooted in social-learning theory (Bandura, 1977) and problem-behavior theory (Jessor & Jessor, 1977).

According to the social-learning theory, individuals learn how to behave according to a four-component model: (1) role modeling, (2) reinforcement, (3) establishment of normative expectations, and (4) coping with social pressure. A fifth component is sometimes employed, i.e., training for generalization. A program entitled "Life Skills Training" based on the social-learning theory was developed by Botvin, Baker, and Renick (1984). The program was taught to 6th and 7th graders, at times led by peers, and resulted in significant improvements.

The problem-behavior theory derives from a sociopsychological framework and recognizes the importance of the complex interaction of personal factors (cognition, attitudes, beliefs), physiological genetic factors, and perceived environmental factors to problems occurring during adolescence, such as drug use, precocious sexual behavior, and delinquency (Donovan & Jessor, 1985). A problem behavior is one that is identified as a problem within the context of a particular value system and that elicits a social response designed to control it. Substance use, therefore, helps the adolescent to achieve personal goals such as peer group approval and alleviation of discomfort in interpersonal or intrapersonal conflicts.

Programs designed to increase awareness of social influence to use drugs, and to reduce anxiety, enhance social and assertive skills, encourage resistance to substance use, and change attitudes and beliefs were reported to reduce smoking initiation up to 50% in 1-year follow-up studies (Botvin et al., 1990). Other reports of substantial reduction in the prevalence of experimental smoking ranging from 42% to 75% cited the use of prevention approaches based on the social-learning theory and the problem-behavior theory (Schinke & Gilchrist, 1983).

A critical review of these results was provided with the addition of two well-designed studies of prevention programs based on the socialization model (Ellickson & Bell, 1990; Pentz et al., 1989). These findings indicated that although previous reports were able to demonstrate reduction of experimental use, they failed to successfully enhance secondary prevention. An earlier review by Flay (1985) is in accord with these findings.

Walter, Vaughan, and Cohall (1991) found that most of the theories aimed at accounting for various aspects of drug-using behavior can be organized into three primary models of substance use: (1) socialization (Huba, Wingard, & Bentler, 1980); (2) stress/strain, known also as self-medication (Khantzian, 1985); and (3) disaffiliation (Jessor & Jessor, 1977). They reported that in a sample of 1091 10th-grade students, the measured risk factors most strongly associated with the use of drugs were derived from these three models (mainly, however, from the socialization model). A similar approach was taken by Weber, Graham, Hansen, Flay, and Johnson (1989). They defined adolescents who are predisposed to more rapid alcohol use onset as Type 2, compared to more normally socialized adolescents termed Type 1. Type 2 adolescents were hypothesized to have a problem-behavior-prone orientation (Jessor & Jessor, 1977).

This study emphasizes that risk status is not necessarily the same for all individuals. It appears that the drawback in prevention programs based on the social-learning theory and the problem-behavior theory is the underlying assumption that these adolescents' characteristics or deficiencies are somehow linked causally to initiation of drug use (Tarter, 1992). This assumption—that drug consumption is prompted by one or more highly salient risk factors such as low self-esteem, lack of social skills, or emotional distress in different individuals—negates the logic for the prevention program implemented (i.e., provide the same menu to all participants). Not surprisingly, these types of prevention programs alone have not yet proven to be effective in follow-up.

So far, it appears that primary prevention programs to defer or prevent initiation of drug use among children and adolescents in the form of experimental or recreational use have had modest success at best, especially among children and adolescents who are not at high risk for substance abuse and dependence. However, in addressing secondary prevention (aimed to deter further use and avoiding abuse) and tertiary prevention (aimed to end abuse and dependence or to ameliorate its effects through treatment), no clinically and statistically meaningful results have been demonstrated.

The reason for the poor success rate in secondary prevention may be that prevention requires individualized intervention due to the adolescent's specific vulnerabilities that predispose him or her to substance abuse. To date, individualized prevention–interventions have not been adopted despite the recognition of drug-abuse etiology as multifactorial (biopsychosocial) in nature. Tarter (1992, p. 4) argues that there are at least three reasons that they have not been:

> 1) the emphasis has been on program content rather than on characteristics of individuals, 2) the state of professional development of prevention specialists has not progressed to a level at which skills are easily adapted for individualized interventions; and 3) institutional and professional environments are neither sensitized to nor prepared for detection of individuals at high risk for drug abuse.

Before starting any individualized program, it is important to identify children and adolescents at risk for APSUDs. Late detection of these youngsters after initiation of substance abuse will require treatment. Children with one or both biological parents diagnosed with PSUD are at up to 10-fold greater risk of developing the same disorder (Tarter, 1992). The transmission of genetic vulnerability to alcoholism Type 2 (male-limited) was presented by Cloninger (1987). This subpopulation of male alcoholics is characterized by early onset of problematic drinking, aggressive behavior, high sensation-seeking behavior, low harm avoidance, and low reward dependence and calls for prevention–intervention as early as possible, preferably before aggressive behavior has been manifested.

Children with conduct disorder (CD) that continues to express itself as antisocial personality disorder (ASPD) in adulthood have an odds ratio of >21 to be diagnosed as substance abusers (Helzer & Pryzbeck, 1988). About 25% of children diagnosed with attention deficit hyperactivity disorder (ADHD) develop CD (Mannuzza, Klein, Bonagura, Malloy, Giampino, & Addalli, 1991) and are therefore at increased risk for substance abuse (Kaminer, 1992). Early-intervention programs are needed to decrease the odds of developing CD and PSUDs in the high-risk population of children and adolescents with ADHD and their families.

Children who themselves are or whose parents are diagnosed with mood disorders, schizophrenia, anxiety disorders, bulimia, and ASPD (adults only) and adolescents with cluster B personality disorders are also at high risk of developing PSUDs (Bukstein, Brent, & Kaminer, 1989). Traumatized children and adolescents who have been exposed to aggression (physical or sexual or both) in the family or in their immediate environment or those who have come from a dysfunctional family are at risk for PSUDs as well.

The intervention in children and adolescents at risk should start by enhancing the motivation of the child or adolescent and the caretakers to participate in a prevention program before the initiation of drug use. The objective of the intervention is to change the specific components of vulnerability within both the individual and the environment. Stable remission of a psychiatric disorder in the adolescent or in the caretaker, or in both, is a key to meaningful intervention. A hypothesis to be tested is that prevention for individuals at risk for PSUDs appears to command the same principles as those for intervention and a curriculum comparable to but less intense than that for treatment of PSUDs. Research has yet to report the results of a study that would aim at prevention–intervention for children at risk for PSUDs and their caretakers. A control group of matched children and caretakers without a known family history of PSUDs and other risk factors for APSUDs may improve the scientific merit of such a study.

9.3. SUICIDE PREVENTION

The efforts to prevent suicide have led to the development of primary, secondary, and tertiary prevention–intervention programs. Primary prevention programs are usually education- or curriculum-based courses. Secondary prevention of suicide focuses on identification and referral of at-risk youth, and the aim of tertiary prevention is to provide crisis intervention and treatment for suicide attempters.

9.3.1. Education Programs

Education- or curriculum-based programs are very popular in schools, and their number increased dramatically in the 1980s and early 1990s. Their main goals, according to Garland and Zigler (1993), are (1) to raise awareness of the problem of adolescent suicide, (2) to train participants to identify adolescents at risk of suicide, and (3) to educate participants about community mental health resources and referral techniques. These programs are most commonly directed to high school students and their teachers and parents.

The curriculum of a program commonly includes a review of the epidemiology of suicidal behavior, identification of "warning signs" of suicidal behavior, and discussion of depression. Referral systems and referral techniques, the importance of confidentiality, and problem-solving as well as stress-reduction skills are also addressed.

Like programs for prevention of substance abuse, suicide-prevention programs that operate mostly at school may never reach the adolescent high-risk population they are targeting. These adolescents are high school dropouts, teens with mental disorders, and others who are also at increased risk for suicide. It has been noted that many suicide victims are likely to have been absent from school before their suicidal act (Hawton, 1986), as compared to students who regularly attend school and are not at high risk for suicidal behavior.

The effectiveness of suicide-prevention programs has been evaluated and published so far only in two large controlled studies that included only self-report measures of knowledge and attitude variables (Shaffer, Garland, Vieland, Underwood, & Busner, 1991; Spirito, Overholser, Ashworth, Morgan, & Benedict-Drew, 1988). Shaffer et al. (1991) found only a few positive effects and a possible negative effect on a minority of students who responded that suicide could be a possible solution to problems. Students most at risk for suicide (those who reported on a previous attempt) found the programs upsetting, and even good attendance in the sessions did not affect their attitude, nor was there a reduction in self-reported suicidal ideations or attempts. Spirito et al. (1988) indicated that the program improved knowledge only minimally and was ineffective in changing attitudes. Boys, who complete suicide more commonly than girls, reported changes in the undesirable direction, such as increased hopelessness and maladaptive coping responses following exposure to the suicide-prevention program (Overholser, Hemstreet, Spirito, & Vyse, 1989).

Garland, Shaffer, and Whittle (1989) revealed that most suicide-prevention programs used a stress model of suicide rather than a mental health model (i.e., construing suicide as a reaction to stress rather than as a result of psychopathology). The rationale for this approach is "destigmatization" of suicide and an emphasis that the vulnerability to suicide is universal. Hoberman and Garfinkel (1988) reported that such an approach is likely to generate ineffective prevention intervention. Garland and Zigler (1993, p. 174) criticize the attempt to destigmatize suicide because "in this way these programs misrepresent the facts and may be, in fact, normalizing the behavior and reducing potentially protective taboos."

Two more aspects of curriculum-based programs have been criticized. The first is the tendency to inflate the reported incidence of adolescent suicide in order to increase awareness and concern about the problem. Garland and Zigler (1993) find this trend unnecessary and risky. They find it unnecessary because surveys of teens indicate that they are aware of the problem. They find it risky because adolescents may perceive suicide as a more common act than previously imagined and therefore may react in one of two ways: They may either view suicidal behavior as acceptable or become overanxious about the possibility of suicide among their peer group.

The second controversial aspect is the use of case histories of adolescents who have attempted or committed suicide. This method may have a paradoxical effect on teens who struggle with various life difficulties and may come to see suicide as a possible solution to their own problems (Garland & Zigler, 1993). Indirect empirical support for this concern was provided by Gibson and Range (1991), although girls responded more positively to help-seeking behaviors while boys responded more positively to suicidal behavior. Further evaluation of curriculum-based programs is needed, and more progressive models assessing behavioral variables and promoting help-seeking behaviors are warranted.

9.3.2. Secondary Prevention

Identification and referral for intervention or treatment of adolescents at risk for suicide is the focus of secondary prevention. Following a suicide or a suicide attempt by an adolescent, there is an increased risk for subsequent outbreaks of suicidal behavior by friends or adolescents from the same school who are at risk (Brent, Kerr, Goldstein, Bozigar, Wartell, & Allan, 1989). Screening and referral for further treatment of students at risk for suicide following two suicides in the same high school proved to be effective (Brent et al., 1989). It is essential that mental health professionals, physicians, nurses, and teachers be trained for increased awareness to suicidal behavior and knowledge about the referral process and system. Professionals who work with youth at risk, such as runaways, juvenile delinquents, and psychiatric patients, must acquire diagnostic and intervention skills. Training programs for settings that host such populations have been developed and have been shown to be effective (Rotheram-Borus & Bradley, 1991).

9.3.3. Tertiary Prevention

The most prevalent types of suicide-prevention programs are crisis-intervention services. Of these, telephone hotlines are the most popular.

There are currently more than 1000 suicide hotlines in the United States that offer services to adolescents (Garland et al., 1989). Garland and Zigler (1993) explained that the rationale behind these centers is based on the need for interpersonal communication as a last-minute "cry for help" of a person who is ambivalent about suicide. On the basis of empirical research, there has been a consensus about the capability of hotlines to reduce suicidal behavior that they are minimally effective, and then only among young white women, who are the most frequent users of these services (Miller, Coombs, & Leeper, 1984).

People who advocate hotline services argue that they have been shown to reach a population not served by any other mental health intervention and that they may appeal to adolescents because of the adolescent-perceived control of the situation as an anonymous caller (Garland & Zigler, 1993).

9.3.4. Suicide-Prevention Policymaking and the Media

The media should be educated about the social-imitation effects of suicide. Responsible reports about suicide by the media and a consensus about what not to expose (preferably following consultation and exchange of information with recognized suicidologists in the community) would be beneficial. Reduced availability of means for suicide, especially firearms, is crucial because the risk of suicide among adolescents has been found to be nearly three times greater in homes where a gun is kept (Brent, Perper, Allman, Moritz, Wartella, & Zelenak, 1991; Sloan, Rivara, Reay, Ferris, Path, & Kellermann, 1990). There is no time to waste in waiting for a stricter Federal gun control law, if and when it is to materialize. Laws ordering safer and separate storage of guns and ammunition, and courses for improved safety measures by gun owners and firearms sellers, are crucial. Garland and Zigler (1993) presented Connecticut's Public Act 90-144 as a model. This act requires gun dealers to provide buyers with trigger locks and makes the unsafe storage of weapons a felony.

9.3.5. Prevention of Adolescent Psychoactive Substance Use Disorders, Suicide, and Other Problem Behaviors

The known risks for suicide among adolescents are also associated with other teen problems/behaviors such as APSUDs, dropping out of school, delinquency, and unplanned pregnancy. APSUD rates are much higher than suicide rates, and therefore any successful intervention aimed at reducing the prevalence of APSUDs would in fact be a preferred preventive intervention for suicide, as well as for other problems that affect youth (Garland & Zigler, 1993). Prevention efforts for suicide could be focused on the underlying constructs that are risk factors for these behaviors, such as depression, lack of social support, or poor problem-solving skills.

Family support programs are important in order to improve primary prevention of deviant behaviors and harmful consequences for children and adolescents. Family support programs are diverse and include grass roots movements, voluntary organizations and a variety of agencies. These programs provide services ranging from empowerment of families by social support and improving parental skills to early interventions with young children at risk for APSUDs, delinquency, and other problems. Parents also need to learn how to identify substance use and APSUDs in their children. Student assistance programs, community groups, and local agencies and school systems should provide an appropriate setting for primary prevention programs for parents and children. Many schools may offer programs on substance abuse, suicide, sex education, and other topics.

The Secretary of Health and Human Services Task Force on Youth Suicide recommended that "suicide prevention activities should be integrated into broader health promotion programs and health care delivery services directed at preventing other self-destructive behaviors, such as alcohol and substance abuse, teen pregnancy, and interpersonal violence" (Alcohol, Drug Abuse, and Mental Health Administration, 1989, p. 3).

As Garland and Zigler (1993) summarize this issue, it seems logical that prevention programs focused at improving the well-being of adolescents will have a wider scope of success than those that address specific behaviors that are multidetermined. Also, they will probably reduce the need for and costs of multiple individual services. Policymakers should support and provide resources for such primary prevention programs. Also, resources should be channeled to prevention-oriented research that will address questions such as these: how to improve resilience of high-risk children for deviant behaviors and psychopathology; how to assess and improve the efficacy of prevention programs and public policies regarding PSUDs, delinquency, suicide reduction, and other related problems; and how to assess the cost-effectiveness of prevention programs, including how to address goal definition within a cost-effectiveness model.

Finally, policy makers and health promotion agencies need to ensure that prevention programs reflect current empirical knowledge of goal-oriented intervention for their targeted population as a prerequisite for financial support.

9.4. CHILDREN OF ALCOHOLICS: CLINICAL UTILITY OF THE CONCEPT FOR PREVENTION AND ETHICS

A large number of American adolescents are the offspring of alcoholic parents. An estimate of more than 6.5 million was reported in a publication by the Children of Alcoholics Foundation (Russell, Henderson, & Blume, 1984). Families of alcoholics were reported to have lower levels of family cohesion, expressiveness, independence, and intellectual orientation and higher levels of conflict than nonalcoholic families (Kumpfer & DeMarsh, 1986). However, many of these characteristics are not specific to alcoholic families and are common across the range of dysfunctional families (Gordis, 1990).

The rich tradition of self-help groups and the Children of Alcoholics movement provided information about the difficulties and life events experienced by individuals who grew up in an alcoholic home. The concept of children of alcoholics (COAs) has gained significant acceptance and has helped many persons who have shared the camaraderie established in the movement. However, there is a growing literature that criticizes the popular diagnostic categorization of COAs, and doubts the clinical utility and benefits attributed to interventions with these individuals. There is also concern that the COAs movement is exploited for political and commercial reasons in a pattern that is similar to the exploitation by religious organizations for profit.

Critics have focused on methodological problems that limit the ability to determine the process by which COAs are affected. The main reason for their criticism is that alcoholism is commonly associated with other stressors in the family, including such factors as divorce, single parenthood, and blended families, and the challenge of disentangling these multiple factors has yet to be addressed (Devine & Braithwaite, 1993).

The fact that most COAs are protected from the adverse effects of alcoholism does not always fit some of the popular models that characterize COAs and even guide intervention programs for these children and adolescents. Black (1979) and Wegscheider (1976) stated that all children are adversely affected by alcoholism and therefore adopt certain dysfunctional roles to protect themselves from additional trauma within the family. These roles do not survive the maturation process of adulthood and lead to a dysfunctional adult life. Devine and Braithwaite (1993) investigated the five types of coping roles described by Black (1979) and Wegscheider (1976): (1) responsible child, (2) lost child, (3) acting-out child, (4) placater, and (5) clown. Their study provided qualified support for the five types of survival roles but could not link them exclusively with parental alcoholism. It is suggested that individual temperament may have an effect in determining reactions to family stress. For example, the extrovert may be more likely to take on the acting-out or clown role, while the introvert may be more likely to become the lost child.

Fulton and Yates (1990) also found only limited support for the validity of the COA concept in adult inpatients treated for substance abuse. Burk and Sher (1990) reported that both mental health professionals and peers labeled known adolescent COAs more negatively than non-COAs regardless of their current behavior. These negative stereotypes were robust and potentially harmful.

In order to recognize the advantages of not viewing a child or adolescent who is a COA as a miniature adult COA, it is helpful to refer to a thoughtful paper published by Wilson and Crowe (1991). The authors suggest that the diagnosis of genetic predisposition to alcoholism and the identification of youth at risk raise several practical and ethical dilemmas: Can those at risk be systematically and effectively identified? What are the possible interventions and the potential consequences of these interventions? An ethical issue is raised as to whether youths at risk should be identified, given the possible negative psychosocial consequences to follow.

Wilson and Crowe (1991) tackled this issue, not with the intention of deterring research on etiology and prevention of alcoholism, but in order to emphasize the human factor involved and put the high-risk individual at center stage. They reassessed two important adoption studies in order to answer some practical questions (Cloninger, Sigvardsson, & Bohman, 1988; Goodwin, Schulsinger, Hermanson, Guze, & Winokur, 1973). Goodwin et al. (1973) reported a 33% incidence of alcoholism among the sons of alcoholic fathers, a rate that is more than 4 times higher than that among sons of nonalcoholics. Another way to examine these results, however, is to conclude that two thirds of the sons of alcoholics investigated in this study *did not* become alcoholics.

Cloninger et al. (1988) reevaluated a cohort that had been assessed at age 11 on personality dimensions relevant to Cloninger's Type 1 and Type 2 classification of alcoholism. The authors confirmed the association between Type 2 and the personality dimensions that were hypothesized to characterize it: high novelty-seeking, low harm avoidance, and low reward dependence (Cloninger, 1987). Moreover, the authors' theory accurately predicted 97% of those at risk from among the persons who had measured at the extreme on all three personality dimensions. However, it is noteworthy that this high success of prediction is reserved for groups and not for individuals. It was recommended that probability of risk, rather than high vs. low risk, should be used when assessing an individual's potential for alcoholism because of the high false-positive individual predictions based on childhood personality (Wilson & Crowe, 1991).

Given the equivocal long-term results of prevention programs (Tarter, 1992) and the fact that most children of alcoholics, according to the Goodwin et al. (1973) study, do not need any intervention, while future alcoholic sons of nonalcoholic parents are overlooked, the purpose of prevention efforts appears dubious and unfocused at best. Children of alcoholics are frequently stigmatized and discriminated against by peers, teachers, and the community (Kumpfer & DeMarsh, 1986). Also, predictions of future development of alcoholism may serve as self-fulfilling prophecies. Consequently, the ethical question regarding the identification of youths at risk is not just a philosophical one of right or wrong. The question has become a risk vs. effectiveness equation wherein the need for intervention should outweigh the risk of harm in order to advocate intervention. It also remains to be determined whose decision it is to place a high-risk individual in a prevention program and what happens if the individual or the family/caretaker disagrees with this decision. Such a scenario could lead to a legal nightmare, especially for poor and disenfranchised populations. This dilemma is not limited to alcoholism, but affects the prevention–intervention efforts vis-à-vis other high-risk problems/behaviors as well.

Even if and when the means to identify and intervene with individuals at risk improve dramatically, concerns regarding autonomy, privacy, and justice will still be valid (Wilson & Crowe, 1991).

9.5. CONCLUSION

Interactions between vulnerability and environmental factors determine pathways to an outcome that, in its worst form, will be an APSUD. Temperament, psychosocial development, personality aspects, family, peer group life-style, sociocultural mores, substance availability, and regulatory policies are the pivotal factors that impact the risk of developing APSUDs (Tarter, 1992). Any intervention to arrest or interfere with the developmental processes that lead to APSUDs must consider these factors, particularly the adolescent life-style as a whole. Finally, the human factor should be carefully considered for the design of an efficacious and yet ethical intervention for the child at risk and his or her family.

REFERENCES

Alcohol, Drug Abuse, and Mental Health Administration (1989). *Report of the Secretary Task Force on Youth Suicide*, Vol. 1, *Overview and Recommendations*. DHHS publication No. ADM89-1621. Washington, DC: U.S. Government Printing Office.

Bandura, A. (1977). *Social Learning Theory*. Englewood Cliffs, NJ: Prentice Hall.

Black, C. (1979). Children of alcoholics. *Alcohol Health and Research, 4*, 23–27.

Board of Trustees of the American Medical Association (1991). Drug abuse in the United States: Strategies for prevention. *Journal of the American Medical Association, 265*, 2101–2107.

Botvin, G., Baker, E., & Filazzola, A. (1990). A cognitive behavioral approach to substance abuse prevention: One year follow-up. *Addictive Behaviors, 15*, 47–63.

Botvin, G., Baker, E., & Renick, N. (1984). A cognitive behavioral approach to substance abuse prevention. *Addictive Behaviors, 9*, 137–147.

Brent, D. A., Kerr, M. M., Goldstein, C. E., Bozigar, J., Wartell, M., & Allan, M. A. (1989). An outbreak of suicide and suicidal behavior in a high school. *Journal of the American Academy of Child and Adolescent Psychiatry, 28*, 918–924.

Brent, D. A., Perper, J. A., Allman, C. J., Moritz, G. M., Wartella, M. E., & Zelenak, J. P. (1991). The presence and accessibility of firearms in the homes of adolescent suicides. *Journal of the American Medical Association, 266*, 2989–2995.

Bukstein, O. G., Brent, D. A., & Kaminer, Y. (1989). Comorbidity of substance abuse and other psychiatric disorders in adolescents. *American Journal of Psychiatry, 146*, 1131–1141.

Burk, J. P., & Sher, K. J. (1990). Labeling the child of an alcoholic: Negative stereotyping by mental health professionals and peers. *Journal of Studies on Alcohol, 51*, 156–163.

Clayton, R. R. (1992). Transitions in drug use: Risk and protective factors. In M. Glantz & R. Pickens (Eds.), *Vulnerability to Drug Abuse* (pp. 15–51). Washington, DC: American Psychological Association.

Cloninger, C. R. (1987). Neurogenetic adaptive mechanisms in alcoholism. *Science, 236*, 410–416.

Cloninger, C. R. Sigvardsson, S., & Bohman, M. (1988). Childhood personality predicts alcohol abuse in young adults. *Alcoholism, Clinical and Experimental Research, 12*, 494–505.

Coate, D., Grossman, N. (1987). Change in alcoholic beverage prices and legal drinking age. *Alcohol Health Research World, 11*, 22–25.

Devine, C., & Braithwaite, V. (1993). The survival role of children of alcoholics: Their measurement and validity. *Addiction, 88*, 69–78.

Donovan, J. E., & Jessor, R. (1985). Structure of problem behavior in adolescence and young adulthood. *Journal of Consulting and Clinical Psychology, 53*, 890–904.

Ellickson, P. L., & Bell, R. M. (1990). Drug prevention in junior high: A multisite longitudinal test. *Science, 16*, 1299–1305.

Flay, B. R. (1985). Psychosocial approaches to smoking prevention: A review of findings. *Health Psychology, 4*, 449–488.

Fulton, A. I., & Yates, W. R. (1990). Adult children of alcoholics: A valid diagnostic group? *Journal of Nervous and Mental Disease, 178*, 505–509.

Garland, A. F., & Zigler, E. (1993). Adolescent suicide prevention: Current research and social policy implications. *American Psychologist, 48*, 169–182.

Garland, A., Shaffer, D., & Whittle, B. (1989). A national survey of adolescent suicide prevention programs. *Journal of the American Academy of Child and Adolescent Psychiatry, 28*, 931–934.

Gibson, J. A. P., & Range, L. M. (1991). Are written reports of suicide and seeking help contagious? High schoolers' perceptions. *Journal of Applied Social Psychology, 21*, 1517–1523.

Goodstadt, M. S. (1980). Drug education: A turn on or a turn off? *Journal of Drug Education, 10*, 89–99.

Goodwin, D. W., Schulsinger, F., Hermanson, L., Guze, S. B., & Winokur, G. (1973). Alcohol problems in adoptees raised apart from alcoholic biological parents. *Archives of General Psychiatry, 28*, 238–243.

Gordis, E. (1990). Children of alcoholics: Are they different? *Alcohol Alert, 9*, 3.

Hawton, K. (1986). *Suicide and Attempted Suicide among Children and Adolescents.* Newbury Park, CA: Sage.

Helzer, J. E., & Pryzbeck, T. R. (1988). The co-occurrence of alcoholism with other psychiatric disorders in the general population and its impact on treatment. *Journal of Studies on Alcohol, 49*, 219–224.

Hoberman, H. M., & Garfinkel, B. D. (1988). Completed suicide in children and adolescents. *Journal of the American Academy of Child and Adolescent Psychiatry, 27*, 689–695.

Huba, G. J., Wingard, J. A., & Bentler, P. M. (1980). Applications of a theory of drug use to prevention programs. *Journal of Drug Education, 10*, 25–38.

Jessor, R., & Jessor, S. L. (1977). *Problem Behavior and Psychosocial Development: A Longitudinal Study of Youth.* New York: Academic Press.

Kaminer, Y. (1992). Clinical implications of the relationship between attention deficit hyperactivity disorder (ADHD) and psychoactive substance use disorders (PSUD). *American Journal on Addictions, 1*, 257–264.

Kandel, D. B. (1982). Epidemiological and psychosocial perspective on adolescent drug use. *Journal of the American Academy of Child and Adolescent Psychiatry, 20*, 328–347.

Khantzian, E. J. (1985). The self-medication hypothesis of addictive disorders: Focus on heroin and cocaine dependence. *American Journal of Psychiatry, 142*, 1259–1264.

Kumpfer, K. L., & DeMarsh, J. (1986). Family environmental and genetic influences on children's future chemical dependency. *Journal of Children in Contemporary Society, 18*, 49–92.

Mannuzza, S., Klein, R. G., Bonagura, N., Malloy, P., Giampino, T. L., & Addalli, K. A. (1991). Hyperactive boys almost grown up: V. Replication of psychiatric status. *Archives of General Psychiatry, 48*, 77–83.

Miller, H. L., Coombs, D. W., & Leeper, J. D. (1984). An analysis of the effects of suicide prevention facilities on suicide rates in the United States. *American Journal of Public Health, 74*, 340–343.

Nathan, P. E. (1990). Integration of biological and psychosocial research on alcoholism. *Alcoholism, Clinical and Experimental Research, 14*, 368–374.

Overholser, J., Hemstreet, A. H., Spirito, A., & Vyse, S. (1989). Suicide awareness programs in schools: Effects of gender and personal experience. *Journal of the American Academy of Child and Adolescent Psychiatry, 28*, 925–930.

Pentz, M. A., Dwyer, J. H., & MacKinnon, D. P. (1989). A multicommunity trial for primary prevention of adolescent drug abuse. *Journal of the American Medical Association, 261,* 3259–3266.

Rotheram-Borus, M. J., & Bradley, J. (1991). Triage model for suicidal runaways. *American Journal of Orthopsychiatry, 61,* 122–127.

Russell, M., Henderson, C., & Blume, S. B. (1984). *Children of Alcoholics: A Review of the Literature.* New York: Children of Alcoholics Foundation.

Schaps, E., Moskowitz, J., & Malvin, J. (1986). Evaluation of seven school based prevention programs: A final report on the Napa project. *International Journal of the Addictions, 21,* 1081–1112.

Schinke, S. P., Botvin, G. J., & Orlani, M. A. (1991). *Substance Abuse in Children and Adolescents: Evaluation and Intervention.* Newbury Park, CA: Sage.

Schinke, S. P., & Gilchrist, L. D. (1983). Primary prevention of tobacco smoking. *Journal of School Health, 53,* 416–419.

Shaffer, D., Garland, A., Vieland, V., Underwood, M., & Busner, C. (1991). The impact of curriculum-based suicide prevention programs for teenagers. *Journal of the American Academy of Child and Adolescent Psychiatry, 30,* 588–596.

Sloan, J.H., Rivara, F. P., Reay, D. T., Ferris, J. A. J., Path, M. R. C., & Kellermann, A. L. (1990). Firearm regulations and rates of suicide: A comparison of two metropolitan areas. *New England Journal of Medicine, 322,* 369–373.

Spirito, A., Overholser, J., Ashworth, S., Morgan, J., & Benedict-Drew, C. (1988). Evaluation of a suicide awareness curriculum for high school students. *Journal of the American Academy of Child and Adolescent Psychiatry, 27,* 705–711.

Swisher, J. D. (1979). Prevention issues. In R. I. Dupont, A. Goldstein, & J. O'Donnell (Eds.), *Handbook on Drug Abuse* (pp. 49–62). Washington, DC: U.S. Government Printing Office.

Swisher, J. D., & Hu, T. W. (1983). Alternative to drug abuse: Some are and some are not. In T. S. Glynn, C. G. Leukefeld, & J. P. Ludford (Eds.), *Preventing Adolescent Drug Abuse: Intervention Strategies* (pp. 93–117). Washington, DC: U.S. Government Printing Office.

Tarter, R. E. (1992). Prevention of drug abuse: Theory and application. *American Journal on Addictions, 1,* 2–20.

Tarter, R., & Mezzich, A. C. (1992). Ontogeny of Substance abuse: Perspectives and findings. In M. Glantz & R. Pickens (Eds.), *Vulnerability to Drug Abuse* (pp. 149–178). Washington, DC: American Psychological Association.

Tobler, N. S. (1986). Meta-analysis of 143 adolescent drug prevention programs: Quantitative outcome results of program participants compared to a control or comparison group. *Journal of Drug Issues, 16,* 537–567.

Walter, H. J., Vaughan, R. D., & Cohall, A. T. (1991). Risk factors for substance use among high school students: Implications for prevention. *Journal of the American Academy of Child and Adolescent Psychiatry, 30,* 556–562.

Weber, M. D., Graham, J. W., Hansen, W. B., Flay, B. R., & Johnson, C. A. (1989). Evidence for two paths of alcohol use onset in adolescents. *Addictive Behaviors, 14,* 399–408.

Wegscheider, S. (1976). *The family trap . . . . No one escapes from a chemically dependent family.* Minneapolis, MN: Johnson Institute.

Wilson, J. R., & Crowe, L. (1991). Genetics of alcoholism: Can and should youth at risk be identified? *Alcohol Health & Research World, 15,* 11–17.

CHAPTER 10

The Assessment Process

A comprehensive, methodical, and objective evaluation of the adolescent with psychoactive substance use disorder (APSUD) is necessary for the development of an effective treatment plan. A detailed assessment of the adolescent, caretakers, and referral systems is important to understanding the functioning of the adolescent in various life domains, his or her motivation for treatment, severity of APSUD, medical and psychiatric comorbidities, and more. This chapter reviews the referral and evaluation process, decisions for triage (patient–treatment matching), and the assessment of APSUDs and other comorbid disorders utilizing rating scales.

10.1. THE REFERRAL PROCESS

In order to develop a referral process for any treatment program for adolescents with PSUDs, the community needs to know the following minimal information: (1) the goals of the treatment program, (2) inclusion and exclusion criteria of the population to be served, and (3) how to communicate with the referral system. Other questions can be answered once communication channels have been established.

The referrals are expected from a wide variety of sources, including: self-referral, parents/family referral, school referral, agency referral (e.g., social services, court system), referral through other substance abuse or psychiatric treatment programs, and physician referral.

Clusters of precipitating factors and psychosocial problems appear to accompany the use of alcohol and other illicit substances among adolescents. However, little is known about the events that precede and are causally related to seeking treatment for APSUDs (Williams, Feibelman, & Moulder, 1989). Some of the most common causes for adolescents with PSUDs to arrive at emergency rooms are: (1) car accidents, falls, near drowning and other associated trauma; (2) panic reaction, "bad trip," or significant intoxication; (3) behavior inappropriate for situations, such as being "stoned" at school or driving while intoxicated (DWI); (4) overdose, either accidental or intentional; (5) drug-seeking behavior; and (6) parents wanting their child checked for substance abuse (Rogers, 1987).

Many adolescents entering treatment for PSUDs report having seen a pediatrician or other physician for illness or injury in the 1-year period before entering treatment. Almost one third report an emergency room visit (Hoffmann, Sonis, & Halikas, 1987). Despite the frequent contacts with health professionals, apparently the nature of the problem is not often recognized.

The reasons for elective referrals to treatment programs are in most cases similar to those found among adults, examples being the threat of loss of a relationship or a job or schooling or a legal problem that results in a forced choice between treatment or placement in a locked facility.

The assessment of an adolescent with PSUD is a difficult task, for several reasons: (1) The state of professional development of intervention–treatment specialists in APSUDs has not fully progressed. (2) The emphasis during the assessment process has been on eliciting information more than on establishing therapeutic alliance and relating to the adolescent. (3) Some adolescents are reluctant to cooperate fully with the assessment process, either because they have been brought to the assessment against their will or because they do not perceive their substance use or PSUD as severe enough to warrant assessment. However, it was reported that self-reports of drug use can provide reliable and valid information (Barnea, Rahav, & Teichman, 1987). (4) Substance abuse is usually not the adolescent's sole problem, and significant others and family members may also suffer from PSUDs and hence may not be fully cooperative during the assessment process. These issues are sometimes neglected during the evaluation process or are covered superficially. (5) Last, it is not common to find clinicians who adopt a behavior-oriented approach as part of the routine evaluation process. Such an approach views the assessment as a continuous and interactive process that occurs before, during, and following the introduction of treatment procedures (Sobell, Sobell, & Nirenberg, 1988). Failure to accept such an approach usually leads to a lack of complete data on the patient.

10.1.1. The Interview Format

There are many elements that may compose a comprehensive assessment of APSUD. The relative urgency of the referral and the setting (e.g., emergency room, outpatient clinic, preliminary interview) may determine the interview format. For example, when a referral is not made via the emergency room and the adolescent is not intoxicated, the referral may start by having an intake coordinator accept phone calls for screening. Even for phone calls, the use of an intake questionnaire (usually not requiring more than 15–20 minutes) is recommended. On the basis of the referral and assessment procedures, a dispositional option can be decided on or an appointment for a more comprehensive assessment can be made.

The first phase of the diagnostic interview is usually a general assessment of the adolescent utilizing information elicited directly from the individual as well as his or her caretakers/referral sources (Table 10.1). Demographic information, presenting complaint, evaluation/treatment expectations, and motivation of the adolescent and of the caretakers/referral source must be noted. Also, the cultivation of a basis for therapeutic alliance should be an objective targeted for the general assessment phase.

Mental status examination and the assessment of APSUD, present and past, will follow the general assessment. The mental status examination will be performed with the knowledge that the patient is or the assumption that the patient may be, under the influence of a recent use of some psychoactive substance or other. Since these substances affect emotional, psychological, and cognitive processes, it is necessary to evaluate the patient carefully and also to obtain urine for screening purposes. The diagnosis and the assessment of the severity of the PSUD must consider present use (i.e., last 30 days, last year) and past use. It is recommended that a checklist of psychoactive substances plus a list of street names of these agents be available.

Present use information includes names of substances used in the last 30 days; number of days used; patterns or context of use (i.e., where, with whom, sources of supply, activities involved in substance-seeking); the physical and psychological effects and side effects (complications included) of the substances; tolerance, withdrawal; and impact on various life domains (e.g., legal, school, relationships, family).

Past use information covers the same questions as in the present use section, with additional necessary information such as age of onset of use, abuse of, or dependence on various psychoactive substances and

Table 10.1

*Recommended Format for Diagnostic Interviews and Severity Assessment
of Adolescent Psychoactive Substance Use Disorders*

I. General assessment
 Obtain demographic information, presenting complaint.
  Assess motivation for treatment.
  Determine what brought the patient in *now*.
  Determine patient and caretaker/referral source goals and time frame (look for
   hidden agendas).
  Conduct mental status examination.
  Evaluate for the presence of concurrent psychiatric disorders.
II. Psychoactive substance use
  Identify the drugs used (use checklist).
  Note the amount and frequency of use (present and past).
  Note the route of administration.
  Obtain data on the amount and time of last use.
  Determine the pattern or context of use (e.g., alone/with friends, family, cult activity).
  Determine the tolerance/dependence/withdrawal status.
III. Effects of the PSUD
  Assess the patient's school or work history.
  Look for the presence of legal problems.
  Explore the nature and quality of interpersonal relationships (peer/social) and family
   interaction.
  Assess the psychological status for subjective distress.
  Explore leisure time and recreational use.
  Determine the presence of physical problems.
  Look for high-risk situations:
   Intrapersonal determinants: negative or pleasant emotional states, negative physical
    state, testing personal control, urges and temptations.
   Interpersonal determinants: interpersonal conflicts, social pressure to drink, positive
    emotional states.
IV. Special considerations
  Review for self-injurious behavior and bulimia.
  Review for suicidal behavior history.
  Review for child abuse history and trauma (sexual and physical).
  Review for involvement in cult activities (e.g., satanism).
V. Treatment considerations
  Identify previous treatment episodes for PSUD and psychiatric disorders.
  Determine whether the patient has been treated with any major drug treatment
   modality (detox, methadone maintenance, antagonist treatment, therapeutic
   communities, outpatient counseling) and evaluate the effects.
  Explore the history of abstinence: how long and under what circumstances.
  Determine the patient's previous attempts at self-treatment.
VI. Establishment of the DSM III-R/IV diagnosis
  Explore one or multiple diagnostic categories to be present on Axis I.
  Explore the personality disorder on Axis II.
VII. Treatment recommendations
  Develop a problem list with the patient according to the following domains: substance
   abuse, school performance (activities, behavior), employment status, family
   function, peer/social relationships, legal status, psychiatric status (T-ASI).
  Review with the patient your suggested treatment plan and attempt to set mutually
   agreeable short-term and long-term goals.

Table 10.2
APSUD: Laboratory Tests on Evaluation

---

 1. Breathalyzer test for recent use of alcohol
 2. Urine toxicology screen
 3. Urinalysis and urine specific gravity
 4. Blood count with differential and platelet count
 5. Bilirubin and liver enzymes such as SGOT, SGPT, GGTP
 6. BUN, creatinine, Na, K, Cl, CO_2
 7. Ca, P, alkaline phosphatase
 8. HCG
 9. Hepatitis B and tuberculosis screen[a]
10. HIV and other sexually transmitted diseases screen[a]
11. Chest X ray[b]
12. Other[a]

---

[a]For suspected IV substance abusers or history of multiple sexual partners or both.
[b]For suspected inhalant abusers.

combinations of them; history of spontaneous remissions and relapses; history of treatment; attendance in self-help groups; high-risk situations (setups) for PSUD; special considerations of high-risk behaviors (e.g., suicidal behavior, sexual activities, self-injurious behavior); history of physical and sexual abuse; and involvement in radical or unusual group activities (e.g., satanism).

Various rating scales reviewed in Section 10.1.2 offer different approaches for comprehensive evaluation of APSUDs.

Medical examination and laboratory work are usually the last procedure in the assessment process (Table 10.2). Medical complications of APSUDs are usually less severe and relatively less common than those in adults; nevertheless, this examination is important. Detailed laboratory work in addition to the urine screening for psychoactive substances is also of great importance.

Finally, the confidential information gathered must now be integrated to comprise a meaningful picture that will determine the most appropriate treatment program and treatment plan.

10.1.2. Rating Scales for the Assessment of Adolescent Psychoactive Substance Use Disorders

The assessment of psychopathology in children and adolescents, including PSUDs, has typically lagged behind that of the general population. Furthermore, many of the measures of psychopathology in child and adolescent psychiatry rely heavily on adult-originated symptomatology, criteria, and rating scales (and PSUDs are no exception).

The introduction of rating scales, usually in the form of self-reports and interviews, is expected to compensate for deficiencies in the recognition of psychopathology in clinical settings based only on observations and nonstructured evaluations. Well-designed instruments with adequate psychometric properties are expected to improve the objectivity, standardization, and accountability of the clinical assessment. A detailed evaluation of the adolescent with PSUD will obtain the information required for integrated, problem-focused, and comprehensive treatment (Tarter, 1990).

The data acquired from an adolescent assessment rating scale must satisfy several fundamental requirements pertaining to validity and reliability. The test that is administered needs to have a proven construct validity and predictive validity. Also, interrater reliability and test–retest reliability are essential.

In essence, the scores obtained must consistently and accurately reflect the process claiming to be measured, must have predictive value, must be stable over time, and should not be an artifact of the assessment context (Tarter, Otto, & Mezzich, 1991).

Tarter (1990, p. 6) summarized the state of the art of assessment scales for APSUDs as follows:

Effective interventions are predicated upon a valid and clinically relevant assessment. Unfortunately, despite the well-known fact that drug use begins typically in early adolescence, there are no standardized instruments available for this age group which objectively link assessments to treatment.

As pointed out by Owen and Nyberg (1983), the majority of treatment facilities servicing adolescent substance abusers either employ locally developed assessment methods or utilize procedures developed for adults. It is also important to note that while there are a variety of drug-use assessment instruments that have been developed for research purposes, their applicability for clinical practice is of dubious validity.

Assessment instruments are devised either for diagnostic use or for recognition of the severity of the problems/disorders measured. Some of the instruments, mainly the diagnostic ones, use a categorical approach. Other rating scales evaluate various problem domains according to a dimensional model (Achenbach, 1990). The latter model follows the paradigm of the etiological and pathogenetic relationships between substance use and maladjustment in each of the problem domains researched. This connection is pivotal in devising and implementing an intervention program (Tarter, 1990).

10.1.2.1. Diagnostic Instruments

Commonly used diagnostic instruments in child and adolescent psychiatry are also designed to capture PSUDs and are reasonably capable of differentiating users from abusers. The instruments to be noted are also helpful in identifying comorbid psychiatric disorders that are very prevalent among adolescents with PSUDs (Bukstein, Brent, & Kaminer, 1989). The rating scales are: the Diagnostic Interview Schedule for Children—Revised (DISC-R) (Costello, Edelbrock, & Costello, 1985), the Kiddie Schedule for Affective Disorders and Schizophrenia—Epidemiological Version (K-SADS-E) (Orvaschel, Puig-Antich, Chambers, Tabrizi, & Johnson, 1982), and the Diagnostic Interview for Children and Adolescents (DICA) (Wellner, Reich, Herjanic, Jung, & Amado, 1987).

Each of these interviews also has a version to be administered to a parent in order to compare the information obtained from multiple informants for ascertaining the degree of consensus. These instruments cover the range of psychiatric disorders in accordance with DSM-III and DSM-III-R (American Psychiatric Association, 1980, 1987), and they have acceptable psychometric support regarding their reliability and validity. It is important to note for practical considerations that a relatively long time is needed for the administration of these instruments (1-2 hours). Given the attention span of adolescents, it may sometimes be necessary to conduct the interview process in two sessions. Also, the administration of these rating scales demands extensive training and understanding of child and adolescent psychopathology.

The K-SADS-E (lifetime version) appears to have a particular advantage over other interviews in that it is flexible and therefore enables the clinician to probe for necessary information to ensure comprehensive diagnosis.

10.1.2.2. Screening Instruments

Screening instruments for substance use/abuse have been available for over two decades, but most were not designed for adolescents. The purpose of utilizing screening instruments is to identify individuals who are at risk or who have already developed symptomatology. These instruments have to be highly sensitive in order to accurately detect the persons with the problem/disorder. Specificity is also important (i.e., the ability to identify individuals without the problem/disorder). Sensitivity and specificity are functions of a screening test's cutoff score. Since it is not possible to simultaneously optimize sensitivity and specificity in a screening instrument, it is preferable to overidentify substance abuse (by increased sensitivity) than to miss individuals with this disorder (by increased specificity). The prevalence of the particular condition in the screened population must be taken into account (Grant, Hasin, & Hartford, 1989). If the base rate of a condition in a population is low, most of the cases identified by a sensitive test will be false-positives (Rice, 1987).

It is helpful to briefly review the advantages and shortcomings of the three most prominent rating scales because many clinicians utilize them regardless of the age of the target population.

10.1.2.2.1. Screening Instruments for Adults. The most widely used screening instruments for alcohol or other substances of abuse are the CAGE (Mayfield, McLead, & Hall, 1974), the Michigan Alcoholism Screening Test (MAST) (Selzer, 1971), and the Drug Abuse Screening Test (DAST) (Skinner, 1982). The acronymic and mnemonic CAGE, which can be self-administered or conducted by a clinician, is a quick four-question screening instrument about alcohol drinking:

C: Have you ever felt the need to Cut down on your drinking?
A: Have other people Annoyed you by criticizing your drinking?
G: Have you ever felt bad or Guilty about your drinking?
E: Have you ever had a drink (Eye-opener) first thing in the morning?

At a cutoff score of two yes answers, the test correctly identified 75% of alcoholics and 96% of nonalcoholics (Bush, Shaw, Cleary, Del Banco, & Aronson, 1987).

The MAST comes in 10-item (b-MAST), 13-item (SMAST), and 25-item versions. It focuses on the consequences of problem drinking and on the subjects' own perceptions of their alcohol problems. In a study of individuals prosecuted for drunk driving, the MAST had 80% sensitivity (Mischke & Venneri, 1987). A cutoff score of 12 or 13 out of 25 items was reported to balance the rates of false-positives and false-negatives (Jacobson & Lindsay, 1980).

The shortened forms of the MAST have been constructed using items from the original test that are highly discriminating for alcoholism. A cutoff score of 3 is suggested for the SMAST; a cutoff score of 6 is recommended for the b-MAST (Pokorny, Miller, & Kaplan, 1972; Selzer, Vinokur, & Van Rooijen, 1975). The MAST has been used in a number of studies of college students and was useful in identifying problem drinkers (Anderson, 1987), but a number of the items are clearly inappropriate for adolescents.

The DAST is an adaptation of items from the MAST to apply to substance abuse in general. The 20-item DAST yields a quantitative index of problems related to PSUDs. The sensitivity reported is 85% according to a cutoff score of 5 or 6 (Gavin, Ross, & Skinner, 1989). Also, Skinner and Goldberg (1986) reported on the emergence of a dependence factor that is characterized by an inability to stop drug use, problems in getting through the week without drugs, and withdrawal symptoms when the drug is stopped.

10.1.2.2.2. Screening Instruments for Adolescents. Some screening instruments have been developed specifically for adolescents. The Adolescent Alcohol Involvement Scale (AAIS) (Mayer & Filstead, 1979) is a 14-item self-report scale. The AAIS was critically examined and not recommended for use due to a lack of common variance among its items (Riley & Klockars, 1984). However, it is still widely used. The Adolescent Drinking Inventory (Harrell & Wirtz, 1989) is a 25-question self-report that focuses on drinking-related loss of control as well as social, psychological, and physical symptoms of alcohol problems. The ADI correctly identified 88% of adolescents with alcohol problems and 82% of those without alcohol problems (Allen, Eckardt, & Wallen, 1988).

The Chemical Dependency Assessment Scale (CDAS) (Oetting, Beauvais, Edwards, & Waters, 1984) and the Personal Experience Inventory (PEI) (Winters & Henly, 1988) are extensively reviewed below because they are the two most developed instruments for the evaluation of suspected adolescent drug users, and their psychometric properties are impressive.

The CDAS is self-administered, but must be computer-scored. Detailed information about drug-use behavior is obtained. Current use (Part I) and past use (Part II) of 11 classes of drugs during the 18-month period before the evaluation are assessed. A 4-point scale (0–3) is applied for the intensity of drug use for each class. Part III of the CDAS describes certain key aspects of the adolescent's psychological profile. A 3-point rating system describes the individual according to emotional adjustment (depression, anxiety, anger, feeling blamed, and excitement-seeking), psychological adjustment (self-esteem, self-consciousness or shyness, feelings of isolation, perception of self as a good person, acceptance of deviance, and deviant behavior), family relationships and socioeconomic status, school adjustment, and peer influences (Tarter, 1990).

The CDAS is currently in wide use, especially in educational settings. Over 100,000 adolescents have been screened, and it is at present the single most standardized and comprehensive method for evaluating drug-use behavior and its consequences in adolescents.

Winters and Henly (1988) have developed an assessment battery that includes the PEI, a comprehensive standardized 260-item self-report measure of chemical involvement and psychosocial use; the Personal Experience Screening Questionnaire (PESQ), a quick 38-item screen; and the Adolescent Diagnostic Interview (ADI), a structured interview based on DSM-III-R diagnostic criteria for PSUD.

The PEI documents the onset, nature, degree, and duration of involvement with 12 classes of psychoactive substances in adolescents. It also identifies the personal use factors that may precipitate or sustain substance abuse. The instrument has a paper-and-pencil-format or a computerized-format questionnaire composed of two parts: (1) Problem Severity Scales that assess symptoms, problem severity, consequences, and patterns of substance use; and (2) Psychosocial Scales, which include assessments of familial, sociodemographic, intrapersonal, social, and environmental influences.

The developmental phase of the PEI covered the assessment of rational scales and empirical scales designed by Winters and Henly (1988). After consideration of psychometric adequacy, the set of Problem Severity Scales enumerated below was identified.

The Basic Scales are (1) Personal Involvement, (2) Effects from Use, (3) Social Benefit Use, (4) Personal Consequences, and (5) Polydrug Use.

The Clinical Scales are (6) Transituational Use, (7) Psychological Benefit Use, (8) Social–Recreational Use, (9) Preoccupation with Use, and (10) Loss of Control.

In addition, there are three Validity Indices: (11) Infrequent Responses, (12) Defensiveness, and (13) Pattern Misfit. These scales evaluate response style to the test items that may point to inattentive responding or suggest an inclination either to be defensive or to present a negative picture of oneself. The revised scales consist of 113 items in 13 scales.

The Clinical Scales, the items of which are largely redundant with the first (Personal Involvement) scale, restructure the information in a way that may be interesting for clinicians. Estimates of internal consistency (Coefficient Alpha) range from 0.80 to 0.97.

The Psychosocial Scales are composed of 147 items that are organized into 8 Personal Adjustment Scales: (1) Negative Self-Image, (2) Psychological Disturbance, (3) Social Isolation, (4) Uncontrolled, (5) Rejecting Convention, (6) Deviant Behavior, (7) Absence of Goals, and (8) Spiritual Isolation.

There are four Family and Peer Environment Scales: (9) Peer Chemical Environment, (10) Sibling Chemical Use, (11) Family Pathology, and (12) Family Estrangement.

Finally, there are two Validity Indices—(13) Infrequent Responses and (14) Defensiveness—and five Screens for other problems: (15) Parent/Sibling Chemical Dependency, (16) Intrafamilial Physical Abuse, (17) Intrafamilial Sexual Abuse, (18) Eating Disorder, and (19) Psychiatric Referral. Internal consistency for the 12 primary scales ranges from 0.74 to 0.90, and estimates of scale redundancy indicate that each scale provides sufficiently unique information to warrant its inclusion.

Interrater reliability and test–retest reliability of the scales of the PEI are good. The instrument was controlled and normed on 1120 adolescents in drug clinics in Minnesota and on 693 high school students (Winters & Henly, 1988). Use of the PEI scales to assist in differential referral and treatment decisions continues to be explored, and they have been selected for inclusion in a national Adolescent Assessment/Referral System.

The 38-item PESQ covers three sections: (1) Problem Severity—psychological and behavioral involvement with chemicals; (2) Psychosocial Risk—personal and environmental problems associated with adolescent substance abuse; and (3) Drug Use History—covers the frequency of use of 12 classes of psychoactive substances in the previous 12 months. Two Validity Scales are included as well. This "mini"-PEI standardized screening test can be completed in about 10–15 minutes and can easily determine whether a patient will be referred for a complete evaluation following a positive finding.

The ADI is a structured interview based on DSM-III-R diagnostic criteria that also evaluates psychosocial stressors, school and interpersonal functioning, and cognitive impairment. The time required for administration depends on the number of different substances that the respondent is using. In addition to the aforenoted diagnostic information evaluated by the ADI, eight psychiatric status screens alert the interviewer to other psychiatric disorders often associated with substance abuse. The ADI is particularly useful in documenting the need for treatment.

In summary, the PEI or the ADI or both provide detailed diagnostic and treatment information, while the PESQ helps in making referrals only. Additional recent study of these instruments has established their reliability and validity (Winters, Stinchfield, & Henly, 1993).

The next two instruments were formulated by the same group of people at the National Institute on Drug Abuse, and they follow the same three-phase paradigm and in essence overlap in many respects: Phase I—screening, Phase II—comprehensive evaluation, and Phase III—treatment. These are the Drug Use Screening Inventory (DUSI) (Tarter, 1990) and the Problem Oriented Screening Instrument for Teenagers (POSIT) (Rahdert, 1991).

The DUSI consists of a multidimensional screening of severity of the adolescent's disturbance in 10 domains: (1) Substance Abuse, (2) Behavior Patterns, (3) Health Status, (4) Psychiatric Disorder, (5) Social Competency, (6) Family System, (7) School Adjustment, (8) Work, (9) Peer Relationships, and (10) Leisure/Recreation. The second phase of comprehensive evaluation utilizes the results of the DUSI, and Tarter (1990) suggests a list of specialized tests that correspond to the DUSI's 10 domains. The third phase in the screening and assessment process formulates a patient's matched treatment, which considers the type and severity of disorders identified in the previous phases.

The DUSI is a 149-item true–false self-report that covers the last 30 days. It is expected to take 30 minutes to complete the form either by pencil and paper or by a personal computer program. Scoring is complex. Severity or problem density is determined by three scores: (1) the absolute problem-density score, (2) the overall problem-index score, and (3) the relative problem-density score. Also, the total number of positive responses in each domain is referred to as a raw score.

For each domain, the problem-density score ranges from 0% to 100%. These scores provide the basis for determining whether treatment is warranted in one or more of the domains. It is important to note that no arbitrary threshold score is advocated for determining appropriateness for treatment; this determination is the responsibility of the treatment provider. Determination of treatment needs should be based on the results of the DUSI in conjunction with other relevant information available.

The overall problem-index score, like the absolute problem-density score, gauges problem density, or severity. The overall score is derived from the total number of positive responses in each domain (raw score) averaged across all domains. This score reflects general severity of disturbance, recognizing that the 10 domains are to some degree interrelated. Also, the score determines the intensity of treatment, such as inpatient or outpatient, that suits the client's overall condition.

The relative problem-density score describes problem density, or severity, in each domain and demonstrates how the 10 domains are distributed with respect to their severity. The score is derived by adding the absolute problem-density scores and dividing the score for each domain into this total. The resulting scores add up to 100% and reflect the relative severity of problems across the 10 domains. This computation reveals the unique intraclient distribution of problem severity across the 10 domains cited. [For a more detailed discussion of scoring procedures, see Tarter (1990).] The DUSI is undergoing studies to assess its psychometric properties, and on the basis of unpublished preliminary findings, these properties appear to be statistically acceptable.

The POSIT is a 139-item questionnaire designed to measure problem severity in 10 generic domains identical to those of the DUSI (although with minimal changes in several titles). The items of the POSIT are randomized and are not organized by domains as in the DUSI. The items of the POSIT are of three types: general-purpose items, general-purpose age-related items, and red-flag items that alone indicate the need for further assessment. Scoring of the POSIT is complex and can be done only by using templates. The cutoff score of each domain was defined arbitrarily by a panel, and no psychometric properties of the instrument have been reported so far. McLaney, DelBoca, and Babor (in press) indicated that the predictive validity of the POSIT was evidenced by significant correlations between scores obtained at baseline and at a 6- to 8-month follow-up evaluation.

The POSIT and the DUSI are expected to serve as screening tools in initial identification systems for adolescents at high risk for PSUDs.

10.1.2.3. Severity-Oriented Rating Scales

The main purpose of severity-oriented scales is to assess pretreatment and posttreatment (aftercare) status. The Addiction Severity Index (ASI) (McLellan, Luborsky, Woody, & O'Brien, 1980) is an interview that yields severity ratings in six domains among individuals already identified with PSUDs. The ASI has been found to be a reliable and valid instrument having a wide range of clinical and research applications in adult substance abusers (Kosten, Rounsaville, & Kleber, 1983; McLellan et al., 1985). Several instruments represent modifications of the ASI for the needs of adolescents, such as the Teen Addiction Severity Index (T-ASI) (Kaminer, Bukstein, & Tarter, 1991), the Adolescent Drug and Alcohol Diagnostic Assessment (ADAD), the Adolescent Problem Severity Index (APSI), and the Comprehensive Addiction Severity Index for Adolescents.

The T-ASI utilizes a dimensional approach to the assessment of the severity of substance abuse in adolescents. Five additional domains are investigated: (1) family function, (2) school or employment status, (3) psychiatric status, (4) peer/social relationship, and (5) legal status. Periodic administration of the T-ASI is recommended in order to assess posttreatment status. The administration time of this semistructured interview is about 25–30 minutes. The T-ASI can be administered to the parent/caretaker following the guidelines of the instruction manual. These collateral data may have important treatment implications. In addition to the instruction manual, there is a useful manual entitled *Follow-up Procedures and Techniques for Locating Out of Treatment Patients.* Preliminary findings regarding the psychometric properties of the

T-ASI indicated good clinical utility and satisfactory interrater reliability (average correlation is 0.78). The T-ASI Validity study indicated that the instrument discriminated between PSUD and non-PSUD adolescents within a group of psychiatric patients, generating a good discriminant validity. This is a stronger test of validity than a comparison of psychiatrically disordered and normal adolescents (a community sample) would provide. Also, the concurrent validity is acceptable (Kaminer et al., 1991; Kaminer, Wagner, Plummer, & Seifer, 1993). The scoring of the T-ASI is based on the clinical impression of the trained rater following a summary of a 5-point scale in each domain.

The ADAD is highly comparable in many respects to the T-ASI, and the interrater reliability and test–retest reliability have been reasonably established. Scoring is complex and follows the ASI approach, which is based on a mathematically derived composite score based on items defined as having a higher relative weight. The ADAD was designed mainly for research purposes.

Two additional interesting adolescent measures are the Inventory of Drug-Taking Situations (IDTS) and the Drug-Taking Confidence Questionnaire (DTCQ). The instruments are the products of the Addiction Research Foundation in Toronto, Canada. These are parallel instruments to the Inventory of Using Situations (IUS) and the Situations Confidence Questionnaire (SCQ) (Annis & Davis, 1988), which were developed on adult alcoholics. However, unlike the IUS and SCQ, the IDTS and DTCQ cover other drug classes in addition to alcohol.

A user's guide for the IDTS containing normative and psychometric data was developed. The data have been collected in a client–computer interactive format that permits the adolescent to choose up to three drugs for which help is being sought. The adolescent then answers on the computer screen the questionnaire for each drug class.

The aforementioned instruments were developed on the basis of empirical findings that provide support for the principles of the self-efficacy theory (Bandura, 1977) in the treatment of alcoholism (Marlatt & George, 1984). Cognitive mechanisms (e.g., efficacy expectations) are proposed as mediating or explaining behavior change, and performance-based treatment procedures (e.g., mastery experiences in high-risk situations) are proposed as the most powerful procedures for producing and maintaining behavior change (Annis & Davis, 1988). The IUS and the IDTS are self-report questionnaires designed to assess high-risk situations for alcohol or other substance abuse. The questionnaires evaluate eight categories of situations divided into two major classes: Intrapersonal and Interpersonal Determinants. Intrapersonal Determinants, in which drinking or substance use involves a response to an event that is primarily psychological or physical in nature, are divided into five categories: (1) Negative Emotional States, (2) Negative Physical States, (3) Positive Emotional States, (4) Testing Personal Control, and (5) Urges and Temptations. Interpersonal Determinants, in which a significant influence of another individual is involved, are distinguished by three categories: (1) Interpersonal Conflict, (2) Social Pressure to Drink, and (3) Positive Emotional States.

Items from the various categories are scrambled within the 100-item questionnaires (a 42-item short format is also available). The IUS and the IDTS are answered on four-point scales (never, rarely, frequently, and almost always). The SCQ and the DTCQ are administered after the intervention to measure its efficacy for the same situations identified in the IUS and IDTS. There are six-point scales in the SCQ and the DTCQ [from 0% ("not at all confident that I would be able to resist the urge to drink or abuse substance") through 20%, 40%, 60%, 80%, and 100% ("very confident")]. These instruments are helpful especially in treatment settings in which relapse-prevention manuals are in use (Monti, Abrams, Kadden, & Cooney, 1989).

10.1.3. Family Assessment

Little work has been done on standardized family assessment of adolescent substance abusers. Bry (1988) provides a review of assessments and treatment techniques based on systems theories and behavior-based family approaches. The last instrument reviewed herein addresses some of the questions regarding the children of an alcoholic family. The Children of Alcoholics Screening Test (CAST) (Jones, 1982) is a scale of 30 true–false items that aims to identify, in order to facilitate early intervention for, individuals who have lived with an alcoholic parent in the past. The test measures responses about the individual's perception of, experience with, and reactions to parent's drinking. A score of 6 or greater (of a possible 30) reliably identified children of alcoholics. The psychometric properties of the CAST for children and adults appear to be acceptable, including test–retest reliability and internal consistency, both in the upper 80s (Dinning & Berk, 1989).

10.1.4. Reliability of the Assessment Process

Finally, regarding the question of the reliability of the information obtained from adolescents about their substance-use pattern, the literature in general confirms an acceptable reliability of the process (Campanelli, Deilman, Shope, 1987; Farrell & Strang, 1991). However, the use of laboratory specimen analyses is important to confirm self-reports independently and to monitor objectively the maintenance of drug-free states.

In summary, it is hoped that assessment packages will serve as an adjunct to clinical assessment of APSUDs. Given that extant assessment practices in the field rely heavily on clinical judgment, there is a crucial need to improve the objectivity of the assessment process. The choice of an instrument should match the expectations from the specific instrument while also taking into consideration the experience accrued in its administration in specific settings, the psychometric properties of the rating scale, and the complexity and costs of scoring.

10.2. PATIENT–TREATMENT MATCHING

Heterogeneity of the population of individuals with PSUDs has been recognized. The transitional shotgun treatment approach appears to be less appropriate to fulfill the needs of the various subpopulations of patients with PSUDs (Craig, 1987). During the 1980s, the patient–treatment matching hypothesis (PTMH) emerged with an aim toward improving dispositional options (triage) while involving a variety of possibilities (depending on service availability). The rapid development of the PTMH was associated with studies reporting that the severity of psychopathologies associated with PSUDs was important in predicting treatment outcome (McLellan, O'Brien, & Kron, 1980). Adult alcoholics with severe psychiatric disorders showed low levels of improvement and significantly less improvement than those with mild and moderate psychiatric problems (Rounsaville, Kosten, Weissman, & Kleber, 1986). Those with additional concurrent family problems showed even poorer outcomes. The patients with middle-severity psychiatric problems achieved significant benefit from patient–treatment matching (Rounsaville et al., 1986). Increased effectiveness of the PTMH was demonstrated in another prospective study (McLellan, Woody, Luborsky, O'Brien, & Druley, 1983). The fewer problems a patient had on admission, the more likely he or she was to benefit from the program. Personality disorders, especially the antisocial type, were correlated with poor treatment outcome in any treatment modality. No such research on APSUD treatment has yet been reported. However, it appears that the matching effect is best seen at the service-provision level and much less at the program, modality, or setting level.

An interesting model for admission, discharge, and transfer criteria for adults and adolescents is the compilation of the Cleveland Criteria

(Hoffmann, Halikas, & Mee-Lee, 1987). The Cleveland Criteria were developed in an effort to find out which patients will benefit most from what type of treatment. Seven domains served as guidelines for assessment: (1) acute intoxication/withdrawal, (2) physical complications, (3) psychiatric complications, (4) impairments in certain areas of life, (5) acceptance of treatment, (6) loss of control, and (7) recovery environment (Hoffmann et al., 1987). A study that examined the validity of the Cleveland Criteria among adults only suggested that they were not fully operationalized properly (McKay, McLellan, & Alterman, 1992). Further research regarding matching treatment and adolescents utilizing the Cleveland Criteria is still warranted.

Youth Evaluation Services (Y.E.S.) is a program for early identification, intervention, and monitoring of adolescents with PSUDs in Connecticut (Babor, Del Boca, McLaney, Jacobi, Higgins-Biddle, & Hass, 1991). This innovative project matches adolescents to appropriate interventions. Data regarding outcome and follow-up have not yet been reported; however, an impressive multidimensional evaluation battery is employed in the matching process and may serve as a model to be adopted by other youth assessment and treatment centers.

10.3. CRITERIA FOR ADMISSION TO VARIOUS HOSPITAL-BASED SETTINGS

Following the completion of the assessment stages, the triage team makes a dispositional decision as delineated in Figure 10.1. Appropriate admissions to an inpatient unit may include: (1) adolescents with PSUDs who have failed or do not qualify for outpatient treatment (e.g., PSUD severity higher than moderate); (2) dually diagnosed adolescents with moderate or severe psychiatric disorders; (3) adolescents who display a potentially morbid or mortal behavior toward themselves or others; (4) adolescents who are IV drug users or who need to be detoxified; (5) patients with accompanying moderate to severe medical problems; (6) adolescents who need to be isolated from their community to ensure treatment without interruptions; and (7) pregnant adolescents who manifest PSUDs that endanger the fetus.

Enrollment criteria to a drug-free outpatient or partial hospitalization include: (1) severity of APSUD and other psychiatric disorders that does not require inpatient treatment (i.e., PSUD severity less than moderate), (2) previous successful outpatient treatment or follow-up after

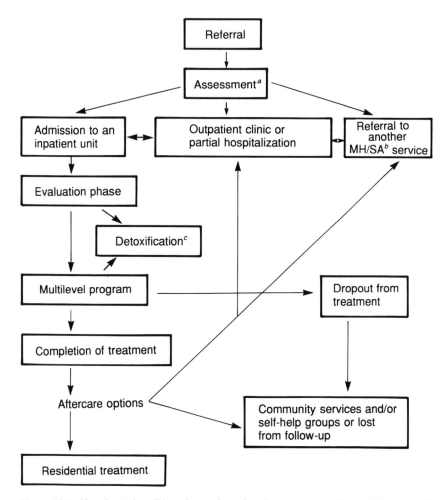

Figure 10.1. Flowchart describing the options for the treatment of an adolescent with psychoactive substance use disorder (dual diagnosis included). [a]Assessment can be done through an assessment coordination team and can combine a preliminary phone evaluation or use of questionnaires or both followed by interviews with the patient and caretaker(s). [b](MH) mental health; (SA) substance abuse. [c]Detoxification is the exception rather than the rule for adolescents.

completion of inpatient treatment, and (3) agreement to a contingency contract that will delineate frequency of visits, compliance with curriculum including random urine screening, consequences of noncompliance and relapse, and participation in the community network including self-help groups.

10.4. CONCLUSION

The careful assessment of the adolescent with PSUD is a process that may utilize clinical skills and rating scales. A careful and comprehensive formulation will be helpful for patient–treatment matching and for the design of an appropriate treatment plan.

REFERENCES

Achenbach, T. M. (1990). Comorbidity in child and adolescent psychiatry: Categorical and quantitative perspectives. *Journal of Child and Adolescent Psychopharmacology, 1,* 271–278.

Allen, J. P., Eckardt, M. J., & Wallen, J. (1988). Screening for alcoholism: Techniques and issues. *Public Health Reports, 103,* 586–592.

American Psychiatric Association (1980). *Diagnostic and Statistical Manual of Mental Disorders,* 3rd ed. Washington, DC: American Psychiatric Association.

American Psychiatric Association (1987). *Diagnostic and Statistical Manual of Mental Disorders,* 3rd ed., rev. Washington, DC: American Psychiatric Association.

Anderson, P. (1987). Early intervention in general practice. In T. Stockwell & S. Clements (Eds.), *Helping the Problem Drinker: New Initiatives in Primary Care* (pp. 150–172). London: Croon Helm.

Annis, H. M., & Davis, C. S. (1988). Relapse prevention. In R. K. Hester & W. R. Miller (Eds.), *Handbook of Alcoholism Treatment Approaches* (pp. 170–182). New York: Pergamon Press.

Babor, T. F., Del Boca, F. K., McLaney, M. A., Jacobi, B., Higgins-Biddle, J., & Hass, W. (1991). Just say Y.E.S.: Matching adolescents to appropriate interventions for alcohol and other drug-related problems. *Alcohol Health and Research World, 15,* 77–86.

Bandura, A. (1977). *Social Learning Theory.* Englewood Cliffs, NJ: Prentice-Hall.

Barnea, A., Rahav, G., & Teichman, M. (1987). The reliability and consistency of self-reports of substance use in a longitudinal study. *British Journal of Addictions, 82,* 891–898.

Bry, B. H. (1988). Family-based approaches to reducing adolescent substance use: Theories, techniques and findings. In *Adolescent Drug Abuse: Analyses of Treatment Research* (pp. 39–68). National Institute on Drug Abuse Monograph 77. Rockville, MD: National Institute on Drug Abuse.

Bukstein, O. G., Brent, D. A., & Kaminer, Y. (1989). Comorbidity of substance abuse and other psychiatric disorders in adolescents. *American Journal of Psychiatry, 146,* 1131–1141.

Bush, B., Shaw, S., Cleary, P., Del Banco, T. L., & Aronson, M. D. (1987). Screening for alcohol abuse using the CAGE questionnaire. *American Journal of Medicine, 82,* 231–235.

Campanelli, P. C., Dielman, T. E., & Shope, J. T. (1987). Validity of adolescents' self-reports of alcohol use and misuse using a bogus pipeline procedure. *Adolescence, 22,* 7–22.

Costello, A., Edelbrock, C., & Costello, A. J. (1985). Validity of the NIMH Diagnostic Interview Schedule for children: A comparison between pediatric and psychiatric referrals. *Journal of Abnormal Child Psychology and Psychiatry, 13,* 579–595.

Craig, J. C. (1987). *Clinical Management of Substance Abuse Programs.* Springfield, IL: Charles C. Thomas.

Dinning, W. D., & Berk, L. A. (1989). The Children of Alcoholics Screening Test: Relationship to sex, family, environment, and social adjustment in adolescents. *Journal of Clinical Psychology, 45,* 335–339.

Farrell, M., & Strang, J. (1991). Substance use and misuse in childhood and adolescence. *Journal of Child Psychology and Psychiatry, 32,* 109–128.

Gavin, D. R., Ross, H. E., & Skinner, H. A. (1989). Diagnostic validity of the drug abuse screening test in the assessment of DSM-III drug disorders. *British Journal of Addiction, 84,* 301–307.

Grant, B. F., Hasin, D. S., & Hartford, T. C. (1989). Screening for major depression among alcoholics: An application of receiver operating characteristic analysis. *Drug and Alcohol Dependence, 23,* 123–131.

Harrell, A. V., & Wirtz, P. W. (1989). Screening for adolescent problem drinking: Validation of a multi dimensional instrument for case identification. *Psychological Assessment, 1,* 61–63.

Hoffmann, N. G., Halikas, J. A., & Mee-Lee, D. (1987). *The Cleveland Admission, Discharge and Transfer Criteria: Model for Chemical Dependency Treatment Programs.* Cleveland: Chemical Dependency Treatment Directors Association.

Hoffmann, N. G., Sonis, W. A., & Halikas, J. A. (1987). Issues in the evaluation of chemical dependency treatment programs for adolescents. *Pediatric Clinics of North America, 34,* 449–459.

Jacobson, G. R., & Lindsay, D. (1980). Screening for alcohol problems among the unemployed. In M. Galanter (Ed.), *Currents in Alcoholism: Recent Advances in Research and Treatment,* V. VII. New York: Grune & Stratton.

Jones, J. W. (1982). *The Children of Alcoholics Screening Test: Preliminary Test Manual.* Chicago: Family Recovery Press.

Kaminer, Y., Bukstein, O. G., & Tarter, T. E. (1991). The Teen Addiction Severity Index (T-ASI): Rationale and reliability. *International Journal of the Addictions, 26,* 219–226.

Kaminer, Y., Wagner, E., Plummer, B., & Seifer, R. (1993). Validation of the Teen Addiction Severity Index (T-ASI): Preliminary findings. *American Journal on Addiction, 2,* 221–224.

Kosten, T. R., Rounsaville, B. J., & Kleber, H. D. (1983). Concurrent validity of the Addiction Severity Index. *The Journal of Nervous and Mental Disease, 171,* 606–610.

Marlatt, G. A., & George, W. H. (1984). Relapse prevention: Introduction and overview of the model. *British Journal of Addiction, 79,* 261–275.

Mayer, J., & Filstead, W. J. (1979). The adolescent alcohol involvement scale: An instrument for measuring adolescent use and misuse of alcohol. *Journal of Studies of Alcohol, 40,* 291–300.

Mayfield, D., McLead, G., & Hall, P. (1974). The CAGE questionnaire: Validation of a new alcoholism screening instrument. *American Journal of Psychiatry, 131,* 1121–1123.

McKay, J. R., McLellan, T., & Alterman, A. I. (1992). An evaluation of the Cleveland Criteria for inpatient treatment of substance abuse. *American Journal of Psychiatry, 149,* 1212–1218.

McLaney, A., Del Boca, B., & Babor, T. (in press). A validation study of the Problem Oriented Screening Instrument for Teenagers. *Journal of Mental Health.*

McLellan, A. T., Luborsky, L., Cacciola, J., Griffith, J., Evans, F., Barr, H., & O'Brien, C. P. (1985). New data from the Addiction Severity Index: Reliability and validity in three centers. *Journal of Nervous and Mental Disease, 173,* 412–423.

McLellan, A. T., Luborsky, L., Woody, G. E., & O'Brien, C. P. (1980). An improved diagnostic evaluation instrument for substance abuse patients. *Journal of Nervous and Mental Disease, 40,* 620–625.

McLellan, A. T., O'Brien, C. P., & Kron, R. (1980). Matching substance abuse patients to appropriate treatments: A conceptual and methodological approach. *Drug and Alcohol Dependence, 5,* 189–295.

McLellan, A. T., Woody, G. E., Luborsky, L., O'Brien, C. P., & Druley, K. A. (1983). Increased effectiveness of substance abuse treatment: A prospective study of patient–treatment matching. *Journal of Nervous and Mental Disease, 171,* 597–605.

Mischke, H. D., & Venneri, R. L. (1987). Reliability and validity of the MAST, Murtiner–Fitkins questionnaire and CAGE in DQI assessment. *Journal for the Study of Alcohol, 48,* 492–501.

Monti, P. M., Abrams, D. B., Kadden, R. M., & Cooney, N. L. (1989). *Treating Alcohol Dependence.* New York: Guilford Press.

Oetting, E., Beauvais, F., Edwards, R., & Waters, M. (1984). *The Drug and Alcohol Assessment System.* Fort Collins, CO: Mountain Behavioral Sciences Institute.

Orvaschel, H., Puig-Antich, J., Chambers, W., Tabrizi, M. A., & Johnson, R. (1982). Retrospective assessment of prepubertal major depression with the Kiddie-SADS-E. *Journal of the American Academy of Child Psychiatry, 21,* 392–297.

Owen, P., & Nyberg, L. (1983). Assessing alcohol and drug problems among adolescents: Current practices. *Journal of Drug Education, 13,* 249–254.

Pokorny, A. D., Miller, B. A., & Kaplan, H. B. (1972). The brief MAST: A shortened version of the Michigan Alcoholism Screening Test. *American Journal of Psychiatry, 129,* 118–121.

Rahdert, E. R. (1991). *The Adolescent Assessment Referral System Manual.* DHHS Publication No. ADM91-1735. Rockville, MD: National Institute on Drug Abuse.

Rice, J. P. (1987). Statistical issues in the interpretation of tests. In *Screening for Alcoholism in Primary Care Settings* (pp. 3–5). Rockville, MD: National Institute on Alcohol Abuse and Alcoholism.

Riley, K., & Klockars, A. J. (1984). A critical reexamination of the Adolescent Alcohol Involvement Scale. *Journal of Studies on Alcohol, 45,* 184–187.

Rogers, P. D. (1987). *Chemical Dependency: Pediatric Clinics of North America.* Philadelphia: W. B. Saunders.

Rounsaville, B. J., Kosten, T. R., Weissman, M. M., & Kleber, H. D. (1986). Prognostic significance of psychiatric disorders in treated opiate addicts. *Archives of General Psychiatry, 43,* 739–745.

Selzer, M. L. (1971). The Michigan Alcoholism Screening Test: The quest for a new diagnostic instrument. *American Journal of Psychiatry, 127,* 1653–1658.

Selzer, M. L., Vinokur, A., & Van Rooijen, L. (1975). A self-administered Short Michigan Alcoholism Screening Test (SMAST). *Journal of Studies on Alcohol, 36,* 117–126.

Skinner, H. A. (1982). The Drug Abuse Screening Test. *Addictive Behaviors, 7,* 363–371.

Skinner, H. A., & Goldberg, B. (1986). Evidence for a drug dependence syndrome among narcotic users. *British Journal of Addiction, 81,* 479–484.

Sobell, L. S., Sobell, M. B., & Nirenberg, T. D. (1988). Behavioral assessment and treatment planning with alcohol and drug abusers: A review with an emphasis on clinical application. *Clinical Psychology Review, 8,* 19–54.

Tarter, R. E. (1990). Evaluation and treatment of adolescent substance abuse: A decision tree method. *American Journal of Drug and Alcohol Abuse, 16,* 1–46.

Tarter, R. E., Otto, Y., & Mezzich, A. (1991). In S. I. Miller & R. Frances (Eds.), *Clinical Textbook of Addictive Disorder* (pp. 237–267). New York: Guilford Press.

Wellner, Z., Reich, W., Herjanic, B., Jung, D., & Amado, K. (1987). Reliability, validity and parent–child agreement studies of the Diagnostic Interview for Children and Adolescents (DICA). *Journal of the American Academy of Child Psychiatry, 26,* 649–653.

Williams, R. A., Feibelman, N. D., & Moulder, C. (1989). Events precipitating hospital treatment of adolescent drug abusers. *Journal of the American Academy of Child and Adolescent Psychiatry, 28,* 70–73.

Winters, K., & Henly, G. (1988). Development of problem severity scales for the assessment of adolescent alcohol and drug abuse. *International Journal of the Addictions, 23,* 65–85.

Winters, K. C., Stinchfield, R. D., & Henly, G. A. (1993). Further validation of new scales measuring adolescent alcohol and other drug abuse. *Journal of Studies on Alcohol, 54,* 534–541.

Treatment Selection and Modalities

The objectives of this chapter are to describe the reported treatment modalities/interventions in different settings of treatment for adolescents with psychoactive substance use disorders (PSUDs). The development of the current state of knowledge concerning relations among patient variables, treatment characteristics, and environmental factors is discussed in light of the treatment-related politics of the era. Consideration is given to selection and planning of individualized treatment menus and review of updated treatment strategies, with special attention to the most commonly diagnosed comorbid psychiatric disorders. Present and future suggestions to decrease attrition and treatment failure and to improve treatment efficacy and aftercare are illuminated.

11.1. INTRODUCTION

The large body of literature on the treatment of PSUDs is replete with descriptive, non-database-oriented publications regarding various treatment philosophies, modalities, and settings. Also, individuals afflicted with PSUDs and their significant others are characterized according to a stereotyped, dogmatic, nonscientific or nonmedical paradigm. These biases have resulted in difficulties concerning generalization and replication of treatment modalities and strategies in different settings and among various subpopulations with a variety of demographic characteristics. Consequently, until the late 1970s, there were still serious doubts in the scientific literature as to the effectiveness of treatment (Edwards, 1979; Wilson, 1980). McLellan, Luborsky, O'Brien, Woody, and Druley (1982) were the first in the United States to put the following issues to the test: (1) Do patients improve after substance abuse treatment? (2) Are improvements specific to the target symptoms of alcohol and drug use, or are they more pervasive? (3) To what extent are improvements due to the effects of treatment?

They came to these conclusions: (1) Treatment contributes significantly to patients' improvement. (2) Major improvements following substance abuse treatment are not limited to alcohol and drug use only; several other areas show moderate to major changes as well. (3) The extent of improvement is not clearly related to the treatment process.

This study heralded the beginning of a new era in the research on treatment outcome and was followed by other studies that have employed rigorous research methodology and have investigated measurable treatment-outcome objectives. Also, subsequent treatment-planning development has had to consider that polysubstance abuse is the rule rather than the exception, that a large proportion of patients with PSUDs are afflicted with a comorbid psychiatric disorder, and that the present classification of PSUDs recognizes these clinical characteristics as occurring along a gradient of severity (Edwards, 1986).

11.2. THE POLITICS OF TREATMENT

Any introduction to the treatment of PSUDs would be incomplete without addressing the politics of addictions. Treatment referrals and assignments of adolescents with PSUDs are too often based on availability of space and not necessarily on the adolescents' needs. Also, there is a strong resistance among many therapists who employ an adult-treatment perspective to recognize the heterogeneity of the subpopulations of adolescents and adults with PSUDs and to identify these special treatment needs. This approach is specifically related to the historical–conceptual roots of substance-abuse treatment according to the disease model (Meyer, 1986) and is also attributable to the relative scarcity of professionals in the field oriented to a child and adolescent developmental perspective (Kaminer, 1991a).

Hoffmann, Sonis, and Halikas (1987) thoughtfully captured the conceptual, political, and territorial disputes in the addictions field as follows (pp. 450–451):

> If treatment is the final common pathway, then is all treatment the same?
> Clearly the answer to this rhetorical question must be no. Substance abuse
> treatment programs vary in their roots of development, philosophical approaches to the patient/client, orientation in treatment, perspective on

problem behaviors, sensitivity to drug use consequences, attention to psychodynamic, family and biological issues, and finally, definition of treatment response and successful management. This heterogeneity must not
be underestimated. The outsider seeking to assess various treatment programs in any particular geographical area may find himself or herself
enmeshed in local territorial disputes, local jargon or code words, local
personality conflicts among elders of the treatment community, and local
philosophic monopolies, all of which thwart objective assessment of treatment adequacy in ways not seen in medicine. . . . There exists a broad
spectrum of philosophies and approaches, none of which has a monopoly
on success or even objective evidence of a higher rate of success than the
other philosophies.

Hoffmann et al. (1987) also refer to the difficulty of self-help groups like
Alcoholics Anonymous (AA) in recognizing and accepting the importance of accurate medical and psychiatric differential diagnoses that
accompany PSUDs. This resistance is rooted in historical issues from the
period when medicine in general and psychiatry in particular were perceived as fully rejecting these patients and the diagnostic concept of
PSUDs and treating only the clearly medical consequences of substance
abuse (e.g., cirrhosis, trauma).

11.3. A DEVELOPMENTAL PERSPECTIVE FOR INTERVENTIONS

In contrast to the convoluted politics of treatment, the increasing
importance and validity of the biopsychosocial etiological and pathogenetic paradigm of PSUDs and the recent conceptual application of the
developmental transactional perspective approach to psychopathology
(Sameroff & Chandler, 1975) have been recognized as a clear advancement in the understanding of adolescent substance use (ASU) and AP-
SUDs. The view that prevention and treatment of PSUDs constitute
interventions on the same continuum and may command a similar menu
of therapeutic strategies/techniques (but a different dosage of specific
interventions has been a significant step toward a fluid conceptualization
of patient–intervention matching (Tarter, 1992).

Theoretical progress in conceptual perceptions of the development
of APSUD treatment-planning strategies has not yet been translated into
a practical application for treatment needs. In the present absence of
true differential treatment and individualized patient–treatment matching in most programs, these paradigms only lay the foundation for
potentially improved future interventions (Hoffmann et al., 1987). Since

adult PSUD research and clinical state of the art are at a more advanced stage than are those for APSUDs, it is sensible to use findings from the adult literature as points of reference. However, it is imperative to recognize their limited potential for generalizability.

11.4. TREATMENT OUTCOME STUDIES: METHODOLOGICAL ISSUES

Studies on adolescents with PSUDs have been especially silent regarding treatment outcome. All the studies that have been published so far suffer from one or more methodological flaws.

Most studies reviewed did not use diagnostic rating scales to assess PSUDs and other psychiatric disorders; others did not employ valid and reliable criteria for the diagnosis of PSUDs. Personal and demographic variables such as sex, age, and race, as well as psychosocioeconomic factors of the adolescents and their first-degree relatives, have not been reported to the extent that would allow a determination of need for specialized treatment-program components. Last, from among the limited available studies enrolling an acceptable number of adolescents within the appropriate age range (12–18 years), the treatment setting, interventions, or time in treatment were neither controlled nor comparable across studies.

11.4.1. Adolescent Psychoactive Substance Use Disorder Treatment Outcome: The Definition Dilemma

It is generally recognized that the criteria for treatment outcome can be defined in relation either to the treatment program or to the individual patient. The two criteria commonly used in program evaluation are attrition rate and length of stay vs. planned stay (Kaminer & Bukstein, 1989). Indeed, dropping out of treatment is perceived as synonymous with failure to achieve even a minimally successful treatment outcome. Arguably, persisting with treatment for at least a brief period of time is essential if any benefits are to be derived (Kaminer, Tarter, Bukstein, & Kabene, 1992b). In defining treatment outcome of the patient with an APSUD, most articles traditionally refer to complete abstinence as the exclusive measure for a successful treatment. The increasing recognition in the adult literature of addiction as a chronic disorder and of the benefit of reduction in severity or improvement in symptoms of PSUDs when it is impractical to achieve abstinence (Meyer, 1992) has not yet been considered as an index for successful adolescent treatment outcome mainly due to the age-related ethical dilemma.

The definition of outcomes is another arena for a clash of treatment philosophies, especially between counselors and other pro-disease-model advocates (Meyer, 1986), on one hand, and, on the other, therapists and other professionals who advocate the self-medication theory or a multidimensional, multidisciplinary model (Kaminer & Frances, 1991).

The issues debated are: Is abstinence an adequate measure of AP-SUD treatment outcome? Are different therapies needed for PSUDs related to a specific drug vs. combinations of psychoactive substances? What is the importance of measuring the functional level of other life domains, especially given reports that severity of drug use is not necessarily the most important factor in predicting treatment outcome in adults with PSUDs (McLellan, Luborsky, Woody, O'Brien, & Druley, 1983; Rounsaville, Kosten, Weissman, & Kleber, 1986)? There is a valid dilemma in how to relate to treatment outcome as perceived by community expectations for the adolescent in treatment to exhibit improved adjustment on completion of treatment and during aftercare/follow-up. These expectations may include reduced disruption of family functions, elimination of delinquency related to substance abuse, improved school or employment function, and others.

11.4.2. Relationship between the Severity of the Adolescent Psychoactive Substance Use Disorder and Treatment Outcome

The introduction of severity measures in studies of PSUDs has facilitated research regarding the relationship of severity to treatment outcome. Investigations focusing on adolescents with PSUDs have not yet been reported. However, the adult-oriented literature and clinical experience indicate that it is timely to raise and test hypotheses regarding this matter.

Empirical studies have suggested that severity of alcohol dependence is a relatively good indication of clinical treatment outcome (Babor, Cooney, & Lauerman, 1987; Rounsaville, Dolinsky, Babor, & Meyer, 1987). Reports on opioid addiction (Babor et al., 1987) and cocaine abuse (Weiss, Griffin, & Hufford, 1992) failed to predict any relationship between the severity of substance-specific PSUD and posttreatment relapse. A study that investigated patient–treatment matching concluded that patients with low to medium severity of alcohol dependence may benefit equally from an outpatient program compared to an inpatient program (Hayashida et al., 1989). It appears that the severity of the PSUD alone has limited predictive validity for treatment outcome.

The severity of comorbid psychopathology and of impairment in other life domains as measured by severity rating scales has been of greater prognostic value. It has been shown that the family, criminal, employment, and psychological problems seen among alcohol and drug abusers are important predictors of response to treatment.

11.4.3. Treatment Outcome Studies: Patient–Treatment– Environment Characteristics of Adolescent Psychoactive Substance Use Disorders

Studies conducted among adults with PSUDs in the 1970s suggested that patient variables are predominantly more predictive of treatment outcome than are characteristics of treatment programs (Holden, 1987). This conclusion could be attributed mainly to the "black box" regimen used in most programs, which was characterized by a shotgun approach to treatment lacking clear differential components (i.e., type of facility, treatment philosophy, and length of treatment appeared to be the pivotal characteristics of the program, without patient–treatment matching).

With the advancement of treatment knowledge, it has become clearer that a substantial proportion of the explained variance is shared between patient-related and program-related variables (Kaminer et al., 1992b). Also, patient–environment interactions are gaining recognition as important determinants that contribute to the maintenance of posttreatment objectives (Sobell, Sobell, & Nirenberg, 1988). The articles on the treatment of APSUDs reviewed herein contribute to the understanding of this issue; however, their methodological limitations must be noted again in order to forestall unconditional generalizing.

Large cohort studies on the treatment of APSUDs emerged in the late 1970s. Rush (1979) conducted treatment-outcome research on a mixed population of adolescents and young adults in the Pennsylvania substance-abuse treatment system. His criteria for successful treatment outcome included complete abstinence in addition to an index score combining education, training, and employment, which he defined as Productivity. Most of the 2,940 adolescents included in this sample were enrolled in outpatient programs. Patient variables that were found to predict treatment completion as well as treatment success in these drug-free outpatient clinics included enrollment in education and employment programs at the time of admission, the abuse of only one psychoactive substance (a nonopioid agent), being white, and being older when the substance of abuse was first used. Delinquency at admission was inversely correlated with successful treatment outcome at discharge. It is important to note that Rush (1979) included other important patient variables under the definition of delinquency used in the study, such as a longer continuous use of psychoactive substances and early initiation of use. It is of interest that a treatment variable such as time in outpatient treatment accounted for very little of the variance and had an inverse relationship with treatment outcome. This finding is perhaps the first report of its kind in a study of APSUD treatment regarding the necessary distinction between "effective" and "effective and least restrictive" treatments (Sobell et al., 1988). This issue is discussed in detail in Section 11.8.1.

Two large-scale national studies have been designed to assess adolescent treatment outcome. The Drug Abuse Reporting Program (DARP) assessed treatment outcomes of 5,405 patients under the age of 19 from a large number of mixed-ages programs. Reduction in the use of opiates but not of alcohol and marijuana was recorded among patients from outpatient clinics and therapeutic communities (Sells & Simpson, 1979). No data that might indicate an optional patient–treatment match were noted. The Treatment Outcome Prospective Study (TOPS) evaluated treatment outcomes for a mixed population of 11,750 adolescents in outpatient clinics and residential treatment facilities (Hubbard, Cavanaugh, Craddock, & Rachal, 1985). The results of this study were compared to those of the DARP study, although lack of an untreated control group in the TOPS study makes it difficult to determine the meaning of treatment (the DARP study employed an "intake only" control group).

Three studies (Benson, 1985; Holsten, 1980; Vaglum & Fossheim, 1980) provided information about overall treatment results and their relation to patient variables. However, lack of information about the specific interventions in treatment in these studies limits their utility in developing matching criteria (Hester & Miller, 1988).

Szapocznik, Kurtines, Foote, Perez-Vidal, and Hervis (1983) reported that adolescents who received a small number of brief strategic family therapy sessions, in addition to individual sessions, reported overall reductions in drug use and delinquent behavior at 6 months follow-up. Also, temporary placement of adolescents with a family of another adolescent who had progressed further in the same day-program appeared to be helpful in reducing PSUDs (Friedman, Schwartz, & Utada, 1989). The rationale for the choice of family interventions is not clearly explained in these reports, nor is it explained in the next two studies cited. Dejong and Henrich (1980) and Langrod, Alksne, and Gomez (1981) published studies that evaluated treatment-program effectiveness among mixed populations of adolescents and young adults. The design of these studies could be classified as "posttest only" follow-up design. As in the study conducted by Rush (1979), no control group was employed and psychiatric comorbidity issues were not investigated.

DeJong and Henrich (1980) conducted a 2-year follow-up study of 89 young addicts in a behavior modification program who attended a rehabilitation center for at least 7 days. They reported that one third of the total sample was drug-free. Langrod et al. (1981) studied a residential, religious intervention program and reported a 24% abstinence rate at outcome. No research methodology on this study was reported.

Amini, Zilberg, and Burke (1982) reported a random-assignment, controlled study of inpatient vs. outpatient treatment of 74 delinquent drug-abusing adolescents. The results at 1-year treatment-effectiveness follow-up showed no significant difference in outcome. Grenier (1985) utilized a waiting-list control group to empirically assess the effectiveness of adolescent residential treatment. The age range of patients in this study was 9–21 years. The abstinence rate for the treatment group (65%) was significantly higher than that for the waiting-list control group (14% spontaneous remissions).

Other studies on the treatment of APSUDs published in the second half of the 1980s indicated the growing awareness of dually diagnosed (DUDI) adolescents and of patient–treatment matching (i.e., individualized treatment objectives). Emphasis on the differences between drop-outs and other patients engaged in treatment illuminated the importance of retention in treatment. One basic difficulty in comparing the findings and rates of attrition reported by the different studies is that attrition occurred at different phases of the referral treatment process.

It is generally realized in child and adolescent psychiatry that drop-out from an outpatient clinic is primarily a function of referral-source expectations and the caretaker's symptomatology (Gould, Shaffer, & Kaplan, 1985). These factors have not yet been emphasized in the outpatient treatment of APSUDs.

The effects of psychiatric symptomatology on treatment outcome for adolescent male drug abusers were studied by Friedman and Glickman (1987). The 130 court-referred substance-abusing delinquent boys of ages 14–18 years were engaged in a day treatment program. The inconclusive findings were that a number of psychiatric symptoms, particularly depression, were positively correlated with treatment outcome. These findings are different from those reported in the adult literature. Patient variables that have been found to predict treatment outcome among the adolescent groups herein reviewed include: age of onset of drug use, race, gender, number of drugs abused, and type of comorbid psychopathology. Friedman and Glickman (1986) also reported on outpatient-program characteristics for successful treatment of adolescent drug abuse, as measured by reduction in drug use. Adolescents in 30 programs were assessed; 50% of them ($N = 5789$) dropped out before completion of treatment. The following characteristics of programs were found to predict outcome to a statistically significant degree: having a special school for school dropouts; employing experienced counselors; providing birth control services; providing vocational, recreational, gestalt, and music/art therapy; employing group confrontation; and being perceived by the client as allowing and encouraging free expression and spontaneous action.

11.4.4. Comorbid Psychiatric Disorders and Treatment Outcome in Adolescent Psychoactive Substance Use Disorders

The recognition of comorbid psychiatric disorder as a key prognostic factor for treatment outcome in the adult literature has influenced the research on this subject in APSUDs (McLellan et al., 1983; Rounsaville et al., 1986).

A large segment of adolescents with PSUDs are DUDI, and this is true for untreated as well as treated populations (Bukstein, Brent, & Kaminer, 1989; Kaminer, 1991b). The two most prevalent Axis I diagnoses according to DSM-III-R are mood disorders and conduct disorders. A comorbid psychiatric disorder may be a reason for adolescents with PSUDs to seek professional help. Indeed, Friedman and Glickman (1986) reported that 28% of the adolescents they examined applied for treatment following emotional and psychiatric problems. The purpose of emphasizing the importance of dual diagnosis (DD) in adolescents is fourfold: (1) to introduce and increase awareness, recognition, and understanding of this concept; (2) to offer treatment and aftercare options for these adolescents and their families; (3) to enhance training designed to improve clinical care and research of these patients; and (4) to advocate allocation of resources and improve reimbursement for the treatment of these youngsters.

A recent study investigated patient variables that may distinguish completers from noncompleters among hospitalized, DUDI adolescents (Kaminer, Tarter, Bukstein, & Kabene, 1992a). About 22% of patients dropped out of the program after the first week (evaluation phase) of treatment. No significant differences between groups were found on any of the following variables: age, parent/caretaker education, socioeconomic status, sex, race, domicile, legal status on admission, and history of past treatment for either psychiatric disorder or substance abuse or both. The two groups did not differ with respect to the prevalence of Axis I psychiatric disorders in their parents. They were distinguishable, however, according to the Axis I psychiatric diagnosis assigned to them. Mood and adjustment disorders were significantly more prevalent among the 50 treatment completers, whereas the noncompleters were more likely to have been assigned a conduct disorder diagnosis. A significantly higher percentage of treatment completers received psychotropic medications.

11.4.5. Motivation in Treatment

Motivation is a term that has usually been used to explain a patient's lack of commitment to treatment as well as a poor outcome (Sobell et al., 1988). Miller (1985) suggested that motivation can be viewed as the probability of engaging in behaviors that are intended to result in beneficial outcomes. He proposed viewing motivation as a dynamic interpersonal process involving the patient, the therapist and treatment program, and the environment. Motivation could be increased by designing intervention strategies.

Wilkinson and LeBreton (1986) studied motivational intervention designed to treat young adult substance abusers. They found that the measures assessing initial levels of motivation for treatment were not associated with outcome. However, motivation during treatment as assessed by not achieving goals and by attrition from treatment was found to be associated with treatment failures. It is concluded that in clinical practice, it is important to ensure setting realistic goals with and for the patients (e.g., use of therapeutic contracts).

11.4.6. Attrition as a Process

Attrition from treatment may be perceived either as a discrete event or as a process. A qualitative *post hoc* examination of adolescents with DD who prematurely terminated treatment was reported by Kaminer et al. (1992a). The results indicated that it is a time-ordered process that can be divided into specific stages: (1) ideas about leaving treatment, (2) threatening to leave treatment, (3) signing the request to leave, and (4) actually leaving. This process, which has strong similarities to the concept of suicidal behavior (Kaminer, 1992c), may end at any one of the first three stages. What, then, is the meaning of progressing to any of the first three phases of the process, but not dropping out? The interpretation offered here, albeit speculative and in need of empirical examination, includes the following: (1) The intention to leave comprises an attempt to neutralize absolute control by the treatment staff regarding the patient's level in the treatment program. (2) It is a way to show off, to put pressure on peers, parents, or staff to gain status or avoid disciplinary actions, or to achieve both ends. (3) It is an impulsive act.

"Motivation" to engage in treatment and "attrition" from treatment are two terms that are not usually defined correctly. Also, level of motivation and attrition rate from treatment are generally perceived to be inversely associated with each other. It is important to continue to clarify the dynamic nature of motivation and the process of attrition.

11.5. ADOLESCENT PSYCHOACTIVE SUBSTANCE USE DISORDERS: LEGAL ASPECTS OF ADMISSION AND TREATMENT

Facilities that treat minors have to follow some basic common rules with slight differences. Consent for admission to an inpatient unit must be provided by the caretaker and child (unless the child or adolescent has been committed). Any patient under 18 years of age who is married, a parent, or emancipated has the right to consent on his or her own behalf. Prior to rendering any care without parental consent, the facility must obtain a written acknowledgment from the minor stating that he or she was: (1) advised of the purpose and nature of such treatment services; (2) told that he or she may withdraw the signed acknowledgment at any time; (3) told that the facility will make attempts to convince the child of the need for involvement of other family members in treatment and the facility's preference for parental consent for the rendering of treatment services; and (4) advised that a medical/clinical record of his or her treatment services will be made and maintained by the facility. For overnight treatment, parental consent is always required unless the parents refuse, in which case the Family Court may substitute its consent.

The provisions of various laws and regulations establish that it is usually, though not always, necessary to obtain parental consent to deliver substance-abuse treatment to minors. However, the release of information regarding such treatment is governed by the strict Federal rules regarding education and medical records. Regardless of state laws granting parents unilateral rights to consent to treatment, the Federal rules require both a parent's and a minor patient's prior consent to the release of medical record information that would identify the patient as an alcohol or drug abuser. Whenever state law does permit a minor to consent unilaterally to treatment, the Federal rules require that only the patient's consent need be obtained prior to the release of medical records information. Also, drug- or alcohol-abusing patients must be notified on admission of the protections afforded by the Federal rules (B. J. Weinberg, personal communication, October 7, 1991).

Methadone maintenance treatment programs for patients under 18 years of age need to consider some legal implications. According to the Food and Drug Administration regulation (State Methadone Maintenance Treatment Guidelines, 1992, p. 284):

A person under 18 is required to have had two documented attempts at short-term detoxification or drug-free treatment to be eligible for maintenance treatment. A 1-week waiting list period is required after such a detoxification attempt; however, before an attempt is repeated, the program physician shall document in the patient's record that the patient continues to be or is again physiologically dependent on narcotic drugs. No person under 18 years of age may be admitted to a methadone maintenance treatment program unless a parent, legal guardian or responsible adult designated by the State authority (e.g., "emancipated minor" laws) completes and signs consent form, Form FDA-2635—Consent to methadone treatment.

11.6. TREATMENT PROGRAMS AND TREATMENT CHARACTERISTICS

Studies conducted in the late 1970s and early 1980s were designed to assess and to characterize types of adolescents in treatment (Beschner, 1985). In these studies, 75% were white and 11.5% were black; also, white adolescents were more likely to abuse multiple drugs than were minority adolescents. Most adolescents (81.5%) are admitted to drug-free outpatient programs (Beschner, 1985). These programs range from unstructured "drop-in" centers to clinics with a more structured environment where a demanding curriculum is followed.

Few substance-abuse treatment programs are designed specifically to serve adolescents. About 20% of all patients in substance-abuse treatment programs are under 19 years of age (Beschner, 1985); only 5% of programs have adolescents as their main clientele. The most prevalent levels of treatment care noted for APSUDs are: outpatient treatment, day or evening treatment known as partial hospitalization, inpatient treatment, and various types of residential treatment (e.g., halfway house, group home). Some or all of the interventions discussed below may be provided to adolescents at any of the levels or settings of treatment depending on philosophy and goals of treatment, resources, accreditation demands, and other factors. Basic components for a drug-free adolescent treatment program may include: individual counseling, individual therapy, self-help groups for the patients and caretakers (e.g., AA, NA, Al-Anon, Al-Ateen), substance-abuse education, random urinalysis for psychoactive substances, Breathaliyzer testing, family therapy or involvement or both, relapse-prevention techniques, educational or vocational counseling, legal assistance, various types of group activities or therapies, contingency contracting, medications, and pencil-and-paper assignments relating to the recovery process.

11.7. THE TWO PIVOTAL THERAPEUTIC MODELS

Substantial variation exists among various models of programs for the treatment of APSUDs. Representing the extreme ends of the spectrum of available programs are two models: the Minnesota model and the multidisciplinary professional model.

The Minnesota model is based on the 12 traditions of AA. This is an intensive 12-step program in which the counselor is the primary therapist who utilizes intensive group processes and self-help group participation as the pivotal therapeutic interventions (Hoffmann et al., 1987). The Minnesota model is also characterized by four short-term goals to be used as indications of progress (Laundergan, 1982). They include the need to: recognize the disease of addiction and its implications; admit the necessity for help; identify specifically what needs to be changed in order to achieve help; make these changes and develop a new life-style. The Minnesota model is not suited to answering the needs of DUDI patients.

The multidisciplinary professional model employs a diverse team of mental health professionals experienced and trained in the evaluation and treatment of APSUDs. This team is usually led by a physician and operates according to a case-management model (Hoffmann et al., 1987). This team may cover some or all of the following domains: PSUDs, psychiatric disorders, family function, legal status, peer–social relationships, school or employment status, and medical problems. Each one of the team's members has one or more specialties that enable him or her to take responsibility for the appropriate domain; however, decisions are made by the entire team. Interventions that are often employed in such a program, regardless of the setting, commonly include individual, family, and various group therapies, self-help groups, and urinalysis for psychoactive-substance detection. Additional interventions such as contracts, cognitive therapy (e.g., individual, family, group), relapse-prevention techniques, social-skills training, medications, and variants of the interventions noted above have been reported (Kaminer & Frances, 1991).

The efficacy of a multidisciplinary professional program for the treatment of APSUDs and the differential contribution of its components were evaluated at an inpatient unit for DUDI adolescents. Kaminer et al. (1992a) investigated the level of agreement between unit staff and patients (treatment completers and noncompleters) regarding the perception of the efficacy of treatment modalities in a program employing ten therapeutic interventions. Results indicated statistically significant and clinically meaningful differences in perception of the value of the following therapeutic modalities: individual treatment contracting, therapeutic community meeting, and educational counseling. The three groups did not differ on the seven following variables: family therapy, self-help group, relapse-prevention group, medication, vocational counseling, social-skills group, and substance-abuse education. These findings suggest the following conclusions: (1) The magnitude of agreement between staff and patients on the efficacy of treatment variables is associated with the likelihood of completing treatment among adolescents with PSUDs. (2) Contracting is very useful for the inpatient treatment of patients who actively negotiate with staff about their treatment objectives. These results should be interpreted cautiously because of the small sample size of noncompleters and staff. (3) The measurement of "treatment dosage" (a descriptive term encompassing frequency, quantity, type, specificity, and quality of the intervention employed) is far from clear. However, since no single strategy appears to be superior to others in dealing with APSUDs, changes in the summation or compilation of components of the "treatment dosage" could affect the patient's threshold for therapeutic change (Kaminer et al., 1992a). (4) The utilization of efficacy-of-treatment and treatment-satisfaction questionnaires has the potential to add a useful dimension to the assessment of treatment outcome.

The Treatment Services Review (TSR) assessment instrument (McLellan, Alterman, Cacciola, Metzger, & O'Brien, 1992) is a recent attempt to assess the quantity of different treatments provided by a program. Instead of focusing on specifying the details of the treatment components provided by a program, it uses the patient's weekly report of treatments received in each of the life areas tapped by the Addiction Severity Index (ASI) (McLellan et al., 1992). The TSR allows quantification of the units and amounts of treatment that a patient receives in a program (Alterman, O'Brien, & McLellan, 1991). A modification of this instrument for the needs of special populations, especially for adolescents with PSUDs, could be beneficial.

11.8. THE TREATMENT PLAN

The development of a treatment plan prepares the patient for the stages of treatment according to the stages of the change model (Prochaska & DiClemente, 1986): (1) Precontemplation—no thought of change; (2) Contemplation—thought but no action, start of intent; (3) Action; (4) Maintenance.

An individual treatment contract was found useful for initiating and maintaining treatment in the adult with PSUD (Rosen, 1978; Vanicelli, 1974) and in the adolescent literature (Kaminer et al., 1992b). Patients who actively negotiate with staff about their treatment objectives show significant improvement and reduction of anxiety. Also, contracting was perceived by adolescent treatment completers to be the most important therapeutic intervention. Indeed, it is suggested that the contract be utilized as the basis for every treatment plan.

This treatment component is based on a contract developed from a problem list conjointly prepared by the patient and the therapist during the evaluation phase. The contract specifies long-term goals according to the Teen ASI (T-ASI) (Kaminer, Bukstein, & Tarter, 1991). The goals are sensible, achievable, and measurable. They are fractioned into periodic objectives according to the following domains: substance abuse, psychiatric symptomatology, family issues, legal status, peer–social relationships, and school or vocational problems. Individual treatment is provided by a team led by the program director or coordinator who supervises the primary therapists/counselors who contract with the patients. Progress of the multilevel system depends on the periodic presentation and review of the contract.

11.8.1. Effective versus Least Restrictive Treatment

Effective treatments are those that help adolescents with PSUDs to achieve treatment and aftercare objectives and have a high probability of maintaining accomplishments. Also, they require the least total life-style change for the client. Sobell et al. (1988, p. 42) summarized this topic as follows:

> Although treatment planning is a process where treatment is designed to meet the needs and resources of each client, sometimes several treatment options may appear viable for a particular client. When this occurs, the cost of the various treatment strategies should be evaluated in relation to the client's lifestyle, values and resources.

A relevant example demonstrating the importance of the distinction between "effective" and "effective and least restrictive" treatment is the choice implicit in a common effective treatment strategy: avoidance of high-risk situations for psychoactive-substance use (e.g., not going to parties). While the tradeoff is a strict limitation of social activities, when the adolescent can master refusal skills to cope with such situations, he or she may choose not to avoid them.

11.8.2. Counselor/Therapist Effectiveness

Assessment of the contribution of treatment variables to treatment outcome often underscores the role of the counselor/therapist. The care provider (e.g., therapist, counselor, case manager, coordinator) has a pivotal role in the treatment process of the individual with PSUD. A review of the literature devoted to evaluating the effectiveness of care providers in treatment programs leads to the conclusion, based on controlled studies, that there are no significant differences in the performance of groups of patients assigned to counselors/therapists on the basis of formal education or past history of addiction (Luborsky, Crits-Cristoph, McLellan, & Woody, 1986; McLellan, Woody, Luborsky, & Goehl, 1988).

Subsequent examination of data within each category group revealed major differences in outcome among the patients of individual therapists (Luborsky et al., 1986). McLellan et al. (1988) also reported large differences among the outcomes obtained by different therapists. The most effective providers appeared to take a more systematic approach to treatment: conducting a careful needs assessment, developing a detailed treatment plan, keeping careful notes, and meeting with patients about twice the minimum required number of sessions. The least effective counselors/therapists had no formal training, kept few or no progress notes, and had fewer formal sessions with patients as compared to effective counselors.

The importance of these staff members as active ingredients in the treatment of adults with PSUDs needs to be confirmed in the treatment of APSUDs. Investigation of the reasons cited by adolescent noncompleters who dropped out of an inpatient unit of adolescents with PSUDs revealed that some adolescents blamed their primary therapist for their having dropped out (Kaminer et al., 1992b). Indeed, therapist characteristics such as hostility, expectancy, and empathy are important in treatment. Failure to develop therapeutic alliance will reduce the chances of agreeing on treatment objectives and preparing a contract (Kaufman & Reaux, 1988).

Training can change the behavior of counselors, as reported by Dennis, Fairbank, & Rachal (1992). Enhanced counselor training may include: counseling skills training, performance feedback, and booster training. It is suggested that future research on retention of APSUDs in treatment focus on therapist variables.

11.9. PSYCHOTHERAPIES AND OTHER INTERVENTIONS

There is consistent and growing evidence that adult patients with PSUDs who receive the most services during treatment have the best outcomes. Also, those substance-abuse treatment programs that provide the most services to their clients have the best programmatic results (Allison & Hubbard, 1985; Ball & Ross, 1991; McLellan et al., 1982, 1988; McLellan, Arndt, Metzger, Woody, & O'Brien, 1993). McLellan et al. (1993) reported that patients in a methadone maintenance program who also received a combination of medical, psychiatric, employment, and family therapy (psychosocial services package) fared better than two other groups of patients who received either counseling in addition to methadone or methadone only.

Empirical research on the contribution of various psychotherapies to abstinence and relapse prevention in APSUDs is virtually nonexistent. However, conceptual papers and descriptive literature on the rationale and implementation of such therapies in adolescent treatment programs are available. The treatment modalities described in the following sections may be utilized individually on the basis of their own merits or in combination with one or more of the others (e.g., multiple family therapy groups, modified psychodynamic group therapy).

11.9.1. Individual Psychotherapy

Viewed from a traditional psychoanalytic approach, a PSUD was perceived as a self-destructive or chronic suicidal behavior (Menninger, 1938). Most of the early psychoanalytic formulations emphasized the instinctive aggressive drives and the pleasurable aspects of drug abuse to explain the compelling nature of addiction (Khantzian, 1980). Khantzian (1980) commented that more recent psychoanalytic formulations have placed greater emphasis on problems in adaptation, ego and self pathologies,* and related psychopathology as etiological factors in drug dependence. Translating psychoanalytic terminology into practical and potentially measurable factors has led to the identification of four areas of self-regulation vulnerability in the individual with PSUD that need to be addressed (Khantzian, Halliday, Golden, & McAuliffe, 1992): difficulties with self-care, relationships, self-esteem, and regulation of affect. These vulnerabilities become more obvious when, as is commonly the case, there is psychopathology—in the form of mood or anxiety disorder, or personality disorder, or both—accompanying the PSUD, regardless of the chronology of the disorders.

The efficacy of individual psychotherapy for substance abusers,

---

*In ego pathology, the emphasis is on disturbances in structure and function in coping with drives and emotions; self pathology relates more to troubled attitudes and experiences about the self and others.

particularly DUDI patients, has been well established (Woody, McLellan, Luborsky, & O'Brien, 1984).

The addition of this modality is more advantageous than drug counseling alone. Khantzian (1985, p. 85) argued in favor of a broadly defined individual psychotherapy that includes "all those interventions and roles a therapist must play in assuring that a substance abuser's physical and psychological needs are understood and managed." This expanded, nontraditional psychotherapy demands that the therapist involve himself or herself in matters of safety and self-care while strengthening the therapeutic alliance with the patient and initiating abstinence. The emphasis in contemporary treatment of APSUDs is on the "here and now." The psychotherapy of patients with PSUDs targets the initiation and maintenance of abstinence as its first goal. This initial phase of early recovery involves a supportive, directive psychotherapeutic approach. A majority of patients are diagnosed with concomitant psychiatric disorder and may need therapy that addresses issues related to it, such as facilitating medication compliance (Kaufman, 1989).

Kaufman (1989) suggested that the therapist should focus on "how" the patient abuses a substance, not on "why," when assessing the history of immediate stressors. Examining "how" (behavioral causes and effects) allows the suggestion of alternative behaviors that can avoid triggering relapse. Following a comprehensive assessment, the therapist develops with the adolescent patient and family a treatment contract that covers their respective commitments to the terms of treatment provision and compliance with required behavior and life-style oriented to abstinence and relapse prevention (e.g., participation in self-help group meetings, family therapy sessions, and medication intake as needed).

During the initial phase, structure, consistency, and maintenance of boundaries in treatment are of tremendous importance, especially for patients who exhibit high levels of novelty-seeking and low levels of harm avoidance. The ability to be a good therapeutic container for an adolescent patient who tends to form intense transitional relationships with the therapist that may rapidly swing from clinging attachment to hostile rejection, and yet to be emphatic, may contribute to progress toward stabilization in a variety of life domains. It is noteworthy that adolescent patients with conduct disorder—antisocial personality disorder continuum (CD-ASPDC) and adults with ASPD do not do well in individual psychotherapy and usually drop out of treatment programs unless they are also depressed (Alterman & Cacciola, 1991; Kaminer et al., 1992a).

Individual therapy with a person with PSUD needs to address commonly used defense mechanisms in concordance with the progress in recovery achieved by the patient. Denial should not be confronted early in therapy because if the patient is left without an alternative means of handling stress, anxiety, and depression, premature reduction of denial may trigger a return to substance abuse (Kaufman, 1989). Other prominent defenses used by substance abusers are projection and rationalization, which aid the individual in attributing uncomfortable and undesirable self-qualities to others. It has been suggested that these defense mechanisms should be shifted to the aim of maintaining abstinence, and previous dysfunctional behavior should be attributed to the disorder rather than to others or to the self. Also, identification with other abstainers can be achieved by a shifting of assimilative projection that assumes that others are like oneself and perceives them as such (Kaufman, 1989). Only much later in therapy, when the patient has been able to maintain long-term abstinence, may a more traditional confrontation and interpretation approach be utilized.

The therapist needs to avoid developing codependency with the patient or becoming a substitute for the addiction. These may be destructive forms of countertransference on the part of the therapist that will lead either to termination of treatment or to therapist burnout (Kaufman, 1989). If more than one person is involved in the treatment of an individual with PSUD, as is usually the case in program settings, the therapist or a case coordinator should prevent the patient from splitting and manipulating other staff members, patients, or relatives. The issue can be addressed in individual therapy as well as in group and family therapy when appropriate. Initiation of the patient's participation in self-help group meetings during the early phase of individual psychotherapy is a challenging approach.

Brown (1985) followed a developmental perspective and compared the early stage of abstinence to infancy. In this view, the substance of abuse is a primary object that provides constant gratification without disappointment, yet gratification is controlled by the individual's voluntary behavior. The provision of other gratifying substitutes may enable the patient to gradually give up to the previous object. Brown (1985) suggests that the most plausible substitutes, in addition to developing a new repertoire of habit patterns and behaviors, are identification with a self-help group and its membership and active participation in the group. In order to gain some control over the PSUD and the environmental stimuli, the patient is given an active role in choosing when and how often to attend the self-help group.

Choosing a sexual partner or a love object as a substitute for a drug at an early stage of treatment is considered to be a diversion from focusing on abstinence (a "setup") and is doomed, in most cases, to result in disappointment that may lead to relapse. The reason is that many of these patients have suffered developmental and maturational arrest in various domains, including the ability to form meaningful relationships and to achieve intimacy. During later phases in treatment, they may be able to address these problems.

The issue of grandiosity and narcissism in the addict has also been known to interfere with abstinence. It has been addressed by the self-help group's ability to become the source for gratification as a "higher power" with which the patient may identify. According to Kaufman (1989, p. 15), "becoming a speaker, or a sponsor, enhances self-esteem and reduces anxiety through helping others, using the more mature defense of altruism."

A patient who has made significant progress in addressing the four areas of self-regulation vulnerability may be able to advance to fulfill mature roles in life, including sustained and meaningful interpersonal relationships, a return to school or vocation, continued participation in 12-step groups and meeting the demands of higher steps, and other forms of recovery-related activity (e.g., sponsorship). Termination of the psychotherapeutic relationship and the ability to handle the separation from the therapist without regression to self-destructive behaviors is the final step in therapy.

Most of the information reviewed in this section is based on adult-oriented literature; however, it appears to be relevant and to have significant clinical utility for adolescents.

11.9.2. Family Therapy

The definition of family has changed during the last few decades. Divorce, single parenthood, adoption, and homosexual parenthood are the most prominent phenomena that have become more normalized through their increased incidence. Children and adolescents are members of family systems and in most cases are dependent on the family unit. Normative ASU is considered to be part of the rebellion against parental authority; however, APSUD is not only a problem of the adolescent as an individual but also a family issue. The adolescent with PSUD and other deviant behaviors may be the family's initial presenting problem in treatment, but other problems of equal or greater magnitude may coexist (Quinn, Kuehl, Thomas, & Joaning, 1988). For example, the existence of PSUD in another family member needs to be detected in order to develop alliance with the therapist. Family therapy sessions may include an individual family or multiple families or both, as is the case in some adolescent substance-abuse treatment programs.

11.9.2.1. Individual Family Therapy

Due to the expansion and diversification of the concept of family in the 1990s, a family may be defined as a social unit that includes people who live in the same household as the adolescent with PSUD, or those with whom he or she has legal, blood, or emotional ties, or both (Bartlett, 1986). Formation of an effective therapist–family relationship is crucial in order to handle potential resistance to treatment. This resistance may be manifested as the family's laying the entire responsibility for change on the adolescent or, in contrast, the adolescent's controlling the family and consequently sabotaging any treatment plan (Quinn et al., 1988). A preliminary meeting between only the parents and the therapist may help to promote parental influence. The therapist may create and improve communication between parents and their offspring by arousing and exposing family conflicts. The therapist may promote the parental role in maintaining relapse prevention by helping them negotiate with the adolescent concerning issues such as curfew, participation in self-help groups, probation, and home detoxification instead of sending the adolescent to another treatment program or "giving up" on the adolescent. Other family members who are identified as having PSUDs must receive treatment.

The therapist needs to be alert to parental or adolescent attempts to sabotage treatment, especially when family secrets are about to be uncovered (e.g., PSUD, child abuse). It is of great importance to be not judgmental but supportive.

11.9.2.2. Multiple Family Therapy

This therapeutic approach includes families whose children participate in a treatment program and may be based either on periodic meetings or on a day, weekend, or even an entire week psychoeducational format, or on both. Bartlett (1986) defined the goals for multiple family therapy: (1) educating the family to the role of the treatment program and the need to plan for relapse prevention and rehabilitation when needed; (2) examining the family relationships and determining what pros and cons could affect treatment and relapse-prevention planning; (3) helping families help one another to cope with the shame and helplessness often related to having an adolescent with PSUD; (4) planning and cooperating with the families regarding treatment techniques for conflict resolution. It is necessary to provide information about various aspects of PSUDs, community resources, and self-help groups for the adolescent and family members.

Groups for adolescent addicted couples were described by Bartlett (1986). Whether they are married or not, these couples may use psychoactive substances together, may become parents together, and usually experience many problems in various life domains, thereby presenting a special challenge for treatment that needs to be explored.

11.9.3. Group Therapy

Therapeutic groups are viewed as social microcosms, which enable members to change and grow while relying on the group to serve as their mirror. Group work with substance abusers is commonly used in a variety of treatment settings. Although the literature contains various theories and techniques of group work, there remains a relative dearth of systematic descriptions concerning the types of groups in use and their relative effectiveness. Groups differ in their aims, inclusion and exclusion criteria, structure, roles of the leaders and participants, therapeutic style employed, and the group process.

Groups are a powerful means to deal effectively with their members' difficulties, especially if the aims and structure are well defined, whether the groups are dynamic, self-help, relapse-prevention, didactic, or focused otherwise (Khantzian et al., 1992). The aims of a group are often not explicit; it is not uncommon to find a cluster of patients going through a group process with leaders who have different goals (Cartwright, 1987). The aims of the group should be made explicit to prevent conflicts between leaders and participants, as well as between participants with different expectations. Some groups focus only on the psychoactive substance of abuse that is the common denominator for the group members (e.g., smoking cessation). However, additional issues and problems may be raised in groups unless the treatment orientation is a highly structured, manual-driven behavioral–cognitive therapy (Kaminer & Frances, 1991).

Harticollis and Harticollis (1980) noted that there seems to be a consensus, even from the psychoanalytic perspectives, that deficient structure in a group may create a degree of anxiety that may hamper the productivity of the group work.

Yalom (1975) advocated a high level of functional homogeneity (which can be determined by, for example, severity of a common psychopathology, level of self-care, or intellectual performance) in the therapy group to enhance effectiveness. This goal can be achieved by designing groups for high- vs. low-functioning individuals, as is the case in treatment programs. However, inclusion and exclusion criteria may be perceived by some patients in a treatment program as discriminatory and could lead to isolation and feelings of low self-esteem. A high level of psychopathological homogeneity could raise difficulties if there is a "critical mass" of borderline or ASPD patients in the group. Sugar (1986) described symbiotic pairing of inpatient borderline adolescents in group therapy and emphasized the necessity to exercise caution and thoroughness in order to avoid possible pitfalls that are inherent in the therapeutic process of such a group. Conduct-disordered adolescents tend to "gang up" on the leader or to scapegoat participants, and the effort to maintain boundaries may exhaust the group and reduce effectiveness. In conclusion, a risk–benefit ratio needs to be considered in selecting group members.

The role of the leader and the extent to which the leader dominates the group appear to be of critical importance. Extreme passivity or dominance is not recommended in groups of individuals with PSUDs. An interpersonal style in which the leader acts as an expert facilitator of communications between members of the group is more effective (Cartwright, 1987).

The quality and quantity of psychosocial support offered by the group to its members are important. The acceptance of individual differences between the participants is in contrast with the confrontational model, in which the member's reluctance to accept the leader's or group's perspective unconditionally is interpreted as denial. Cartwright (1987, p. 952) commented that "such groups unwittingly encourage unauthentic and compliant behavior because the only way in which the members can gain support is by adopting the group's views about themselves."

Information regarding group style and its relationship to outcome is limited. A classic study suggested that a patient-centered style is more beneficial than a reward–punishment oriented group interaction (Ends & Page, 1957). Another study of a change in group style revealed that a facilitative role rather than a rigid and didactic one increased the rate of success in a smoking-cessation clinic (Hajek, Belcher, & Stapleton, 1985).

Cartwright (1987) suggested that openness and flexibility of the group moderator to the group needs, in addition to meeting goals and facilitating the interpersonal process, may improve treatment outcome. For example, helping members who have difficulties in joining and staying in groups due to social anxiety or shame-related anxiety (following difficult sessions) should be emphasized. Further research is required to advance the knowledge of group processes.

11.9.3.1. Selected Therapeutic Groups

11.9.3.1.1. Relapse-Prevention Group. Relapse prevention groups most commonly rely on behavioral–cognitive therapy (a detailed discussion of which is presented in Section 11.9.4). The group empowers the participants to believe in their potential to control their behavior, to regulate their emotions, and to handle interpersonal relationships. The members of the group learn how to recognize and cope with external cues and with high-risk situations that may lead to drug cravings (Kaminer & Bukstein, 1992).

11.9.3.1.2. Psychodynamic Group. Psychodynamic group psychotherapy rests on the assumption that the unstructured nature of the group experience allows natural unfolding of individuals' behaviors, emotions, affects, and styles of relating with people (Khantzian et al., 1992). This therapeutic model is designed to expose salient themes of psychological vulnerability and characteristic defensive styles that may promote PSUDs and make relapse likely.

Modified dynamic group therapy (MDGT) is a contemporary conceptualization of dynamic psychotherapy designed by Khantzian et al. (1992). In contrast to concepts of traditional psychotherapy that emphasize subconscious conflicts, greater emphasis is placed on developmental and structural deficits that have affected the patients' capacities for self-regulation. The four primary dimensions examined are self-care, relationship conflicts, self-esteem, and affect. A supportive group approach encourages the members to examine, recognize, and regulate these dimensions in order to initiate and maintain abstinence and acquire greater flexibility in their lives (Khantzian et al., 1992). MDGT is also applicable for adolescents with PSUDs who have reached the stage of Formal Operational Thinking (a full cognitive capacity), which enables them to understand abstract values and concepts that are needed for treatment and relapse prevention (Kaminer, 1991a).

11.9.3.1.3. Self-Help Group. A self-help group is a voluntary program that operates to promote mutual aid among its members (Galanter, 1990). Support or self-help groups are known to emerge when existing professional approaches to a problem are either slow in responding or are not effective (Khantzian, 1985). Khantzian (1985, p. 83) noted that "this is a natural evolutionary process in which at best the self-help community draws attention to and legitimizes a problem and creates a context for professionals to take up the challenge for understanding and dealing with it." Also, according to a community-psychiatry approach, self-help groups and professionals need not and should not compete with each other (Caplan, 1974).

Alcoholics Anonymous (AA) paved the way for other self-help groups in the addictions field, such as Narcotics Anonymous (NA), Cocaine Anonymous (CA), Gamblers Anonymous (GA), and more. Most of these groups have incorporated the 12-Step program and the 12 traditions of AA, with some modifications to meet the specific needs of their membership. The recognition of DD patients led to the emergence of "double-trouble" self-help groups in order to meet the needs of DUDI individuals who take prescribed psychotropic medications. These individuals had problems finding a sponsor who would be supportive of such treatment, which is unacceptable in many AA chapters.

Adolescents may benefit from participating in AA meetings; however, it is recommended that they be assisted in cautiously examining different chapters and in finding appropriate sponsors in order not to repeat morbid patterns of relationships or abuse they have experienced in their families or in the community. Supervised meetings are the rule during the period that they are in treatment. Two specific groups are of critical importance for adolescents with PSUDs: Al-Anon and Al-Ateen.

Al-Anon is comprised of family members and friends of alcoholics and addicts who meet regularly for mutual support. Most members are spouses of alcoholics, many of whom are members of AA. Al-Ateen is another group focusing on adolescents with PSUDs or parents with PSUDs, or both. Al-Atot is a group for younger children of alcoholics. Al-Ateen and Al-Atot chapters may be formed in schools. Khantzian (1985) expressed concerns that due to political, economic, and control issues, self-help groups and professional health providers have failed to learn from each other about the advantages, limitations, and complementarity of the two approaches. This situation must change, for the benefit of the public and the ones in need of support.

11.9.4. Behavioral and Cognitive Therapy

Behavioral and cognitive (BC) therapy processes play a possible role in the etiology and pathogenesis of PSUDs. The drug dependence syndrome proposed by Edwards and Gross (1976) implicates both biological processes and learning. The rapid reinstatement of tolerance and withdrawal symptoms with resumption of substance abuse in afflicted individuals suggests a biological process, whereas the use of psychoactive agents to relieve withdrawal symptoms and craving in response to internal or external cues seems more consistent with a learning process composed of behavioral and cognitive elements (Meyer, 1986).

Pavlovian conditioning models of tolerance and relapse incidence based on animal as well as human data indicate that environmental cues present at the time of substance administration contribute to tolerance (Kaminer & Bukstein, 1992). Stimuli associated with drug-seeking behavior followed by substance abuse precede the onset of drug effects and establish anticipatory responses (cognitive, physiological, and emotional). These external cues, such as places, situations, people, and drug paraphernalia, can serve as "paired" conditioning stimuli. These stimuli can provoke conditioned responses even in the absence of the drug. Because these conditioned responses are often drug-opposite (or "drug-compensatory") in nature, they may often mimic the effects of withdrawal symptoms (Childress, McLellan, & O'Brien, 1986). Psychoactive substances may serve as positive reinforcement (e.g., euphoria) or negative reinforcement (e.g., relief of withdrawal symptoms or unpleasant affects), and these characteristics contribute to the maintenance of PSUDs.

The recognition of the importance of the relations among the host, agent, and environment to the initiation and maintenance of PSUDs led to the development of experimental BC strategies for the treatment of PSUDs (Kaminer & Bukstein, 1992).

Recent challenges to the effectiveness of various treatment modalities of PSUDs suggest that many of the modalities are modestly effective at best. The introduction of BC interventions has contributed to the available treatment strategies and was reported to reduce rates of "lapse" (the initial episode of psychoactive substance use following a period of recovery) and "relapse" (a process in which indicators or warning signs appear prior to the individual's actual resumption of psychoactive substance use) (Daley & Marlatt, 1992, p. 533).

Cognitive therapy is an active, short-term, symptom-reduction-oriented system of psychotherapy. The therapy is based on an information-processing model that aims toward correcting cognitive distortions and specific habitual errors in thinking (Beck & Rush, 1989). The overall strategy in the wide variety of specific therapeutic techniques available is a blend of verbal procedures and behavior modification techniques. The most common variants are rational emotive therapy, stress inoculation training, and BC therapy.

According to cognitive therapy, early experiences in life result in underlying "schemas"—i.e., subconscious avenues—that assign meaning and organization to events. Thinking errors may result from such schemas and lead to stereotyped unreasonable ideas that overtake a person's approach to life. These ideas are termed "automatic thoughts." Automatic thoughts and faulty schemas lead to self-fulfilling prophecies.

The purpose of therapy is to make patients aware of their automatic thoughts, schemas, and reasoning errors, then develop and exercise new ways of thinking. These strategies and techniques have been implemented in a variety of psychiatric disorders and maladaptive behaviors including depression, anxiety, suicidal behavior, aggressive behavior, and PSUDs.

11.9.4.1. Behavioral and Cognitive Therapeutic Processes for Adolescent Psychoactive Substance Use Disorders

It is important to define the goals of BC therapies for APSUDs as well as to inform the adolescents about the process of change that subsequently occurs. The process is composed of three stages: (1) initial commitment to change, (2) cessation of psychoactive substance abuse, and (3) maintenance of abstinence. The role of the therapeutic environment is to facilitate and consolidate the patient's initial commitment to change (whether as an inpatient or an outpatient). An inpatient setting or a residential treatment program is very effective though not exclusive for the implementation of BC interventions as part of a highly structured curriculum. There are two dimensions to the BC therapeutic process in such programs. The first one is inherent within the structure of the program, since the highly demanding and structured program keeps the adolescent constantly occupied by a busy and demanding schedule. On admission, after the rules and regulations of the program are explained to the patient, a contract is usually prepared and signed by both patient and therapist, assuring the commitment to comply with the program. A level system (a bidirectional graded evaluation system) is usually implemented in order to monitor and respond to the patient's progress toward the treatment program objectives. The adolescent is aware of the relationship between behavior and consequences, and, for example, reinforcement and punishment in a token economy system are commonly used in treatment programs for APSUDs to modulate compliance.

The second dimension of BC treatment is less related to the therapeutic framework and is more qualitative in nature. It may include interventions with BC components appropriate to adolescents, such as contingency contracting, extinction of conditioned responses, social and cognitive skills training, relapse-prevention techniques, and more.

Some of these interventions can be used by the adolescent with PSUD as part of a self-management treatment program or in treatment groups in which role playing, behavioral rehearsal, feedback, written assignments, and exercises are used. The use of a daily inventory or journal aims at getting patients to continuously monitor their daily life events so as to identify high-risk factors and relapse-warning signs (Daley & Marlatt, 1992).

Daley and Marlatt (1992) identified the following key themes in relapse prevention: First, help patients identify their high-risk relapse factors and develop strategies to deal with them. Interpersonal and intrapersonal determinants were identified as responsible for the behavior that will lead to alcohol and substance abuse. Annis and Davis (1989) developed rating scales to measure these high-risk factors pre- and post-BC therapy (see Chapter 10 for details). Second, help patients understand relapse as a process. Third, help patients recognize and cope with cues and cravings. Fourth, help patients deal with social pressure to use substances. Fifth, help patients develop a supportive network (e.g., self-help groups). Sixth, help patients to cope with cognitive distortions. Seventh, help patients work toward a drug-free, balanced life-style. Finally, help patients develop a plan to interrupt a lapse or relapse.

Application of the general coping-skills training approach to treatment of PSUDs has grown out of the principles of the social-learning theory proposed by Bandura (1977). A major focus is on the functional analysis of the relationship between and among antecedents, behaviors, and consequences (Monti, Abrams, Kadden, & Cooney, 1989). Monti et al. (1989) developed a treatment manual for adults with alcohol dependence that has been found to be appropriate, with some modification, for adolescents with PSUDs. A major thesis of this treatment program is that social-skills deficits may restrict alternatives of actions in a social situation, minimize an individual's control over the situation, and decrease his or her access to desired resources. Therefore, the patient needs to improve, acquire, or learn how to utilize special coping skills according to structured self-efficacy expectations. The manual written by Monti et al. (1989), which, as noted, may be modified or utilized in a manner that will meet the needs of adolescents, includes more than 20 sessions that aim to promote social skills and alcohol-refusal skills, such as drink refusal, receiving criticism, managing thoughts about alcohol, awareness and management of negative thinking, planning for emergencies, and anger control. The format for each session is uniform and includes introduction and rationale sections, skill guidelines, modeling, behavior rehearsal role play, and a written practical exercise as homework.

My clinical experience with the manual and the adolescents' responses has been very positive. Social-skills training and relapse-prevention techniques are beneficial in a group format and generate constructive feedback from members of the group to each other during an active, goal-oriented, and time-limited exercise. The use of rating scales designed to measure changes in the patient's perception regarding self-efficacy potential has been found helpful (Annis & Davis, 1989).

Also, either other treatment modalities may utilize BC therapeutic principles or these techniques may be incorporated in rituals that characterize specific models of treatment. For example, family therapy may incorporate patient-management training and functional family therapy for the treatment of APSUDs as well as of CD-ASPDC (Kazdin, 1987).

Support groups, such as AA and Al-Ateen, have inherent behavioral elements in their rituals and therapeutic interventions. As an example, AA members undergo cognitive restructuring. In this charismatic group, the forces of group cohesiveness, shared beliefs, behavioral conformity, and shared jargon are heavily tooled with BC interventions (Galanter, 1990). An AA meeting follows a specific ritual and communication style between members and between speakers and the audience. This behavior is rewarded by the membership at the meeting. AA and NA use the acronym HALT (which stands for "don't get too Hungry, Angry, Lonely, or Tired") to represent the effort to prevent experience of emotional states that are seen as high-risk factors (Daley & Marlatt, 1992). Efforts are made to help members develop a schema that will generate procedures to intervene between the conditioned stimuli (e.g., places, people) that may expose them to the triggering of craving and the conditioned response (e.g., use of alcohol or other substance). Coping skills include delay tactics, calling or meeting the designated sponsor, or going to a self-help group meeting.

11.10. EMERGENCY TREATMENT OF THE SUBSTANCE-ABUSING ADOLESCENT

Adolescent referrals to the emergency department for substance use/abuse-related emergencies were listed by Felter, Izsak, and Lawrence (1987). The most common reasons were (1) overdose of one or more psychoactive substances either accidentially or intentionally; (2) associated trauma, motor vehicle accident, falls, near drowning; (3) intoxication, idiosyncratic (pathological) intoxication, "bad trip," or panic reaction; (4) drug-seeking behavior; and (5) parents wanting their child checked for "drug use."

11.10.1. Overdose or Severe Intoxication

The first priority in emergency treatment of overdose or severe intoxication, particularly in the unconscious patient, is to follow the ABC mnemonic: Assure that the Airway is patent, that Breathing (ventilation) is adequate and regular, and that Circulation-related vital signs, such as pulse and blood pressure, are sufficient for life support. Consideration must be given to differential diagnoses for the comatose adolescent (e.g., hypoglycemia or ketoacidosis). A thorough physical examination is essential to identify signs and symptoms of trauma. Also, clues for the psychoactive substance(s) responsible for a toxic state and possible trauma may be found by meticulous assessment of the eyes (e.g., nystagmus), pupils (e.g., dilation), skin (e.g., needle marks), odors, and a search of the patient's clothing (Felter et al., 1987). The patient and accompanying parties may also provide the necessary information, following a comprehensive anamnestic history. It is noteworthy that street drugs are often misrepresented, and what the adolescent thinks he swallowed, injected, snorted, or smoked may be altogether different from what he actually took (Felter et al., 1987). A list of street names of drugs could help improve communication with the patient and identification of the abused agents by accompanying parties (see Table 11.1). Examples of substance-specific physical findings include these: Needle marks may be visible in the case of injection of heroin or stimulants, as may bullae usually secondary to barbiturate injection. Pustular dermatosis or rash around the mouth is a sign of a chronic solvent abuser, as are telltale smells of hydrocarbons and solvents on the patient's breath. Signs of paint on the hands or on the patient's face might be clues to the use of cans of spray paint for inhalation "bagging."

Table 11.2 lists neurological findings of toxic overdose symptoms and the substances that may induce them. Table 11.3 lists other systemic signs and symptoms that may be seen in intoxication and emergencies resulting from psychoactive substance abuse. These tables do not list withdrawal symptoms.

Laboratory work should include an immediate analysis of bodily fluids such as urine and blood, and of gastric contents if a gastric lavage has been done. Clinical personnel must take proper precautions against contamination by the patient's body fluids to prevent an HIV or hepatitis infection.

Emergency treatment for overdose of unknown substances usually involves beginning an intravenous infusion once airway, breathing, and circulation are assessed. Dextrostick to assess for hypoglycemia caused by or mimicking alcohol intoxication is necessary. IV naloxone (Narcan), 2 mg, with repeat dose every half hour as necessary should be given if the patient is unconscious. This dose should be repeated every 1–2 hours after the patient regains consciousness if there is a response suggesting that a narcotic is present. Long-acting opiates, particularly methadone, will outlast the antagonist effects of single doses of Narcan. Cardiovascular support, artificial respiration, keeping the patient warm, and elevating the legs to avoid signs and symptoms of shock are part of the immediate management of an undefined overdose until laboratory testing can be obtained.

Noncomatose adolescents who are intoxicated and who have not ingested tart or caustic materials (such as lye, acid, or hydrocarbons) may

Table 11.1
A List of Some Street Drug Names

Heroin

Above the Law	Caballo	High Class	Public Enemy
Airborne	Cash	High Power	Shit
American Eagle	C.O.D.	Hitman	Shoot Out
Bad Boy	Crash	Horse	Smack
Beetle Juice	Dope	Hurricane	Square Biz
Best Seller	Excalibur	Hypnotic	The System
Big Red	Five Star	Lights Out	This Is It
Black Bird	Flag	New York	Top Court
Blue Bag	Goldstar	Nightmare	Up North
Body Bag	Goodyear	Obsession	Valentine
Body Heat	Halloween	Porsche	Yellow Bag
Brown		Power	

Other opioids

Opium	Methadone	Morphine	Paregoric
Black	Dollies	M	Blue Velvet
Poppy		Microdots	PG
Tar			Po

Depressants

Blues	Goofballs	Sleepers	Yellows
Downs	Rainbows	Tranqs	

Cocaine

Batman	Destroyer	Less Than	Snow
Blood Red	Flake	Zero	Uptown
Bunny	Gold Dust	Maneo	White Lady
Clear Bag	High Class	Pony Pak	White Lightning
Coke	Kelly Boys	Scarface	Yeyo
Crazy Eddie		Seven-Up	

Crack

Bases	Blue Caps	Jelly Beans	Rock Attack
Beautiful Boulders	Capital	Kangaroo	Rocks of Hell
Black Rock	Demolish	Red Caps	Rocky III

Heroin mixed with cocaine (IV): Speedballs

Heroin mixed with crack (smoked): Moonrock

(continued)

Table 11.1   (*Continued*)

Marijuana			
Black Dot	Get Your Head Together	Out of Sight	White Stripe
Blue Square	House of Lollipop	Pink Bag	

Amphetamines			
Dexies	Oranges	Pinks	Uppers
Meth	Peaches	Speed	Whites

Ice[a]			
Batu	Crystal Meth	L.A.	Rock Candy
Crystal Crank	Hawaiian Salt		

Crank[b]			
Fast	Quick	Speed	Ups

Ectasy[c]			
Adam	Euphoria	X	XTC

PCP			
Angel Dust	Death Wish	Lumberjack	Milk
Daze	Funeral Home	Madman with a Hatchet	Sudden Impact

LSD			
Acid	Blots	Copilot	Goofy
Batman	Blue Dots	E.T.	Truck-drivers

[a]Ice is a common street name for methamphetamine, a synthetic stimulant. Like crank, it can be snorted, injected, or taken orally. However, smoking is the most popular route.
[b]Crank is crystal methedrine, which is a powerful amphetamine.
[c]Ectasy is a designer drug, chemically known as 3,4-methylenedioxy-methamphetamine or MDMA. The substance represents a combination of synthetic amphetamine with mild hallucinogenic properties.

be administered syrup of ipecac, 30 ml, to induce vomiting prior to being seen in the emergency room. Following emesis (or for patients for whom ipecac is contraindicated) and only after gastric contents have been aspirated for analysis, ingestion or gastric infusion of 50–100 g activated charcoal in 4–8 oz of water is suggested. Gastric lavage should be performed meticulously only after protection of the airway has been

Table 11.2
Possible Neurological Findings in Psychoactive Substance Use Emergencies

Finding	Possible agent
Conjunctival injection	Marijuana, inhalants
Hallucinations	Alcohol, stimulants, hallucinogens, belladonna alkaloids
Coordination and gait impaired	Depressants
Memory and attention impaired	Depressants
Nystagmus	Depressants, inhalants, PCP
Pain sensation diminished	PCP
Pupillary constriction	Opioids
Pupillary dilation	Stimulants
Reflexes increased	Stimulants
Reflexes decreased	Depressants
Seizures	Stimulants, codeine, methaqualone, propoxyphene
Slurred speech	Depressants, inhalants
Dysarthria	PCP
Tremor	Stimulants, hallucinogens, inhalants
Vision blurred, diplopia	Inhalants

established and by trained emergency room personnel. If a patient vomits the first dose of activated charcoal, the dose can safely be repeated. Multiple doses of charcoal are indicated for drugs that are recirculated enterohepatically, such as glutethimide.

Most substances are well absorbed by activated charcoal, including volatile substances such as alcohol, kerosene, and other hydrocarbons; barbiturates; opioids; cocaine; and amphetamines.

11.10.2. Alcohol

Alcohol-intoxicated patients should be questioned and evaluated for trauma, multiple chemical ingestions, and hypoglycemia. Alcohol is absorbed rapidly, and emesis, lavage, and activated charcoal are seldom useful alone unless other substances have been ingested. Blood alcohol levels of 0.4 mg% are usually considered toxic, but death may occur at lower doses. Correction of metabolic abnormalities and supportive care of respiration, circulation, and body temperature are necessary in the alcohol-unconscious adolescent until the patient regains consciousness. Alcohol is metabolized by a zero-order metabolism at a steady rate of somewhere between 10 and 100 m/liter per hour. The use of stimulants such as coffee to so-called "sober up" an intoxicated individual with alcohol is contraindicated. Tactile stimulation of a partially comatose

Table 11.3
Possible Systemic Findings in Psychoactive Substance Use Emergencies

Finding	Possible agents
Tachycardia	Stimulants,[a] alcohol, marijuana, PCP
Bradycardia	Gasoline, opioids, depressants, hallucinogenic mushrooms
Ventricular arrhythmias	Stimulants, cocaine and ethanol mixed[b] inhalants
Hypertension	Stimulants, LSD, PCP
Hypotension	Depressants,[c] opioids
Pulmonary edema	Opioids, depressants
Respiration decreased	Opioids, stimulants
Body temperature increased	Stimulants, belladonna alkaloids[d]
Body temperature decreased	Opiates, depressants

[a]Examples of stimulants are cocaine, amphetamine, and stimulant "look-alike."
[b]Cocaine and ethanol consumed together produce a cardiotoxic metabolite—cocaethanol.
[c]Examples of depressants are barbiturates, ethanol, and benzodiazepines.
[d]An example of a belladonna alkaloid is atropine.

patient can be of help. When the patient is conscious, forced liquids, exercise, and fresh air can help toward speeding return to full consciousness.

11.10.3. Stimulants

Overdose of a stimulant (e.g., amphetamine) is a medical emergency because of the risk of seizures and cardiac arrhythmias. Antiarrhythmia drugs and intravenous benzodiazepine, carbamazepine, or phenytoin may be necessary. A review of physical examination and laboratory tests for trauma is necessary. Gastric lavage with acidic solution and acidification of the urine with ascorbic acid or ammonium chloride may enhance excretion of the amphetamines. A hypertensive crisis is treated with antihypertensives and α-adrenergic blockers. Haloperidol is used to manage psychotic reactions. Anxiety reactions may be managed with reassurance and occasionally small doses of a short-acting benzodiazepine such as lorazepam (Ativan).

11.10.4. Cocaine

The biphasic problems of acute cocaine overdose are notorious. The first phase of high stimulation may require "talking down" therapy and reassurance. The patient may experience panic, paranoia, agitation, and visual and tactile hallucinations ("coke bugs," "coke lights," or "trails"). This visual–tactile phenomenon is also associated with acute amphetamine overdose. Seizures may require intravenous diazepam or phenytoin. Arrhythmias may require propanolol, lidocaine, or phenytoin.

The second phase of cocaine overdose may present with profound depression, suicidal ideation, drug-seeking, hypertension, respiratory depression, and shock. Intravenous fluids, reassurance, and prevention of further ingestion are part of the treatment. Amphetamines and cocaine may trigger psychotic episodes requiring psychiatric attention and may be treated with small doses of neuroleptic such as haloperidol.

11.10.5. Barbiturates

Ingestion of barbiturates, since they are central nervous system (CNS) depressants, requires hospitalization and emergency management of sedation. Barbiturate withdrawal can be associated with rebound seizure and other signs of CNS stimulation. Cardiorespiratory and hospital emergency room support may be required for the former condition and carbamazepine may be used for the latter.

11.10.6. Inhalants

Inhalants follow a biphasic course with initial euphoria and CNS stimulation followed by depression. The stimulated and excited inhalant user should be prevented from self-harm. When possible, an attempt should be made to use assurance, rather than physical restraints. A complete medical evaluation is necessary to rule out organ damage, such as hepatic damage, and upper airway complications, such as chemical pneumonitis.

11.10.7. Hallucinogens

Most acute toxic reactions of hallucinogens such as LSD, mescaline, and psilocybin are treated supportively and nonpharmacologically. A quiet, supportive, and nonthreatening environment is recommended. The first phase of toxicity usually occurs within 6 hours and often includes frightening visual imagery. The degree of "bad trip" is highly related to the lack of a positive mental state and environmental setting. The patient may forget having taken the drug and believe that this phase will continue forever. This situation requires reassurance that it will not.

In the second stage of psychedelic ingestion, unpleasant, obsessionally recurring thoughts or feelings may be overwhelming to the adolescent, and it may be helpful for the therapist or health worker to suggest new trains of thought. A positive, supportive, and calm approach to the patient can be extremely reassuring. If the therapist cannot achieve contact with the patient and anxiety persists, oral administration of a benzodiazepine may be useful to calm the youth, although paradoxical effects may occur in some instances.

During the third phase of intoxication, a toxic psychosis or break with reality may occur. A neuroleptic such as haloperidol, 1–4 m, may be given orally or intramuscularly and repeated if necessary during psychotic reactions. As soon as rapport and verbal communication can be reestablished, further medication is usually not necessary. Rest and a darkened room with low stimulation are also extremely helpful.

Chronic effects of hallucinogens include persistent flashbacks, initiation of psychosis, or exacerbation of preexisting psychosis. All these sequelae will require psychiatric care. Also, permanent visual damage in an adolescent following chronic use of LSD was recently reported (Kaminer & Hrecznyj, 1991).

11.10.7.1. Jimson Weed

This agent is often used as a hallucinogen. It contains the belladonna alkaloids atropine and scopolamine. The patient may be confused and disoriented and pick at himself or herself. A mnemonic for the telltale symptoms of atropine poisoning is "High as a kite, hot as a pistol, red as a rose, dry as a bone." Other anticholinergic effects include blurred vision, dilated pupils, and hoarse voice. Excitation, euphoria, stupor, and coma may result. Severe hallucination and arrhythmias may be treated with physostigmine. Urinary retention may require catheterization.

11.10.7.2. Phencyclidine (PCP)

This drug is often laced into marijuana, cocaine, and other stimulant preparations sold on the street. Overdoses may result in hypertension or hypotension, cardiarrythmias, and coma. PCP coma may be identified if the patient's eyes are open when the patient is comatose. Seizures from PCP ingestion may require intravenous diazepam, carbamazepine, or phenytoin. Hypertension may require intravenous propranolol or another antihypertensive. Behavioral disinhibition may require a neuroleptic such as haloperidol. Generally, PCP has three types of acute toxicity:

1. Combativeness, catatonia, convulsions, and coma. Users often look as though they were trying to walk in a space suit ("moon walking"). Grand mal seizures may require hospitalization and anticonvulsants during this phase.
2. Toxic psychosis occurs especially after a high dose of PCP or repeated PCP use. PCP psychosis may last 1–7 days or more and requires psychiatric intervention.
3. PCP-induced depression may mimic major depressive symptoms and may require prolonged psychiatric attention. The recurrence of PCP intoxication or "flashbacks" may be caused by PCP being retained within the system and recirculated through the enterohepatic or gastrohepatic circulation.

Since PCP is a disassociative anesthetic, PCP users are insensible to pain, often feel that they have superhuman strength and power, are capable of breaking out of restraints, and are likely to burn or bruise themselves during violent reactions and to suffer simple or compound fractures, internal organ damage, and bleeding. Because PCP is fat-soluble, it may remain dormant in fat cells for days or even weeks after its use and retain its potency. It may periodically reenter the user's spinal fluid and cause another toxic reaction.

11.10.7.3. Morning Glory Seeds, Hawaiian Woodrose, Nutmeg, and Mace

These short-acting hallucinogens have low potency; however, tolerance and toxicity effects develop rapidly. Adverse reactions usually require supportive, comforting personnel who reassure the patient that overall effects may not last more than 6 hours. Rest, and decrease of sensory input by medical support in the form of small doses of a sedative hypnotic, may help allay anxiety.

11.10.8. Opioids

Opioids are used intranasally or intravenously (IV). Overdose is common in the IV drug user. Doses of naloxone, 0.4–2 mg, in repeated doses every 1/2–1 hour depending on the degree of sedation, is the treatment of choice. The classic signs of opiate overdose are pinpoint pupils and hypoventilation. Cardiorespiratory support and intravenous infusion are often necessary. Pulmonary edema may require emergency hospital treatment. For long-acting opioids such as methadone or propoxyphene (Darvon), repeated doses of naloxone may be necessary. Long-term signs and symptoms of opioid withdrawal may be managed with oral clonidine or clonidine transdermal patches.

11.10.9. Marijuana

Marijuana generally has low toxicity, although panic attacks induced by marijuana are not uncommon. Bad trips from marijuana laced with PCP or cocaine may include paranoid or psychotic reactions. A talking-down therapy is the treatment of choice, with additional therapeutic isolation as needed.

11.10.10. Anabolic Steroids

Prolonged abuse of steroids can result in dependence syndrome. Regular anabolic steroid use has also been associated with psychiatric problems/disorders such as aggressive behavior, manic states, depression, and psychosis. Heart attack, stroke, hypertension, testicular atrophy, and liver disease are medical complications reported among steroid abusers. Immediate abstinence is required and is commonly sufficient. Acute psychiatric symptoms may be treated on the basis of the severity of their clinical presentation.

11.11. PHARMACOTHERAPY

Studies on the pharmacotherapy of APSUDs are rare and yet important. The high prevalence of dually diagnosed adolescents demands pharmacological interventions for the treatment of comorbid psychiatric disorders by psychotropic agents that have not been proven useful as primary therapeutic tools for PSUDs.

There are four main pharmacological treatment strategies for substance abuse: (1) make drug administration aversive (e.g., disulfiram for alcohol abuse); (2) substitute for the drug (e.g., methadone for heroin abuse); (3) block the reinforcing effects of the drug (e.g., naltrexone for opioid abuse); and (4) relieve craving/withdrawal (e.g., clonidine for heroin abuse) (Kaminer, 1992b). To employ one of these current approaches, there is a need not only to identify an appropriate agent but also to increase its appeal by maintaining a feeling of well-being that will encourage the patient to comply with the chosen pharmacotherapy.

11.11.1. Detoxification and Acupuncture

Lack of empirical studies on adolescents with PSUDs regarding detoxification from opioids, alcohol, barbiturates, and other psychoactive substances prevents a reliable and valid comment on this issue. However, clinical experience suggests that there is no reason to assume that this therapeutic process should be any different from that of adults as long as legal consent is obtained.

Acupuncture has become a well-established method of treating various health disorders in Western medicine. Acupuncture offers an option for the treatment of PSUDs. The following functions of acupuncture have been observed among adults with PSUD: (1) detoxification, relief of withdrawal symptoms, and craving; (2) general relaxation; and (3) enhancement of mental and physical functioning (Smith & Khan, 1988). Patients should be provided with acupuncture as part of a comprehensive treatment plan. There is a risk of infection if the needles are not cleaned or sterilized properly.

11.11.2. Other Pharmacological Treatments

11.11.2.1. Methadone and Other Opioid Maintenance

This is a common form of opioid substitution therapy that is usually researched for the treatment of adult heroin addicts. The desired response from methadone maintenance (MM) is threefold: (1) to prevent the onset of opioid abstinence syndrome, (2) to eliminate drug hunger or craving, and (3) to block the euphoric effects of any illicitly self-administered opioids (Jaffe, 1986).

MM and not opioid detoxification is the treatment of choice for pregnant adolescents who abuse heroin. MM eliminates the danger of contracting AIDS from a contaminated needle and also assures a relatively stable plasma level of methadone, which reduces the fetus's risk of developing intrauterine distress (compared to heroin, which has a short half-life and causes abrupt changes in plasma level) (Finnegan & Kandall, 1992).

Other individuals under 18 years of age are required to have two documented detoxification attempts before MM is offered. No person under 18 years of age may be admitted to an MM treatment program unless an authorized adult signs an official consent form.

Two additional oral pharmacotherapies are examined in therapeutic trials and are expected to expand the arsenal of opioids available for maintenance treatment.

LAAM (L-acetyl-methadol) is an opioid that is quite similar to methadone in its pharmacological actions. It is converted into active metabolites that have longer biological half-lives than methadone. Opioid withdrawal symptoms are not experienced for 72–96 hours after the last oral dose; therefore, LAAM can be given only 3 times per week as compared to daily administration of methadone. LAAM has been shown to have effects equivalent to those of methadone in terms of suppressing illicit opioid abuse and encouraging a more productive life-style (Jaffe, 1986).

Buprenorphine is a partial opioid agonist–antagonist available also as an analgesic due to its ability to produce morphine-like effects at low doses. This agent relieves opioid withdrawal, diminishes craving, and does not produce euphoria. It is more difficult to overdose on buprenorphine than on methadone because of the antagonist effects of the former in high doses (Rosen & Kosten, 1991).

Many heroin addicts also abuse cocaine, which "speeds" the rush from heroin injected alone (e.g., a speedball). MM fails to reduce cocaine abuse for many patients. On the basis of preliminary data, buprenorphine may reduce cocaine use in opioid addicts (Kosten, Kleber, & Morgan, 1989). The mechanism of action in combination with cocaine remains to be clarified.

11.11.2.2. Alcohol

There is no information regarding aversive pharmacological therapy for alcohol APSUD, e.g., disulfiram for alcohol abuse. This antidipsotropic agent produces a drug–ethanol reaction by inhibiting the liver enzyme aldehyde dehydrogenase, which catalyzes the oxidation of aldehyde (the major metabolic product of ethanol) to acetate (Alterman et al., 1991). The resulting accumulation of acetaldehyde is responsible for the symptoms of drug–ethanol reaction that follow alcohol consumption.

Recent findings regarding the impact of alcohol drinking on opioid receptors include: (1) alcohol stimulates opioid receptor activity; (2) alcohol drinking is affected by opiate agonists; and (3) an opiate antagonist such as naltrexone blocks the reinforcing properties of alcohol and therefore decreases alcohol drinking days and severity of alcohol-related problems and improves abstention and relapse rates (O'Malley, Jaffe, Chang, Schottenfeld, Meyer, & Rounsaville, 1992).

11.11.2.3. Cigarette Smoking (Nicotine)

Nicotine dependence is common among adolescents. The pharmacotherapy of nicotine dependence utilizes the strategy of finding a substitute for the psychoactive substance. The invention of nicotine gum and its successor, the nicotine transdermal patch, as self-administering agents was a breakthrough in the treatment of cigarette dependence. The efficacy of these agents doubled success rates (validated long-term abstinence) of treatment programs from about 15% to about 30% (West, 1992). Furthermore, their success in reducing nicotine craving improved even more when behavioral or cognitive therapy sessions were also part of a comprehensive treatment plan (Lichtenstein & Glasgow, 1992).

Only one study (Johnson, Stevens, Hollis, & Woodson, 1992), of 612 subjects who had received a prescription for nicotine gum, included adolescents, an unknown number of 15- to 18-year-olds. No special reference was made to the characteristics and treatment outcome of these adolescents in the outpatient clinic sample studied.

Side effects of nicotine gum include bad taste and, because it is hard to chew, sore mouth and jaws. The patch may increase nicotine toxicity, particularly if the person continues to smoke, or it can irritate the user's skin and disrupt sleep if left on for 24 hours. Some people find it difficult to wean themselves off it (Lichtenstein & Glasgow, 1992). Neither one should be used by an active smoker. Unfortunately, advertisements by pharmaceutical companies recommend these agents for decrease as well as for smoking cessation, which may induce nicotine intoxication.

No specific contraindications for the use of nicotine gum or the patch by adolescents with nicotine dependence are known. It appears that any therapeutic trial should start as a carefully designed case study on an individual basis for consenting adolescents with severe dependence.

11.11.2.4. Cocaine and Other Stimulants

Stimulants have proven to be useful for the treatment of children and adolescents diagnosed with attention deficit hyperactivity disorder (ADHD). The pharmacokinetic similarities between cocaine (an illegal stimulant) and therapeutic stimulants such as methylphenidate, pemoline, and dextroamphetamine led to the assumption that they might be useful for the treatment of cocaine abuse. Also, it was suggested that adult abuse of cocaine could be attributed to a residual type of attention deficit disorder. Neither assumption was solidly confirmed (Kaminer, 1992a). The abuse potential of therapeutic stimulants deserves a comment. Regardless of the common perception that these agents may be abused by children and adolescents, only two cases of methylphenidate abuse by patients diagnosed with ADHD were reported (Kaminer, 1992a). However, there is a potential for abuse by siblings, parents, or peers who are manifest ASPD or who are substance abusers. The substantial overlap between ADHD and ASPD in adolescents and adults may influence physicians' decision to prescribe stimulant medications to such patients (Carroll & Rounsaville, 1993).

There has been only one reported case of facilitation of cocaine abstinence in an adolescent by the tricyclic antidepressant desipramine, with 6-month follow-up that confirmed continued abstinence (Kaminer, 1992b). It is noteworthy that cocaine addicts show more conditioned responses than any other drug addicts. It is hypothesized that many repetitions cause release of the neurotransmitter dopamine (which is suggested to be responsible for the reinforcing effects of cocaine and for craving and withdrawal phenomenology) even with no cocaine present. The memory of the experience alone may initiate dopamine release, which equals cocaine effect and may lead to subsequent craving and withdrawal (C. P. O'Brien, personal communication, December 2, 1993). A combination of pharmacological intervention and BC therapy should be further explored especially, although not exclusively, in the treatment of cocaine abuse.

11.12. TREATMENT OF COMORBID PSYCHIATRIC BEHAVIORS AND DISORDERS

11.12.1. Mood Disorders

11.12.1.1. Major Depressive Disorder

Clinical experience suggests that many patients with PSUDs are diagnosed as depressed, especially on admission to inpatient treatment programs. This predominance could be attributed to various factors other than primary depression, such as substance abuse or withdrawal, loss of the availability of psychoactive substances and related life-style, or a reaction to the loss of freedom, friends, and family following the admission (Kaminer, 1991a). Most of the patients experience a gradual and spontaneous lifting of the depressive symptomatology within 2 weeks.

The adolescents who are diagnosed with major depressive disorder (MDD) are most commonly treated with antidepressants such as imipramine, amitriptyline, or other tricyclics, or by selective serotonin-reuptake inhibitors (SRIs) such as fluoxetine, sertraline, paroxetine, and fluvoxamine (Ambrosini, Bianchi, Rabinovich, & Elia, 1993a). Clinical improvement is usually expected after 3–4 weeks of pharmacotherapy with tricyclics (Kaminer, Seifer, & Mastrian, 1992). It is noteworthy that a new antidepressant was recently approved by the Food and Drug Administration. Venlafaxine (Effexor) is a member of a new class that selectively inhibits the uptake of both norepinephrine and serotonin. Following controlled trials, it was concluded that venlafaxine has efficacy and safety equal or superior to other antidepressants, including SRIs and tricyclics (Montgomery, 1993).

It is important to note the following: (1) No relation of plasma levels of tricyclics with clinical response in adolescent MDD was found (Ryan et al., 1986). (2) The synergistic effect of BC therapy with antidepressants appears to be beneficial in the treatment of MDD. (3) Amitriptyline abuse has been reported recently by addicts, and its street value is rising due to its sedative effects.

Antidepressants generate side effects similar to those reported in adults. The tricyclics may be lethal in overdose situations, primarily because of cardiovascular toxicity (Ambrosini, Bianchi, Rabinovich, & Elia, 1993b). Four cases of sudden death related to the use of Norpramin (desipramine) by children 8–12 years old were reported (Riddle, Geller, & Ryan, 1993). The speculated pathophysiological mechanism is that desipramine may increase noradrenergic neurotransmission, which leads to increased cardiac sympathetic tone and could predispose vulnerable persons to ventricular tachyarrhythmias, syncope, and sudden death.

Neurotoxicity of antidepressants includes seizures, behavioral changes, and delirium. Data on adolescents' exposure to tricyclic neurotoxicity are limited to sporadic case reports. Anticholinergic effects are usually correlated with plasma tricyclic levels and most commonly include dry mouth, drowsiness, nausea, constipation, urinary retention, tremor, flushed face, and excessive sweating. Antidepressants can induce behavioral toxicity, primarily precipitation, induction, or rapid cycling of manic symptomatology (Strober & Carlson, 1982).

Abrupt discontinuation of tricyclics may produce withdrawal symptoms. The most common symptoms are cholinergic effects. Coadministration of SRIs with tricyclic antidepressants or even a few weeks later is contraindicated because it may raise the plasma level of these agents to a toxic level, most likely due to interference with their hepatic oxidative metabolism. Side effects of SRIs in adolescents have been reported in case studies and in preliminary studies. Ambrosini et al. (1993b) reviewed and classified these effects into gastrointestinal, neuropsychiatric, and behavioral.

The risk of suicide among adolescents with PSUDs is high (Kaminer, 1992c). SRIs are less cardiotoxic with overdoses and they lack sedative potentiation with alcohol as compared with tricyclic antidepressants; therefore, their use is preferable for MDD in impulsive or suicidal adolescents.

Current experience suggests that before initiating treatment of any psychopathology in adolescents with tricyclic medication, a baseline ECG needs to be done. Also, the medical examination and medical history should emphasize the cardiovascular system of the patient and family members in order to detect any cardiac vulnerability. Prolongation of the P-R interval on the ECG should not exceed 0.21 second, the QRS complex should not be prolonged by more than 30% over baseline, and the QTc interval should be within normal limits. Resting pulse should not exceed 130 beats/minute, and blood pressure should not exceed 140/90 mm Hg.

11.12.1.2. Bipolar Disorders

Bipolar disorders in adolescents respond favorably to lithium, which is the drug of choice (Carlson, 1990), alone or in combination with anticonvulsants such as carbamazepine and valproic acid. DeLong and Aldershof (1987) reported that of their 59 bipolar children and adolescent patients, two thirds were considered favorable responders to lithium. Poor responders consisted of subjects with ADHD or CD or both.

Lithium effectivity for acute symptomatology and for long-term management of bipolar disorder has been well established in the adult literature; however, the failure rate for lithium in prevention of bipolar disorder is approximately 33% (Prien & Gelenberg, 1989). Lithium side effects in adolescents are similar to the symptoms manifested in adults; tremor, urinary frequency, nausea, and diarrhea are the most common ones. Relative contraindications for the use of lithium include heart and kidney disease, diuretic use, chronic diarrhea, and electrolyte imbalance. Basic laboratory studies include blood electrolytes, urea, and nitrogen levels, blood count with differential, thyroid function tests, and pregnancy test due to the potential teratogenic effects of lithium.

The recommended therapeutic blood level is within the therapeutic range of 0.7–1.2 meq/liter. A level of more than 1.4 meq/liter should not be exceeded due to a risk of toxicity. Signs of toxicity include severe neurobehavioral and gastrointestinal symptoms.

The recommended blood levels and the contraindications and side effects of anticonvulsants are similar along age groups. Compared to lithium, monitoring of fluid and electrolyte intake is not required, and the risk of toxicity is lower should serum levels exceed the recommended therapeutic range. In some cases, bipolar disorder may be refractory to all these agents. One alternative, verapamil (a calcium channel antagonist), has been used without consistently proving clear effectiveness in the treatment of adults with a bipolar disorder. In addition, verapamil is associated with depression (Barton & Gitlin, 1987). However, successful use of verapamil and valproic acid in the treatment of prolonged mania in an adolescent was reported by Kastner and Friedman (1992). Another alternative based on a single case report of an adolescent with a rapid cycling bipolar disorder was described by Berman and Wolpert (1987). The authors noted that the disorder, which was precipitated by a tricyclic antidepressant, responded to electrocurrent therapy.

The adolescent with PSUD and a comorbid bipolar disorder is at very high risk for suicide and aggressive behavior and should be followed carefully. The need for blood level monitoring of lithium is a special challenge, particularly at the outpatient level.

11.12.2. Anxiety Disorders

Panic and obsessive–compulsive disorders (OCDs) in youth share phenomenological similarities with the adult patterns; however, avoidant disorder, overanxious disorder, separation anxiety, and school phobia are unique to children and adolescents as delineated in DSM-III-R (American Psychiatric Association, 1987). The use of medications with addictive properties such as benzodiazepines for the pharmacotherapy of anxiety disorders in adolescents with PSUDs is not recommended. Furthermore, benzodiazepines that are commonly used among adults with anxiety disorders, such as alprazolam (Xanax), have not been unequivocally proven to be more efficacious than tricyclic antidepressants.

Panic disorder and OCDs among adolescents with PSUDs are rare. No studies regarding the pharmacological treatment of panic disorder in adolescents have been reported. The psychopharmacological treatment of OCDs has been studied and reviewed extensively (Rapoport, 1987). Antianxiety agents appear to be ineffective, and the tricyclic antidepressant clomipramine was reported to have significant superiority over placebo in lessening OCD symptomatology in children and adolescents (DeVeaugh-Geiss et al., 1992). Clomipramine appears to have better results than desipramine; however, this conclusion remains to be tested in future studies. Open studies with SRIs, such as that with fluoxetine as reviewed by Ambrosini et al. (1993b), suggest that they may be effective in adolescent OCDs with or without clomipramine.

Separation anxiety and school phobia have been studied for more than 20 years. In contrast to the early report regarding a positive response to imipramine compared to placebo (Gittelman-Klein & Klein, 1971), recent studies have failed to show superiority of tricyclic antidepressants (e.g., imipramine, clomipramine) to placebo (Bernstein, 1990; Klein, Koplewicz, & Kanner, 1992). It is noteworthy that these disorders were found to be associated with adult forms of panic and depressive disorders (Gittelman & Klein, 1984; Weissman, Leckman, Merikangas, Gammon, & Prusoff, 1984).

A study on the effects of alprazolam on children and adolescents with overanxious and avoidant disorders was reported by Simeon et al. (1992). The authors' findings failed to show efficacy of the medication in comparison to placebo. This finding stands in marked contrast to the favorable effects reported in studies with adults. Simeon et al. (1992) intend to increase the dosage of alprazolam and the length of pharmacotherapy in a future study. The authors did not discuss the implications of the addictive potential of alprazolam in this study. It is noteworthy that these diagnoses have been dropped from DSM-IV (American Psychiatric Association, 1994). Avoidant disorder has been included in the modified social phobia diagnosis, and overanxious disorder has been subsumed by generalized anxiety disorder. Buspirone hydrochloride (Buspar) is a relatively new anxiolytic drug, pharmacologically different from the benzodiazepines. This agent has been marketed as a less sedative anxiolytic that does not potentiate alcohol effects and has a low, if any, abuse potential. Buspar has been used to successfully treat an adolescent with overanxious disorder who did not tolerate treatment with desipramine (Kranzler, 1988). Buspar may be particularly useful for clinical trials with teens with PSUDs and anxiety symptoms.

The studies reviewed in this section have significant importance for the treatment of adolescents with PSUDs and anxiety disorders. Moreover, they have unequivocal implications for the treatment and detoxification of benzodiazepine abuse and dependence, respectively. Tricyclic antidepressants are useful substitutes for these medications, which are abused for their sedative properties.

11.12.3. Eating Disorders

Since the mid-1980s, pharmacological trials among adult patients with bulimia nervosa have demonstrated the short-term efficacy of several antidepressants in diminishing binging frequencies in bulimic patients. These agents include imipramine, desipramine, phenelzine (MAOI), and fluoxetine (Ambrosini et al., 1993b). The bulimic symptomatology improved even in the absence of coexistent depression and was not correlated with pretreatment severity or plasma medication levels. These findings do not support early epidemiological and family studies linking the etiology of mood disorders and eating disorders (Hudson, Pope, Jonas, & Yurgelum-Todd, 1983).

Anorexia nervosa and PSUD is a rare dual diagnosis. No effective pharmacotherapy for anorexia nervosa has been reported.

11.12.4. Schizophrenia

No studies on the comorbidity of PSUDs and schizophrenia among adolescents have yet been reported. However, there are no data even among adult patients to suggest that there should be any difference between the pharmacotherapeutic regimens for schizophrenic patients with and those without accompanying PSUDs. Therefore, neuroleptics remain the category of medications of choice.

11.12.5. Attention Deficit Hyperactivity Disorder

The effectiveness of stimulant therapy for ADHD in childhood has been extensively documented (Greenhill, 1990). Methylphenidate (ritalin), dextroamphetamine (dexedrine), and pemoline (cylert) are the most commonly used medications. Antidepressants have also been found to be effective in the treatment of the aggression, inattention, and hyperactivity that characterize the heterogeneous population of children diagnosed with this disorder (Ambrosini et al., 1993b). Desipramine, clomipramine, and MAOI should remain a second line to stimulants that have less severe side effects and produce a more consistent response from patients (Pliszka, 1987). However, these antidepressants should be used when an ADHD patient is manifesting a comorbid anxiety or depressive disorder. Side effects of stimulants include weight loss, decreased appetite, possible mood liability, and a potentially reversible growth suppression once the medication is discontinued. This issue still generates debate.

Neuroleptics, carbamazepine, and clonidine (including a patch form) have been tested as treatments for childhood ADHD. However, only equivocal reports about a certain level of efficacy were noted in uncontrolled studies of neuroleptics and carbamazepine and in controlled studies of clonidine, especially in patients with comorbid tic disorders (Steingard, Biderman, Spencer, Wilens, & Gonzalez, 1993). These medications are characterized by serious side effects that limit their use in this group.

Stimulant therapy for adolescents with ADHD has also been found to be effective (Klorman, Brumaghin, Fitzpatrick, & Borgstedt, 1990). Abuse of therapeutic stimulants by patients with ADHD is rare; however, peers and relatives may abuse the medication, either because it is available or because they have PSUDs.

11.12.6. Conduct Disorder and Aggression

Aggressive behaviors are frequently seen by clinicians working with adolescents with PSUDs. These behaviors may be directed toward others or toward self. Any pharmacological treatment of aggression as part of a conduct disorder (CD) must be integrated with a comprehensive treatment plan.

Anticonvulsants and stimulants were used for the treatment of aggression in the 1970s with negative or ambiguous results (Stewart, Meyers, Burket, & Lyles, 1990). The efficacy of antidepressants in the treatment of antisocial behavior as a form of "masked depression" was questioned and negated (Cytryn & McKnew, 1972).

Studies addressing the use of neuroleptics and lithium (Campbell et al., 1984; Werry & Aman, 1975) generally have yielded positive findings. These studies support the use of these agents for patients with such characteristics as unmanageability, aggressiveness, and impulsivity. Treatment of aggressive patients aged 5–15 years with clonidine in an open pilot study showed some promise (Kemph, Devane, Levin, Jarecke, & Miller, 1993). Also, β-blockers manifested some usefulness in a small group of subjects with aggressive behavior and additional disruptive or organic disorders (Kuperman & Stewart, 1987).

The use of antianxiety medication is not indicated, since there is a substantial risk of disinhibition and subsequently more aggressive or impulsive behavior (Biederman & Jellinek, 1984).

11.12.6.1. Treatment of Adolescent Psychoactive Substance Use Disorders Associated with Conduct Disorder

CD is one of the most prevalent diagnoses in children and adolescents. Antisocial behaviors are evident in one third to one half of clinically referred youth, but they are also seen in varying degrees in most children and adolescents over the course of normal development (Kazdin, 1987). CD relates to antisocial behavior that is clinically and socially significant (e.g., violence, acts against others, lying, truancy). Kazdin (1987) noted that progress in identifying effective treatments has been relatively slow. Furthermore, antisocial behavior tends to be relatively stable over time and continues to manifest itself in adolescence and adulthood as antisocial personality disorder (CD–ASPD continuum). There is a strong association between ASPD and PSUD (a specific odds ratio >21 between alcoholism and ASPD) as reported by Helzer and Pryzbeck (1988). The treatment of this dually diagnosed (DUDI) population of adolescents is difficult; poor prognosis appears to be the rule rather than the exception.

Due to the sparse empirical literature on the relationship between CD-APSUD and treatment outcome and the commonly held categorical approach to CD-ASPD diagnosis, it becomes important to carefully examine the heterogeneity and differential responses to intervention if this is possible.

It was reported in the adult literature that lifetime diagnosis of depression differentiated patients with ASPD who were able to benefit from psychotherapy from those who showed no gains (Gerstley, McLellan, Alterman, Woody, Luborsky, & Prout, 1989). Kaminer et al. (1992a) reported that DUDI adolescents with CD who also received a comorbid diagnosis of mood disorder were more likely to complete an inpatient treatment program than were those without a mood disorder.

Gerstley et al. (1989, p. 508) examined the hypothesis that

> there are primary antisocial individuals whose antisocial behaviors are the results of an underlying personality structure, and that there is a more healthy group whose antisocial behaviors are secondary. Because the distinction between these groups cannot be made based on their behavior it should be found according to their ability to empathize, to experience guilt and their potential to develop meaningful relationships.

Indeed, they found that there was a significant association between the ability of patients with ASPD to develop working relationships with their therapists and treatment outcome.

The increased recognition of the heterogeneity within patients diagnosed along the CD-ASPDC may influence the choice of patient–treatment matching. Alterman and Cacciola (1991) discussed the differential effectiveness of specific treatments for adults with PSUD and comorbid ASPD. They suggested that compared with non-ASPD addicts, these patients showed lesser relapse after a 26-week treatment period when treated with training in behavioral coping skills. Psychotherapy was less beneficial to this group.

A cautious speculation regarding adolescents like the cohort studied by Kaminer et al. (1992a) would suggest that (1) adolescents with PSUD also diagnosed with CD could be better served in a therapeutic facility other than a psychiatric hospital and (2) due to their special needs, specialized interventions may be necessary to increase the retention of this population in treatment and to improve their chances for successful treatment outcome.

11.12.6.2. Heterogeneity of Antisocial Behaviors and Treatment Issues

CD encompasses a wide array of behaviors, from overt or confrontational antisocial behaviors to concealed or covert ones. The different types and combined patterns of behavior may vary in their onset, etiologies, and risk factors. The clinical course can vary for any given behavior along several dimensions, such as frequency, intensity, repetitiveness, and chronicity (Kazdin, 1987). Treatment may need to address a package of deviant behaviors, and a single technique or procedure may be inherently limited in its effect (Patterson, 1986). As delineated by the problem-behavior theory (Jessor & Jessor, 1977), these adolescents manifest additional deficiencies and problems in the academic domain, in interpersonal relationships, and in other areas.

The adolescent with PSUD and comorbid CD-ASPDC may benefit from four techniques in particular: parent management training, functional family therapy, problem-solving skills, and community-based treatment (Kazdin, 1987).

The first three have strong BC components. Community-based treatment offers a complementary component for treatment as well as for prevention and relies heavily on the assumption that segregation of deviant youths will lead to increased severity and versatility of maladaptive behavior. Consequently, mixing with nonreferred (normal) youths in the community and participation in shared activities will reduce antisocial behavior (Feldman, Caplinger, & Wodarski, 1983; Offord, Jones, Graham, Poushinsky, Stenerson, & Weaver, 1985).

Amenability to treatment is an important predictor for a successful treatment outcome. The literature of CD-ASPD tries to identify alternative models that might be used to identify effective treatments that increase amenability to treatment. Additional research in this direction is warranted.

11.13. MONITORING PROGRESS DURING TREATMENT

In order to assess the progress made by the patient during treatment, it is important to consider the following variables: (1) treatment dosage and the therapeutic alliance with therapist/staff, (2) treatment integrity—the operationalization of the treatment plan as designed, and (3) measurement of the treatment as it is delivered.

The following questions, adapted from Sobell et al. (1988, pp. 44–45), are intended as guidelines for assessing difficulties in making therapeutic progress and accomplishing the treatment goals:

1. Is the client attempting to engage in the treatment plan (contract)? If not, why are the strategies failing?
2. Were the adolescent's strengths and resources correctly evaluated?

3. Are there necessary supports in the adolescent's environment to promote behavior changes?
4. Are the treatment goals appropriately specified? Are they achievable? Were early success experiences built in to help the client later accomplish more difficult goals?
5. Were the high- and low-risk relapse situations properly evaluated?
6. Do the positive benefits of substance use outweigh the negative consequences?

11.14. TREATMENT COMPLETION AND CONTINUED AFTERCARE

During the last phase of treatment, a strong emphasis on preparation for termination of treatment and separation from staff and other patients involved in treatment is needed regardless of specificity of setting and therapeutic interventions. It is important to summarize treatment gains as well as remaining deficiencies and weaknesses that may put the patient in high-risk situations for relapse.

It is generally agreed that aftercare is necessary to solidify and maximize treatment gains and to minimize relapse. Aftercare also ensures the transfer and generalization of treatment results to the adolescent's community. The environment has to be conducive to continued maintenance of behavioral and cognitive changes accomplished in treatment and provide ready access to care in the event of relapse. Lack of follow-up services may essentially nullify treatment gains.

A postdischarge contract (from an inpatient program) or a follow-up contract (in an outpatient clinic) that delineates what the adolescent may and may not do is helpful.

For example, in such a contract, the patient agrees to maintain a drug-free life-style, to attend self-help meetings in a specific location at a certain frequency for a fixed period of time, to continue therapy meetings (e.g., family group), and to ask for help in case of relapse. Contingencies may vary according to the terms negotiated between the patient, therapist, and caretakers. Tracking patients after discharge on a periodic basis is warranted. A follow-up manual is part of the T-ASI package (Kaminer et al., 1991).

Resources in the community for aftercare may include self-help groups for adolescents, school-based counseling, and a support system for caretakers. The impact of social support and self-esteem improvement was found necessary to maintain the major life-style changes necessary for continued abstinence (Richter, Brown, & Mott, 1991). Social resources for abstention may be critical to the coping process because the majority of adolescent relapse occurs in social settings with pressure to drink alcohol or use drugs (Myers & Brown, 1990).

Little is known concerning the typical stay in aftercare; however, it is well known that only a small proportion of those who start aftercare complete it. The extent to which failure to complete aftercare is associated with relapse is undetermined and needs to be investigated (Alterman et al., 1991).

11.15. ASSESSMENT OF THE RELATIVE EFFICACY OF TREATMENT PROGRAMS

Evaluation of the efficacy of treatment programs for APSUDs is complex. Hoffmann et al. (1987) provide a set of guidelines for the clinician to do so.

First, the differential referral sources must be considered. Second, the differential characteristics of the patient population must be assessed. Third, the differential characteristics of treatment programs should be delineated. Fourth, the presence or absence of differential treatment strategies responsive to the particular needs of adolescents has to be categorized. Fifth, the differential response of the adolescent with PSUD to the treatment process must be able to be assessed. Sixth, appropriate outcome and aftercare variables have to be identified and used.

11.16. TREATMENT OUTCOME RESEARCH AND THE FUTURE

The National Institute of Alcohol Abuse and Alcoholism—Alcohol Alert (1992) covered the issue of treatment outcome research, which is designed to answer several basic questions: Is treatment better or worse than no treatment? Is one treatment better than another? If a treatment is effective, is a little just as good as a lot? Are the benefits of treatment worth the cost? These questions close a cycle that was started at the beginning of this chapter with a reference to the seminal article by McLellan et al. (1982) questioning the effectiveness of treatment conducted 15 years ago. Improved methodology in the form of controlled trials, randomization, blinding, follow-up, and outcome measures will increase efficiency based on "correct" research, the results of which would be generalizable.

Ethical and legal implications of treatment and education about PSUDs and comorbid psychiatric disorders, improved communication with the public and especially parents of patients regarding the efficacy of pharmacotherapy in specific disorders, and promotion of the concept of treatment dosage as a summation of the effects of comprehensive treatment modalities based on patient treatment matching will improve the perceptions of treatment programs.

The importance of the age of onset of a disorder (e.g., mood disorder, PSUD) and the age-specific response to medications has been recognized because it may represent a biological marker. This marker may facilitate and improve identification of heterogeneous clinical subpopulations, course of disorders, and long-term morbidity and may potentiate future research for specific biological treatments designed for the identified groups.

It is still premature to abandon conventional models of treatment due to lack of appropriate treatment alternatives. However, it is hoped that while we continue to illuminate the many difficulties and prospects that designing and implementing treatment programs for APSUDs impose, a healthy skepticism about current treatment strategies will accompany us. Continued efforts for the exploration of new and improved models of treatment should pursue more research.

REFERENCES

Allison, M., & Hubbard, R. L. (1985). Drug abuse treatment process: A review of the literature. *International Journal of the Addictions, 20,* 1321–1345.

Alterman, A. I., & Cacciola, J. S. (1991). The antisocial personality disorder diagnosis in substance abusers: Problems and issues. *Journal of Nervous and Mental Disease, 179,* 401–409.

Alterman, A. I., O'Brien, C. P., & McLellan, A. T. (1991). Differential therapeutics for substance abuse. In R. J. Frances & S. I. Miller (Eds.), *Clinical Textbook of Addictive Disorders* (pp. 369–390). New York: Guilford Press.

Ambrosini, P. J., Bianchi, M. D., Rabinovich, H., & Elia, J. (1993a). Antidepressant treatments in children and adolescents. I. Affective disorders. *Journal of the American Academy of Child and Adolescent Psychiatry, 32,* 1–6.

Ambrosini, P. J., Bianchi, M. D., Rabinovich, H., & Elia, J. (1993b). Antidepressant treatments in children and adolescents. II. Anxiety, physical, and behavioral disorders. *Journal of the American Academy of Child and Adolescent Psychiatry, 32,* 483–492.

American Psychiatric Association (1987). *Diagnostic and Statistical Manual of Mental Disorders,* 3rd ed., rev. Washington, DC: American Psychiatric Association.

American Psychiatric Association (1994). *Diagnostic and Statistical Manual of Mental Disorders,* 4th ed. Washington, DC: American Psychiatric Association.

Amini, F., Zilberg, N. J., & Burke, E. L. (1982). A controlled study of inpatient vs. outpatient treatment of delinquent drug abusing adolescents. *Comprehensive Psychiatry, 23,* 436–444.

Annis, H. M., & Davis C. S. (1989). Relapse prevention training: A cognitive–behavioral approach based on self-efficacy theory. *Journal of Chemical Dependency Treatment, 2,* 81–104.

Babor, T. F., Cooney, N. L., & Lauerman, R. J. (1987). The dependence syndrome concept as a psychological theory of relapse behavior: An empirical evaluation of alcoholics and opiate addicts. *British Journal of Addiction, 82,* 393–405.

Ball, J. C., & Ross, A. (1991). *The Effectiveness of Methadone Maintenance Treatment.* New York: Springer-Verlag.

Bandura, A. (1977). *Social Learning Theory.* Englewood-Cliffs, NJ: Prentice-Hall.

Bartlett, D. (1986). The use of multiple family therapy groups with adolescent drug addicts. In M. Sugar (Ed.), *The Adolescent in Group and Family Therapy* (pp. 262–282). Chicago: University of Chicago Press.

Barton, B., & Gitlin, M. J. (1987). Verapamil in treatment-resistant mania: An open trial. *Journal of Clinical Psychopharmacology, 7,* 101–103.

Beck, A. T., & Rush, A. J. (1989). Cognitive therapy. In H. I. Kaplan & B. J. Sadock (Eds.), *Comprehensive Textbook of Psychiatry IV* (pp. 1541–1550). Baltimore: Williams & Wilkins.

Benson, G. (1985). Course and outcome of drug abuse and medical and social condition in selected young drug abusers. *Acta Psychiatrica Scandinavica, 21,* 48–66.

Berman, E., & Wolpert, E. A. (1987). Intractable manic–depressive psychosis with rapid cycling in an 18-year-old depressive adolescent successfully treated with electroconvulsive therapy. *Journal of Nervous and Mental Disease, 175,* 236–239.

Bernstein, G. A. (1990). Anxiety disorders. In B. D. Garfinkel, G. A. Carlson, & E. B. Weller (Eds.), *Psychiatric Disorders in Children and Adolescents* (pp. 64–83). Philadelphia: W. B. Saunders.

Beschner, G. M. (1985). The problem of adolescent drug abuse: An introduction to intervention strategies. In A. S. Friedman & G. M. Beschner (Eds.), *Treatment Services for Adolescent Substance Abusers* (pp. 1–12). NIDA-DHHS Publication No. ADM 85-1342. Rockville, MD: National Institute on Drug Abuse.

Biederman, J., & Jellinek, M. S. (1984). Psychopharmacology in children. *New England Journal of Medicine, 310,* 968–972.

Brown, S. (1985). *Treating the Alcoholic, a Developmental Model of Recovery.* New York: Wiley.

Bukstein, O. G., Brent, D. A., & Kaminer, Y. (1989). Comorbidity of substance abuse and other psychiatric disorders in adolescents. *American Journal of Psychiatry, 146,* 1131–1141.

Campbell, M., Small, A. M., Green, W. H., Jennings, S. J., Perry, R., Bennett, W. G., & Anderson, L. (1984). A comparison of haloperidol and lithium in hospitalized aggressive conduct disordered children. *Archives of General Psychiatry, 41,* 650–656.

Caplan, G. (1974). *Support Systems and Community Mental Health.* New York: Behavioral Publications.

Carlson, G. A. (1990). Bipolar disorders in children and adolescents. In B. D. Garfinkel, G. A. Carlson, & E. B. Weller (Eds.), *Psychiatric Disorders in Children and Adolescents* (pp. 21–36). Philadelphia: W. B. Saunders.

Carroll, K. M., & Rounsaville, B. J. (1993). History and significance of childhood attention deficit disorder in treatment seeking cocaine abusers. *Comprehensive Psychiatry, 34,* 75–82.

Cartwright, A. (1987). Group work with substance abusers: Basic issues and future research. *British Journal of Addiction, 82,* 951–953.

Childress, A. R., McLellan, A. T., & O'Brien, C. P. (1986). Role of conditioning factors in the development of drug dependence. *Psychiatric Clinics of North America, 9,* 413–425.

Cytryn, L., & McKnew, D. (1972). Proposed classification of childhood depression. *American Journal of Psychiatry, 129,* 148–155.

Daley, D. C., & Marlatt, G. A. (1992). Relapse prevention: Cognitive and behavioral interventions. In J. H. Lowinson, P. Ruiz., R. B. Millman, & J. G. Langrod (Eds.), *Substance Abuse: A Comprehensive Textbook* (pp. 533–542). Baltimore: Williams & Wilkins.

DeLong, G. R., & Aldershof, A. L. (1987). Long-term experience with lithium treatment in childhood: Correlation with clinical diagnoses. *Journal of the American Academy of Child and Adolescent Psychiatry, 26,* 389–394.

DeJong, R., & Henrich, G. (1980). Follow-up results of a behavior modification program for juvenile drug addicts. *Addictive Behaviors, 5,* 49–57.

Dennis, M. L., Fairbank, J. A., & Rachal, J. V. (1992). Measuring substance abuse counseling: The methadone enhanced treatment study approach. Presented at the American Psychological Association's 100th Annual Meeting, August. Washington, DC.

DeVeaugh-Geiss, J., Moroz, G., Biederman, J., Cantwell, D., Fontaine, R., Griest, J. H., Reichler, R., Katz, R., & Landau, P. (1992). Clomipramine hydrochloride in childhood and adolescent obsessive–compulsive disorder—a multicenter trial. *Journal of the American Academy of Child and Adolescent Psychiatry, 31,* 45–49.

Edwards, G. (1979). British policies on opiate addiction: Ten years working on the revised response, and options for the future. *British Journal of Psychiatry, 134,* 1–13.

Edwards, G. (1986). The alcohol dependence syndrome: A concept as a stimulus for enquiry. *British Journal of Addiction, 81,* 171–183.

Edwards, G., & Gross, M. M. (1976). Alcohol dependence: Provisional description of a clinical syndrome. *British Medical Journal, 1,* 1058–1061.

Ends, E. J., & Page, C. W. (1957). A study of three types of group psychotherapy with hospitalized male inebriates. *Quarterly Journal of Studies on Alcohol, 18,* 263–277.

Feldman, R. A., Caplinger, T. E., & Wodarksi, J. S. (1983). *The St. Louis Conundrum: The Effective Treatment of Antisocial Youths.* Englewood-Cliffs, NJ: Prentice-Hall.

Felter, R., Izsak, E., & Lawrence, H. S. (1987). Emergency department management of the intoxicated adolescent. *Pediatric Clinics of North America, 34,* 399–421.

Finnegan, L. P., & Kandall, S. R. (1992). Maternal and neonatal effects of alcohol and drugs. In J. H. Lowison, P. Ruiz, R. B. Millman, & J. G. Langrod (Eds.), *Substance Abuse: A Comprehensive Textbook* (pp. 628–656). Baltimore: Williams & Wilkins.

Friedman, A. S., & Glickman, N. W. (1986). Program characteristics for successful treatment of adolescent drug abuse. *Journal of Nervous and Mental Disease, 174,* 669–679.

Friedman, A. S., & Glickman, N. W. (1987). Effects of psychiatric symptomatology on treatment outcome for adolescent male drug abusers. *Journal of Nervous and Mental Disease, 175,* 425–430.

Friedman, A. S., Schwartz, R., & Utada, A. (1989). Outcome of a unique youth drug abuse program: A follow-up study of clients of Straights, Inc. *Journal of Substance Abuse Treatment, 6,* 259–268.

Galanter, M. (1990). Cults and zealous self-help movements: A psychiatric perspective. *American Journal of Psychiatry, 147,* 543–551.

Gerstley, L., McLellan, A. T., Alterman, A. I., Woody, G. E., Luborsky, L., & Prout, M. (1989). Ability to form an alliance with the therapist: A possible marker of prognosis for patients with antisocial personality disorder. *American Journal of Psychiatry, 146,* 508–512.

Gittelman, R., & Klein, D. F. (1984). Relationship between separation anxiety and panic and agoraphobic disorders. *Psychopathology, 17,* Supplement 1, 56–65.

Gittelman-Klein, R., & Klein, D. F. (1971). Controlled imipramine treatment of school phobia. *Archives of General Psychiatry, 25,* 204–207.

Gould, M. S., Shaffer, D., & Kaplan, D. (1985). The characteristics of dropouts from a child psychiatric clinic. *Journal of the American Academy of Child Psychiatry, 24,* 316–328.

Greenhill, L. L. (1990). Attention deficit hyperactivity disorder in children. In B. D. Garfinkel, G. A. Carlson, & E. B. Weller (Eds.), *Psychiatric Disorders in Children and Adolescents* (pp. 149–182). Philadelphia: W. B. Saunders.

Grenier, C. (1985). Treatment effectiveness in an adolescent chemical dependency treatment program: A quasi-experimental design. *International Journal of Addictions, 20,* 381–391.

Hajek, P., Belcher, M., & Stapleton, J. (1985). Enhancing the impact of groups: An evaluation of two group formats for smokers. *British Journal of Clinical Psychology, 124,* 289–294.

Harticollis, P., & Harticollis, P. (1980). Alcoholism borderline and narcissistic disorders: A psychoanalytic overview. In W. Fann (Ed.), *Phenomenology and the Treatment of Alcoholism* (pp. 93–110). New York: Spectrum Publications.

Hayashida, M., Alterman, A. I., McLellan, A. T., O'Brien, C. P., Purtill, J. J., Volpicelli, J. R., Raphaelson, A. H., & Hall, C. P. (1989). Comparative effectiveness and costs of inpatient and outpatient detoxification of patients with mild-to-moderate alcohol withdrawal syndrome. *New England Journal of Medicine, 320,* 358–365.

Helzer, J. E., & Pryzbeck, T. R. (1988). The co-occurrence of alcoholism with other psychiatric disorders in the general population and its impact on treatment. *Journal on Studies of Alcohol, 49,* 219–224.

Hester, R. K., & Miller, W. R. (1988). Empirical guidelines for optimal client–patient matching. In E. Rahdert & J. Grabowski (Eds.), *Adolescent Drug Abuse: Analyses of Treatment Research* (pp. 27–39). NIDA Research Monograph 77. Rockville, MD: National Institute on Drug Abuse.

Hoffmann, N. G., Sonis, W. A., & Halikas, J. A. (1987). Issues in the evaluation of chemical dependency treatment programs for adolescents. *Pediatric Clinics of North America, 34,* 449–459.

Holden, C. (1987). Is alcoholism treatment effective? *Science, 236,* 20–22.

Holsten, F. (1980). Repeat follow-up studies of 100 young Norwegian drug abusers. *Journal of Drug Issues, 10,* 491–504.

Hubbard, R. L., Cavanaugh, E. R., Craddock, S. G., & Rachal, J. V. (1985). Characteristics, behaviors, and outcomes for youth in the TOPS. In A. S. Friedman & G. M. Beschner (Eds.), *Treatment Services for Adolescent Substance Abusers* (pp. 49–65). NIDA-DHHS Publication No. ADM-85-1342. Rockville, MD: National Institute on Drug Abuse.

Hudson, J. I., Pope, H. G., Jonas, J. M., & Yurgelum-Todd, D. (1983). Phenomenologic relationship of eating disorders to major affective disorder. *Psychological Research, 9,* 345–354.

Jaffe, J. H. (1986). Opioids. In A. I. Frances & R. E. Hales (Eds.), *Annual Review,* Vol. 5 (pp. 137–159). Washington, DC: American Psychiatric Association Press.

Jessor, R., & Jessor, S. L. (1977). *Problem Behavior and Psychosocial Development: A Longitudinal Study of Youth.* New York: Academic Press.

Johnson, R. E., Stevens, V. J., Hollis, J. F., & Woodson, G. T. (1992). Nicotine chewing gum use in the outpatient care setting. *Journal of Family Practice, 34,* 61–65.

Kaminer, Y. (1991a). Adolescent substance abuse. In R. J. Frances & S. I. Miller (Eds.), *Clinical Textbook of Addictive Disorders* (pp. 320–346). New York: Guilford Press.

Kaminer, Y. (1991b). The magnitude of concurrent psychiatric disorders in hospitalized substance abusing adolescents. *Child Psychiatry and Human Behavior, 22,* 89–95.

Kaminer, Y. (1992a). Clinical implications of the relationship between ADHD and PSUD. *American Journal of Addiction, 1,* 257–264.

Kaminer, Y. (1992b). Desipramine facilitation of cocaine abstinence in an adolescent. *Journal of the American Academy of Child and Adolescent Psychiatry, 31*, 312–317.

Kaminer, Y. (1992c). Psychoactive substance abuse and dependence as a risk factor in adolescent attempted and completed suicide. *American Journal on Addictions, 1*, 21–29.

Kaminer, Y., & Bukstein, O. (1989). Adolescent chemical dependency: Current issues in epidemiology, treatment and prevention. *Acta Psychiatrica Scandinavica, 79*, 415–424.

Kaminer, Y., & Bukstein, O. G. (1992). Inpatient behavioral and cognitive therapy for substance abuse in adolescents. In D. J. Kolko & U. B. Van Hasselt (Eds.), *Inpatient Behavior Therapy for Children and Adolescents* (pp. 313–339). New York: Plenum Press.

Kaminer, Y., Bukstein, O. G., & Tarter, R. E. (1991). The Teen Addiction Severity Index: Rationale and reliability. *International Journal of the Addictions, 26*, 219–226.

Kaminer, Y., & Frances, R. J. (1991). Inpatient treatment of adolescents with psychiatric and substance abuse disorder. *Hospital and Community Psychiatry, 42*, 894–896.

Kaminer, Y., & Hrecznyj, B. (1991). LSD induced chronic visual disturbances in an adolescent. *Journal of Nervous and Mental Disease, 179*, 173–174.

Kaminer, Y., Seifer, R., & Mastrian, A. (1992). Observational measurement of symptoms responsive to treatment of major depressive disorder in children and adolescents. *Journal of Nervous and Mental Disease, 180*, 639–643.

Kaminer, Y., Tarter, R. E., Bukstein, O. G., & Kabene, M. (1992a). Comparison between treatment completers and noncompleters among dually-diagnosed substance-abusing adolescents. *Journal of the American Academy of Child and Adolescent Psychiatry, 31*, 1046–1049.

Kaminer, Y., Tarter, R. E., Bukstein, O. G., & Kabene, M. (1992b). Staff, treatment completers' and noncompleters' perception of the value of treatment variables. *American Journal on Addictions, 1*, 115–120.

Kastner, T., & Friedman, D. L. (1992). Verapamil and valproic acid treatment of prolonged mania. *Journal of the American Academy of Child and Adolescent Psychiatry, 31*, 271–275.

Kaufman, E. (1989). The psychotherapy of dually diagnosed patients. *Journal of Substance Abuse Treatment, 6*, 9–18.

Kaufman, E. R., & Reaux, O. (1988). Guidelines for the successful psychotherapy of substance abusers. *Drug and Alcohol Abuse, 14*, 199–209.

Kazdin, A. E. (1987). Treatment of antisocial behavior in children: Current status and future directions. *Psychological Bulletin, 102*, 187–203.

Kemph, J. P., Devane, C. L., Levin, G. M., Jarecke, R., & Miller, R. L. (1993). Treatment of aggressive children with clonidine: Results of an open pilot study. *Journal of the American Academy of Child and Adolescent Psychiatry, 32*, 577–581.

Khantzian, E. J. (1980). An ego/self theory of substance dependence, a contemporary psychoanalytic perspective. In D. J. Lettieri, M. Sayers, & H. W. Pearson (Eds.), *Theories on Drug Abuse: Selected Contemporary Perspectives* (pp. 29–33). Rockville, MD: National Institute on Drug Abuse.

Khantzian, E. J. (1985). Psychotherapeutic interventions with substance abusers—the clinical context. *Journal of Substance Abuse Treatment, 2*, 83–88.

Khantzian, E. J., Halliday, K., Golden, S., & McAuliffe, W. E. (1992). Modified group therapy for substance abusers. *American Journal on the Addictions, 1*, 67–76.

Klein, R. G., Koplewicz, H. S., & Kanner, A. (1992). Imipramine treatment of children with separation anxiety disorder. *Journal of the American Academy of Child and Adolescent Psychiatry, 31*, 21–28.

Klorman, R., Brumaghin, J. T., Fitzpatrick, P. A., & Borgstedt, A. D. (1990). *Journal of the American Academy of Child and Adolescent Psychiatry, 29*, 702–709.

Kosten, T. R., Kleber, H. D., and Morgan, C. (1989). Treatment of cocaine abuse with buprenorphine. *Biological Psychiatry, 26,* 637–639.

Kranzler, H. R. (1988). Use of Buspirone in an adolescent with overanxious disorder. *Journal of the American Academy of Child and Adolescent Psychiatry, 27,* 789–790.

Kuperman, S., & Stewart, M. A. (1987). Use of propranolol to decrease aggressive outbursts in younger patients. *Psychosomatics, 28,* 315–319.

Langrod, L., Alksne, L., & Gomez, E. (1981). A religious approach to the rehabilitation of addicts. In J. H. Lawison & P. Ruiz (Eds.), *Substance Abuse Clinical Problems and Perspectives* (pp. 408–420). Baltimore: Williams & Wilkins.

Laundergan, J. C. (1982). *Easy Does It.* Center City, MN: Hazelden Foundation.

Lichtenstein, E., & Glasgow, R. E. (1992). Smoking cessation: What have we learned over the past decade? *Journal of Consulting and Clinical Psychology, 60,* 518–527.

Luborsky, L., Crits-Christoph, P., McLellan, A. T., & Woody, G. E. (1986). Do psychotherapists vary in their effectiveness? Findings from four outcome studies. *American Journal of Orthopsychiatry, 20,* 14–25.

McLellan, A. T., Alterman, A. I., Cacciola, J. S., Metzger, D., & O'Brien, C. P. (1992). A new measure of substance abuse treatment: Initial studies of the Treatment Survey Review. *Journal of Nervous and Mental Disease, 180,* 101–110.

McLellan, A. T., Arndt, I. O., Metzger, D. S., Woody, G. E., & O'Brien, C. P. (1993). The effects of psychosocial services in substance abuse treatment. *Journal of the American Medical Association, 269,* 1953–1959.

McLellan, A. T., Luborsky, L., O'Brien, C. P., Woody, G. E., & Druley, K. A. (1982). Is treatment for substance abuse effective? *Journal of the American Medical Association, 247,* 1423–1428.

McLellan, A. T., Luborsky, L., Woody, G. E., O'Brien, C. P., & Druley, K. A. (1983). Predicting response to alcohol and drug abuse treatment: Role of psychiatric severity. *Archives of General Psychiatry, 40,* 620–628.

McLellan, A. T., Woody, G. E., Luborsky, L., & Goehl, L. (1988). Is the counselor an "active ingredient" in substance abuse rehabilitation? *Journal of Nervous and Mental Disease, 176,* 423–430.

Menninger, K. (1938). *Man Against Himself.* New York: Harcourt Brace Jovanovich.

Meyer, R. E. (1986). Old wine, new bottle: The alcohol dependence syndrome. *Psychiatric Clinics of North America, 9,* 435–453.

Meyer, R. E. (1992). New pharmacotherapies for cocaine dependence revisited. *Archives of General Psychiatry, 49,* 900–904.

Miller, W. R. (1985). Motivation for treatment: A review with special emphasis on alcoholism. *Psychological Bulletin, 98,* 84–107.

Montgomery, S. A. (1993). Venlafaxine: A new dimension in antidepressant pharmacotherapy. *Journal of Clinical Psychiatry, 54,* 119–126.

Monti, P. M., Abrams, D. B., Kadden, R. M., & Cooney, N. L. (1989). *Treating Alcohol Dependence.* New York: Guilford Press.

Myers, M. G., & Brown, S. A. (1990). Coping and appraisal in potential relapse situations among adolescent substance abusers following treatment. *Journal of Adolescent Chemical Dependency, 1,* 95–115.

National Institute on Alcohol Abuse and Alcoholism. (1992, July). Treatment outcome research of alcoholism. *Alcohol Alert.* Rockville, MD: Author.

Offord, D. R., Jones, M. B., Graham, A., Poushinsky, M., Stenerson, P., & Weaver, L. (1985). *Community Skill-Development Programs for Children: Rationale and Steps in Implementation.* Ontario, Canada: Canadian Parks and Recreation Program.

O'Malley, S. S., Jaffe, A. J., Chang, G., Schottenfeld, R. S., Meyer, R. E., & Rounsaville, B.

(1992). Naltrexone and coping skills therapy for alcohol dependence. *Archives of General Psychiatry, 49,* 881–887.

Patterson, G. R. (1986). Performance models for antisocial boys. *American Psychologist, 41,* 432–444.

Pliszka, S. R. (1987). Tricyclic antidepressants in the treatment of children with attention deficit disorder. *Journal of the American Academy of Child and Adolescent Psychiatry, 26,* 127–132.

Prien, R. E., & Gelenberg, A. J. (1989). Alternative to lithium for preventive treatment of bipolar disorder. *American Journal of Psychiatry, 146,* 840–848.

Prochaska, J. O., & DiClemente, C. (1986). Toward a comprehensive model of change. In W. R. Miller & N. Heather (Eds.), *Treating Addictive Behaviors: Processes of Change* (pp. 3–27). New York: Plenum Press.

Quinn, W. H., Kuehl, B. P., Thomas, F. N., & Joaning, H. (1988). Families of adolescent drug abusers: Systematic interventions to attain drug-free behavior. *American Journal of Drug and Alcohol Abuse, 14,* 65–87.

Rapoport, J. L. (1987). Pediatric psychopharmacology: The last decade. In H. Y. Meltzer (Ed.), *Psychopharmacology: The Third Generation of Progress* (pp. 1211–1214). New York: Raven Press.

Richter, S. S., Brown, S. A., & Mott, M. A. (1991). The impact of social support and self-esteem on adolescent substance abuse treatment outcome. *Journal of Substance Abuse, 3,* 371–385.

Riddle, M. A., Geller, B., & Ryan, N. (1993). Another sudden death in a child treated with desipramine. *Journal of the American Academy of Child and Adolescent Psychiatry, 32,* 792–797.

Rosen, B. (1978). Written treatment contracts: Their use in planning treatment programs for inpatients. *British Journal of Psychiatry, 133,* 410–415.

Rosen, M. I., & Kosten, T. R. (1991). Buprenorphine: Beyond methadone. *Hospital and Community Psychiatry, 42,* 347–349.

Rounsaville, B. J., Kosten, T. R., Weissman, M. M., & Kleber, H. D. (1986). Prognostic significance of psychiatric disorders in treated opiate addicts. *Archives of General Psychiatry, 43,* 739–745.

Rounsaville, B. J., Dolinsky, Z. S., Babor, T. F., & Meyer, R. E. (1987). Psychopathology as a predictor of treatment outcome in alcoholics. *Archives of General Psychiatry, 44,* 505–513.

Rush, T. V. (1979). Predicting treatment outcome for juvenile and young adult clients in the Pennsylvania substance abuse system. In G. M. Beschner & A. S. Friedman (Eds.), *Youth Drug Abuse* (pp. 629–656). Lexington, MA: Lexington Books.

Ryan, N. D., Puig-Antich, J., Cooper, T., Rabinovich, H., Ambrosini, P., Davis, M., King, J., Torres, D., & Fried, J. (1986). Imipramine in adolescent major depression: Plasma level and clinical response. *Acta Psychiatrica Scaninavica, 73,* 275–288.

Sameroff, A. J., & Chandler, M. J. (1975). Reproductive risk and the continuum of caretaking casualty. In F. D. Horowitz (Ed.), *Review of Child Development Research,* Vol. 4 (pp. 187–244). Chicago: University of Chicago Press.

Sells, S. B., & Simpson, D. D. (1979). Evaluation of treatment outcome for youths in the drug abuse reporting program (DARP): A follow-up study. In G. M. Beschner & A. S. Friedman (Eds.), *Youth Drug Abuse* (pp. 571–628). Lexington, MA: Lexington Books.

Simeon, J. G., Ferguson, H. B., Knott, V., Roberts, N., Gauthier, B., Dubois, C., & Wiggins, D. (1992). Clinical, cognitive, and neurophysiological effects of alprazolam in children and adolescents with overanxious and avoidant disorders. *Journal of the American Academy of Child and Adolescent Psychiatry, 31,* 29–33.

Smith, M. O., & Khan, I. (1988). An acupuncture program for the treatment of the drug-addicted person. *Bulletin of Narcotics, 40,* 35–41.

Sobell, L. C., Sobell, M. B., & Nirenberg, T. D. (1988). Behavioral assessment and treatment planning with alcohol and drug abusers: A review with an emphasis on clinical applications. *Clinical Psychology Review, 8,* 19–54.

State Methadone Maintenance Treatment Guidelines (1992). Washington, DC: Food and Drug Administration.

Steingard, R., Biderman, J., Spencer, T., Wilens, T., & Gonzalez, A. (1993). Comparison of clonidine response in the treatment of attention-deficit hyperactivity disorder with and without comorbid tic disorders. *Journal of the American Academy of Child and Adolescent Psychiatry, 32,* 350–353.

Stewart, J. T., Meyers, W. C., Burket, R. C., & Lyles, W. B. (1990). A review of the pharmacotherapy of aggression in children and adolescents. *Journal of the American Academy of Child and Adolescent Psychiatry, 29,* 269–277.

Strober, M., & Carlson, G. (1982). Bipolar illness in adolescents with major depression: Clinical, genetic, and psychopharmacologic predictions in a three-to-four prospective follow-up investigation. *Archives of General Psychiatry, 39,* 549–555.

Sugar, M. (1986). The inpatient borderline adolescent in group therapy. In M. Sugar (Ed.), *The Adolescent in Group and Family Therapy* (pp. 235–241). Chicago: University of Chicago Press.

Szapocznik, J., Kurtines, W. M., Foote, F., Perez-Vidal, A., & Hervis, O. (1983). Conjoint versus one person family therapy: Some evidence of the effectiveness of conducting family therapy through one person. *Journal of Consulting Clinical Psychology, 51,* 881–889.

Tarter, R. E. (1992). Prevention of drug abuse: Theory and application. *American Journal on Addictions, 1,* 2–20.

Vaglum, P., & Fossheim, I. (1980). Differential treatment of young abusers: A quasi-experimental study of therapeutic community in a psychiatric hospital. *Journal of Drug Issues, 10,* 505–516.

Vanicelli, M. (1974). Treatment contracts in an inpatient alcoholism setting. *Journal of Studies on Alcohol, 40,* 457–471.

Weiss, R. D., Griffin, M. L., & Hufford, C. (1992). Severity of cocaine dependence as a predictor of relapse to cocaine use. *American Journal of Psychiatry, 149,* 1595–1596.

Weissman, M. M., Leckman, J. F., Merikangas, K. R., Gammon, G. D., & Prusoff, B. A. (1984). Depression and anxiety disorders in parents and children: Results from the Yale family study. *Archives of General Psychiatry, 41,* 845–852.

Werry, J. S., & Aman, M. G. (1975). Methylphenidate and haloperidol in children. *Archives of General Psychiatry, 32,* 790–795.

West, R. (1992). The "nicotine replacement paradox" in smoking cessation: How does nicotine gum really work? *British Journal of Addiction, 87,* 165–167.

Wilkinson, D. A., & LeBreton, S. (1986). Early indicators of treatment outcome in multiple drug users. In W. R. Miller & N. Heather (Eds.), *Treating Addictive Behaviors: Processes of Change* (pp. 239–261). New York: Plenum Press.

Wilson, S. (1980). Can drug abuse treatment be adequately evaluated? *Acta Psychiatrica Scandinavica, 67,* 52–57.

Woody, G. E., McLellan, A. T., Luborsky, L., & O'Brien, C. P. (1984). Severity of psychiatric symptoms as a predictor of benefits from psychotherapy: The Veterans Administration —Penn Study. *American Journal of Psychiatry, 141,* 1172–1177.

Yalom, I. D. (1975). *The Theory and Practice of Group Psychotherapy.* New York: Basic Books.

Index